THE GUIDE TO EATING HEALTHY
IN ANY RESTAURANT

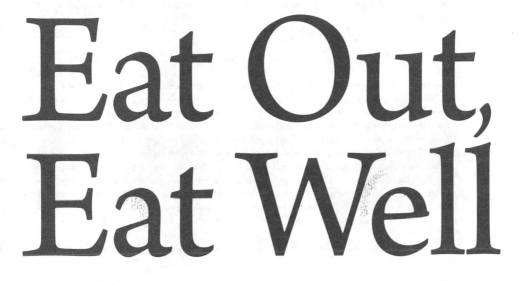

Eat Out, Eat Well

HOPE S. WARSHAW, MMSc, RD, CDE

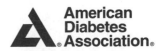

American
Diabetes
Association.

Director, Book Publishing, Abe Ogden; Managing Editor, Greg Guthrie; Acquisitions Editor, Victor Van Beuren; Editor, Lauren Wilson; Production Manager, Melissa Sprott; Composition, Circle Graphics; Cover Design, Sport Creative; Printer, Marquis Imprimeur

Printed in Canada
1 3 5 7 9 10 8 6 4 2

The suggestions and information contained in this publication are generally consistent with the *Clinical Practice Recommendations* and other policies of the American Diabetes Association, but they do not represent the policy or position of the Association or any of its boards or committees. Reasonable steps have been taken to ensure the accuracy of the information presented. However, the American Diabetes Association cannot ensure the safety or efficacy of any product or service described in this publication. Individuals are advised to consult a physician or other appropriate health care professional before undertaking any diet or exercise program or taking any medication referred to in this publication. Professionals must use and apply their own professional judgment, experience, and training and should not rely solely on the information contained in this publication before prescribing any diet, exercise, or medication. The American Diabetes Association—its officers, directors, employees, volunteers, and members—assumes no responsibility or liability for personal or other injury, loss, or damage that may result from the suggestions or information in this publication.

♾ The paper in this publication meets the requirements of the ANSI Standard Z39.48-1992 (permanence of paper).

ADA titles may be purchased for business or promotional use or for special sales. To purchase more than 50 copies of this book at a discount, or for custom editions of this book with your logo, contact the American Diabetes Association at the address below, at booksales@diabetes.org, or by calling 703-299-2046.

American Diabetes Association
1701 North Beauregard Street
Alexandria, Virginia 22311

DOI: 10.2337/9781580405423

Library of Congress Cataloging-in-Publication Data

Warshaw, Hope S., 1954-
 Eat out, eat well : the guide to eating healthy in any restaurant / Hope S. Warshaw.
 pages cm
 Summary: «This book will help the reader find healthier foods and mealswhen eating out at restaurants. We>ve got more nutrition facts at our fingertips than ever before and due to regulations, we>ll see more calorie counts for restaurant foods in front of our eyes. For people with diabetes or care givers, this is all particularly good news!»-- Provided by publisher.
 Includes bibliographical references and index.
 ISBN 978-1-58040-542-3 (paperback)
 1. Diabetics--Nutrition. 2. Diabetes--Diet therapy. 3. Restaurants--United States--Guidebooks. I. American Diabetes Association. II. Title.
 RC662.W312 2014
 641.5>6314--dc23
            2014025794

Dedication

To people with diabetes and their caregivers who, day in and day out,
strive to eat healthy, to stay healthy, and to prevent or delay diabetes
complications. May the knowledge and counsel you gain from
this resource make eating healthy just a bit easier and help you or
your loved one stay complication-free for many years to come.

— HSW

Contents

Acknowledgments

This book came to reality with the assistance of many individuals.

I'd like to acknowledge the masterful and dedicated assistance of two registered dietitian colleagues, Laura Chalela Hoover, MPH, RDN, and Carlene Thomas, RD. I'd like to thank FoodCare, Inc., and particularly Elizabeth Turner, RD, who knew exactly what I needed to compile the nutrient data for *Health Busters* and *Healthier Bets*.

Thanks to the staff from the American Diabetes Association—who took my words, and in this case numbers, and edited and designed them into an easy-to-use resource—including Greg Guthrie, Managing Editor, Melissa Sprott, Production Manager, and Abe Ogden, Director of Book Publishing, and Lauren Wilson of Boldface LLC.

On behalf of people with diabetes and their caregivers, as well as diabetes care clinicians, who will all benefit from this knowledge, I give my thanks to many large national and regional restaurant chains for making their nutrition information available and ever more accessible. And for slowly but surely making more healthy restaurant foods available. Kudos!

Lastly, thanks to my professional colleagues in diabetes care and weight management who consistently lend their ears and ideas. They continue to be an endless source of inspiration and encouragement.

SECTION 1

Healthy Restaurant Eating with Diabetes: The Basics

CHAPTER 1

Trends in Restaurants, Foods, and Eating

Never before have Americans eaten more meals in restaurants or ordered more restaurant meals to take out or have delivered to, well, wherever they may be. The number of restaurant chains and independent restaurants in our midst is at an all-time high. We have access to a wider array of cuisines, foods, and ingredients than ever before. Experts in the prediction business expect these restaurant growth trends to continue due to our dual quests for convenience and flavor as we deal with the hustle and bustle of daily life.

Yet, as the consumption of restaurant meals has skyrocketed, we've witnessed an epidemic of the diseases exacerbated by carrying around excess weight—prediabetes, type 2 diabetes, heart disease, high blood pressure, certain cancers, sleep disorders, fatty liver problems, and more. Is there a connection? Researchers and nutrition experts say "yes!" Why? The simple answer is that unhealthy foods surround us while healthier foods are harder to find. All things considered, it's simply tougher to eat healthy when you eat away from home.

But on to the good news—yes, there's plenty! There are more healthy foods and meals to choose from at restaurants than ever before. Plus, it's becoming easier to help your children eat healthier restaurant meals. We have more nutrition facts at our fingertips than ever before due to regulations, and more are on the way. For people with diabetes and their caregivers, this is all good news. With this book in hand, you'll be a pro at healthy restaurant eating in no time.

A Few Statistics:

▶ There are nearly one million restaurants within our borders.*

▶ Americans spend about $1.8 billion a day on restaurant foods.*

▶ Restaurant sales were projected at over $660 billion, equal to 4% of the U.S. gross domestic product.*

▶ More than 7 out of 10 eating and drinking locales are independently owned, single-unit restaurants.*

▶ Consumers spend 47% of their food dollars away from home. (That's 47% of food dollars, not food consumption. Generally, restaurant foods cost more than foods purchased for preparation or assembly at home or another non-restaurant location.)*

▶ On average, American adults eat about 5 of the 21 traditional weekly meals away from home.*

▶ Americans eat roughly one-third of their calories from foods purchased away from home.

▶ Nutritionally speaking, restaurant meals tend to be higher in fat and calories than home-prepared meals. Higher, in fact, than most people guess. And these meals, as you would guess, are light on vegetables, fruit, whole grains, and low-fat dairy foods—just what we should be eating more of.

A Historical Refresher

What a difference a few hundred years makes! Taverns and boarding houses of the 1700s, where food was often an afterthought to alcohol-containing refreshments, preceded restaurants. Taverns, mainly inhabited by men, morphed into the first restaurants, such as Delmonico's in New York City, which opened in the mid-1800s. Two hundred years ago it was a novelty and a rarity to sit down to dine on a hot meal away from home. Restaurant dining was done mainly by the wealthy residing in metropolitan areas.

Fast forward another hundred years to the mid-1900s. Restaurant meals were mainly enjoyed by the wealthy and relished only on special occasions—to celebrate a birthday or anniversary. Oh yes, and on Mother's Day, when moms around the country got to hang the "kitchen's closed" sign.

From National Restaurant Association, Pocket Factbook.

Fast food was born in the mid-1900s and relatively quickly became fully integrated into our eating-away-from-home culture. In 1954 Ray Kroc discovered the San Bernardino, California, restaurant being run by brothers Dick and Mac McDonald. In 1955, he became president of the McDonald's Corporation and 6 years later bought out the brothers McDonald. The rest, as they say, is history.

In 1950, according to the National Restaurant Association, the average American spent about a quarter of their food dollars eating away from home.

Restaurant Eating Today

Americans spend nearly half of our food dollars eating away from home today. In 60 years, restaurant meals have catapulted from a special-occasion treat to a major way Americans get the job of eating done. According to the National Restaurant Association, 45% of Americans say restaurants are an essential part of their lifestyle.

Let's face it, it's just so darn easy to eat restaurant meals. Restaurants are everywhere in metropolitan areas and small towns and cities. Restaurant foods are available from morning until night, if not 24 hours a day, in plenty of urban centers. Why bother doing the daily grunt work of planning, shopping, food preparation, and cooking with this amount of access to ready-to-eat foods and meals? (Actually there are plenty of good reasons. One good reason is nutrition, another is your health.)

We also order takeout regularly. We pick up and tote restaurant foods for breakfast or lunch to our places of employment, traveling from here to there, or to school. We grab a ready-to-serve dinner on the way home or order a pizza for delivery to the sports field, social events, or meetings. And it's not just meals being purchased at restaurants, plenty of snacks are purchased too. Perhaps it's an afternoon coffee drink, a piece of fruit, a sweet treat, a crunchy favorite, or a nutrition bar. Yes, procuring restaurant foods is one big way we get the job of eating done today.

Restaurant and Food Trends in Sight

Restaurants and Service:

▶ Burgers and fries are just the tip of the iceberg when it comes to the types of fast food available now. Today, many restaurants serve food fast, from chicken restaurants, to pizza and sub shops, to plenty of ethnic restaurants. This book refers to this genre of restaurants as "walk up and order." (Just so you know, in the restaurant industry they're known as Quick Service Restaurants, abbreviated as QSRs).

► Coffee and bagel shops and bakery cafes appear to be on nearly every street corner in metro areas. And they want to serve you drinks, foods, and snacks all day long, not just for breakfast.

► Frozen yogurt shops have made a comeback.

► Chain restaurants serving you sit-down style are on a growth curve, too, with a hefty dose of the all too similar fusion of American fare mixed with a scattering of popular ethnic favorites.

► Plenty of ethnic restaurants—from the common Chinese, Mexican, and Italian, to less common Korean, Vietnamese, and Peruvian—are open for your business.

► Fine dining establishments have exploded in the last decade. They celebrate a myriad of cuisine fusions and their celebrity chefs, who might also double as a TV cooking star.

Foods in Vogue:

► The use of locally grown ingredients or those purchased at nearby farmers markets has become common. Some restaurants even tout their own outside or rooftop garden. This is known as hyper-local food sourcing.

► The use of organically grown ingredients, grass-fed meats, non GMO foods, and hormone-free poultry is also gaining in popularity.

► Chefs sleuth out uncommon ingredients and serve lesser-known foods. When it comes to vegetables, they've slowly but surely put kale, Brussels sprouts, and cauliflower steak (a full slice of the whole cauliflower) on the "in" list. They've introduced us to pork belly and raised interest in venison, Kobe beef, and quail.

► With an increase in diners going vegetarian, restaurants, from upscale to mainstream, regularly list at least one or two vegetarian options, and many restaurants are testing the waters with vegan offerings.

Meal Sizes and Styles:

► Many people are "grazing" instead of eating full meals. They'll have a snack here and a nibble there.

▶ Our appetite for handheld foods that fit our on-the-go lifestyles is at an all-time high and will likely continue. To satisfy our desires, you see items like smoothies, wrap sandwiches, fruit and cheese snack packs, and pretzel bites with hummus. These foods are plentiful at airports. That's good news because there's not much to eat, even peanuts or pretzels, on most flights today.

▶ Tapas, the famous little plates served in Spanish restaurants, have gone mainstream and multiethnic. Some restaurants build their whole menu, or a large section of it, around small plates. They can be a boon to the health- and calorie-conscious diner as long as you choose wisely and limit the number of plates you order.

▶ Value meals tout plenty of volume for your dollars. Meal deals, such as kids eat free, two for the price of one, and all-you-can-eat buffets, encourage overeating.

Health and Healthy Eating Factors:

▶ There's pressure on restaurants to offer healthier foods and tighten their belts on portions. (Though many seem to find this very hard to do.)

▶ Healthier kids' meals, both in fast food and some sit-down restaurants, are now available due, to an extent, to public health concerns and pressure on restaurants to take actions to help prevent childhood obesity.

▶ More fruits, vegetables, and whole grains as well as fat-free milk, yogurt, and bottled water are available in fast food restaurants and some sandwich shops.

▶ Fast-food restaurants and other types of chains are aware of possible allergens and let consumers know if foods do or do not contain nuts, wheat, dairy, gluten, or others.

▶ Nutrition information for foods served in chain restaurants is plentiful and will become even more available

Environmentally Friendly Focus:

▶ Many restaurants, particularly upscale restaurants, pride themselves on serving only sustainable seafood and locally sourced meats and produce.

▶ Some large chains serve takeout in eco-friendly containers and ask you to place your recyclables in their recycling containers.

Conveniences for the Fast-Paced and Frequent Diner:

▶ Drive-up and to-go windows go well beyond just fast-food burger chains today.

▶ Diners can explore various restaurants' menus via desktop computers or smartphones.

▶ You can place an order, either by phone, on the restaurant's website, or on an app, and some restaurants can deliver directly to your GPS coordinates.

▶ Several restaurants feature new ordering technology: you sit down at a table and order on a tablet-based device in place at every table, or your server places your order with a handheld device.

▶ Many restaurants have frequent diner reward programs and they're in constant contact with you.

▶ You can stay connected with your favorite restaurants using social media.

▶ Diners can rate a restaurant, good or bad, on the restaurant's website, TripAdvisor, Yelp, or plenty of other websites/apps.

Let's face it, restaurant meals—whether you eat them in or out—are, and will continue to be, part of dealing with our fast-paced lifestyle. Eating restaurant meals is time-efficient and one of the ways we socialize. According to the National Restaurant Association, nearly 80% of American adults say that restaurant meals with family or friends give them an opportunity to socialize and they'd rather spend leisure time in a restaurant than at home cooking and cleaning up. Restaurant meals are and, even more so, will continue to be part of our children's reality.

Knowing the large role that restaurant eating plays in our reality and recognizing the pitfalls of restaurant foods, it might seem like a person with diabetes will have to strictly limit restaurant meals and significantly change his or her lifestyle. But this is not a workable solution for many. While you can certainly tweak your lifestyle in a healthier direction, it's hard for most people to make wholesale changes and make these stick long term. The challenge for people with diabetes, as for anyone and everyone who wants to eat healthy, is to learn to make healthier choices and eat reasonable portions … at least most of the time.

This book is designed specifically to help you do just that, step by step. For starters, take a look at the table of contents on page 1. As you see, the book is divided into three sections. Section 1 focuses on helping you master the basics of healthy restaurant eating. You'll read about how to apply today's *Nutrition Therapy Recommendations for the Management of Adults With Diabetes* to restaurant eating. You'll delve into the pitfalls of restaurant eating and gather strategies to conquer each pitfall. You'll learn how to deal with diabetes-specific restaurant dilemmas in Chapter 5. If you've got celiac disease or a gluten sensitivity as well as diabetes, be sure to read Chapter 6. If you're raising or caring for a child or children with diabetes, you can pick up some tips and tactics in Chapter 7. Get the ins and outs of ordering both alcoholic and nonalcoholic beverages in Chapter 9. Then in Sections 2 and 3 you'll learn all about the different types of fare and ethnic cuisine. Look to Chapter 10 for an in-depth rundown of everything you'll find in Sections 2 and 3.

Good luck on your journey towards eating and enjoying healthier restaurant meals! Make sure this book tags along with you on your journey and becomes your restaurant companion!

CHAPTER 2

Today's Healthy Eating Goals for Diabetes

The saying, "We've come a long way," certainly applies to the changes made over the years to the nutrition and eating guidelines for diabetes … and that's not even going all the way back to the pre-insulin days before 1921.

During the 1990s diabetes nutrition and eating goals underwent a major revolution. In fact, the phrase "a diabetic diet" is now outdated, actually extinct. People with diabetes should no longer be told to axe sugary foods and sweets from their list of acceptable foods. If you so desire and it fits into your overall healthy eating plan, you can savor the taste of a few slices of pizza at your local pizza parlor or cruise to the drive-thru for a hamburger or grilled chicken sandwich when time is not on your side. The bottom line: the *Nutrition Therapy Recommendations for the Management of Adults With Diabetes* (available at http://care.diabetesjournals.org/content/37/Supplement_1/S120.full.pdf+html), published by the American Diabetes Association, echoes the healthy eating goals for *everyone*—as outlined by the federal government, in the *Dietary Guidelines for Americans*, and by health associations like the American Heart Association and American Cancer Society.

For people with diabetes, eating healthy can help you achieve both your short- and long-term health goals. Staying healthy for the long haul with diabetes is no longer just about blood glucose control. It's about what's called "metabolic control." Metabolic control includes glucose control (also called glycemic control), control of your blood lipids/fats, and blood pressure. One of the goals of the American Diabetes Association's *Nutrition Therapy*

Recommendations for the Management of Adults With Diabetes is achieving and maintaining target ranges for these three categories (also known as the diabetes ABCs) in people with diabetes.

Target ABC Goals		
A is for ...	**B is for ...**	**C is for ...**
A1C or blood glucose	Blood pressure	Cholesterol or blood lipids (fats)
American Diabetes Association Recommendations*		
A1C: <7%[†]	<140/80 mmHg	LDL: <100 mg/dl
Glucose: Fasting and before meals: 70–130 mg/dl[†]		HDL: >40 mg/dl (men) >50 mg/dl (women)
Glucose: 1–2 hours after the start of a meal: <180 mg/dl[†]		Triglycerides: <150 mg/dl

*Based on American Diabetes Association: Standards of medical care in diabetes: 2014. *Diabetes Care* 37 (Suppl. 1): S14–S80, 2014 (http://care.diabetesjournals.org/content/37/Supplement_1/S14.full.pdf+html)
[†] Based on your age, years with diabetes, other medical issues, and personal considerations you and your health-care provider may decide on slightly lower or higher goals.

Another major goal of the *Nutrition Therapy Recommendations for the Management of Adults With Diabetes* is to help people with diabetes reach or maintain a healthy weight. Today, roughly two-thirds of American adults are overweight or obese (about one-third of adults are overweight and one-third are obese). Overweight is defined as the weight range between normal body weight and 30% above normal weight. Obesity is defined as a weight more than 30% above normal body weight. Many children and adolescents are also overweight. Being overweight or obese becomes a significant risk factor for many chronic diseases, including prediabetes—the precursor to type 2 diabetes. Roughly 80% of people with prediabetes and type 2 diabetes are overweight. Research has shown over and over again that losing 5–7% of body weight and, even more critical, keeping as much of this weight loss off over time as possible, goes a long way toward helping people hit those target ABC goals and stay healthy. For people with prediabetes this amount of weight loss has been shown to help them reverse the condition or slow its progression towards type 2 diabetes.

A good diabetes eating plan should be designed to be in sync with your glucose-lowering medications (most people with type 1 require insulin, most people with type 2 require one or more medications) and work around your needs and lifestyle, not vice-versa. Factors to consider include your restaurant eating habits, food preferences, and life schedule. Today, and even more so in the future, health-care providers have (and will have) many glucose-lowering medications, medication delivery devices (like pens and pumps), and monitoring tools (like glucose meters and continuous glucose monitors) available to help you formulate a diabetes plan that fits your lifestyle and enables you to make important behavioral changes. (Be in the know about these newer tools and ask your providers about them!)

The end goal, of course, is to help you stay healthy and prevent or slow down the long-term complications of diabetes, such as heart disease and certain cancers. (Yes, cancers! There's solid evidence now that people with type 2 diabetes who are overweight are at higher risk of developing certain cancers.)

Diabetes Eating Goals in a Nutshell

Here is an overview of the overarching goals of the American Diabetes Association's *Nutrition Therapy Recommendations for the Management of Adults With Diabetes:*

► To promote and support healthful eating patterns, emphasizing a variety of nutrient-dense foods in appropriate portion sizes, in order to improve overall health and specifically to:
  ▷ Attain individualized blood glucose, blood pressure, and lipid goals (see above Target ABC Goals)*
  ▷ Achieve and maintain healthy body weight
  ▷ Delay or prevent the complications of diabetes

*A1C, blood pressure, and cholesterol goals may need to be adjusted for the individual based on age, duration of diabetes, health history, and other present health conditions. Further recommendations for individualization of goals can be found in American Diabetes Association: Standards of medical care in diabetes: 2014, Diabetes Care 37 (Suppl. 1): S14–S80, 2014 (http://care.diabetesjournals.org/content/37/Supplement_1/S14.full).

► To maintain the pleasure of eating by providing positive messages about food choices while limiting food choices only when indicated by scientific evidence.

► To provide practical tools for day-to-day meal planning. (That's exactly the goal of this book!)

How Much Should You Eat?

Even if you're trying to make the long-term changes in your eating habits that can help you stay healthy, you can continue to eat and enjoy many of the foods you have loved for years, albeit perhaps less often or in smaller quantities. But you also want to enjoy *more* of the healthier foods, such as fruits, vegetables, legumes, and whole grains. The quantities of food you eat and how often you eat need to match your lifestyle and schedule. Another critical element of planning your meals is to determine which foods and which times for meals and snacks (if you need or want them) work best to help you keep your glucose, blood lipids, and blood pressure under control.

There is no set number of calories or amount of food or nutrients (carbohydrate, protein, and fat) that is right for everyone with diabetes. Today there are far fewer nutrition "rules" for people with diabetes than ever before. Research shows that there is a range of eating styles—from following a vegan lifestyle to following a diet that includes a low to moderate amount of carbohydrate with lean protein foods and healthy fats—that can help people with diabetes achieve both their short- and long-term health goals. What is critical, however, is that you get all of the nutrients, vitamins, and minerals you need while following your eating plan.

Your individual characteristics, such as your height, age, current weight, your daily activity level, the type of physical activity you do, whether you want to lose weight or maintain your weight, how difficult it is for you to lose weight, and more, will dictate your calorie and nutrient needs. Word to the wise: find an eating plan and style that works for you for the long haul.

To be successful with a healthy eating plan and to adopt a healthy lifestyle, it might be helpful to work with a registered dietitian nutritionist/registered dietitian (RDN/RD) with diabetes expertise or with a certified diabetes educator (CDE). A dietitian can help you learn how to work almost any food or type of restaurant cuisine into a healthy eating plan. These experts can coach you and support your efforts to change your eating habits over time. Several books published by the American Diabetes Association on the topic of food, nutrition, and meal planning, including *Diabetes Meal Planning Made Easy*, give more in-depth information about what and how much you should eat. Check out these books at store.diabetes.org.

Singing the Same Healthy Eating Verse

The healthy eating guidelines in this book reflect today's American Diabetes Association *Nutrition Therapy Recommendations for the Management of Adults With Diabetes*. As noted, these recommendations echo those from the federal government, as published in the *Dietary Guidelines for Americans*, and several health-related organizations. In essence, all of these organizations are singing the same healthy eating verse. In fact, the American Diabetes Association collaborates with the American Heart Association and the American Cancer Society on an initiative called the Preventive Health Partnership. These three large organizations have created this partnership and a program called Everyday Choices (everydaychoices.org), which encourages healthy living, because eating healthfully and living a healthy lifestyle reduces the risk of all three diseases—some cancers, heart and circulatory diseases, and type 2 diabetes.

As more people strive to eat healthier and as healthier restaurant foods become available, this effort will become easier. By no means is healthy restaurant eating simple; at times you will feel like a fish swimming upstream because so many Americans chow down on downright unhealthy foods and large portions of them. It's not always easy to eat healthfully. And that's particularly true when it comes to restaurant foods—whether you eat in or take out. You'll gather plenty of tips, tactics, and tricks through the pages of this book and before long you'll be a pro. Yes, practice makes, well, almost perfect.

The Top 10 Healthy Eating How-Tos

The following chart explains the top 10 healthy eating goals for all Americans, including people with diabetes. You'll see the Dietary Guidelines in the center column accompanied by a translation of each guideline. In the right column you'll see a few tips to help you implement this dietary guideline when you eat restaurant meals. The BIG challenge is putting these seemingly straightforward and simplistic nutrition guidelines into practice in your hurried and harried daily life amongst a sea of less than healthy foods.

Number	The Dietary Guideline*	Tips to Implement Healthy Eating Goals in Restaurants
1	*Guideline:* Control total calorie intake to manage body weight. For people who are overweight or obese, this will mean consuming fewer calories from foods and beverages. *Translation:* To lose weight you'll need to eat fewer calories than your body uses. Keeping the lost weight off requires constant vigilance to calorie intake and regular daily exercise. To stay at a healthy weight (if you've not been overweight) shoot for the goal of equalizing the number of calories you eat and the number of calories you burn.	▶ Choose your calories and fats wisely. Be on the lookout for ways that fats creep into your restaurant foods. Fats are concentrated forms of calories and send the calorie count up. ▶ Portion control is king when it comes to controlling restaurant calories. Split and share to your heart's content. Order half portions or take half home for another meal. ▶ To fill up without filling out, try to fill your plate with a healthy dose of vegetables. Just make sure they're not doused in fats. ▶ Get out of your comfort zone. Use the variety of foods served in restaurants to test your palate with unfamiliar healthy foods you'd like to try (and should be eating more of)—whole grains, beans and peas, and vegetables.
2	*Guideline:* Reduce daily sodium intake to less than 2,300 milligrams (mg). *Translation:* Your sodium count should be no higher than 2,300 milligrams per day. Though this is a challenge to accomplish, particularly when eating restaurant foods, try to eat fewer processed and prepared foods. They contribute about three-quarters of the sodium Americans eat. Hold the salt. That's about 10% of the sodium we eat.	▶ Realize that a large percent of sodium intake comes from frequent consumption of foods with a moderate amount of sodium. The American Heart Association identifies these foods as "The Salty Six:" 1) breads and rolls 2) cold cuts and cured meats 3) pizza (often topped with high-sodium meats and cheese) 4) poultry (mainly processed products) 5) soups 6) sandwiches (made with poultry products, cold cuts, cured meats, and "special" sauces). (Learn more about "The Salty Six" at http://www.heart. org/HEARTORG/General/Salty-Six–Common-Foods-Loaded-with-Excess-Sodium_UCM_446090_Article.jsp)

Number	The Dietary Guideline*	Tips to Implement Healthy Eating Goals in Restaurants
		▶ Beware of ingredients and sauces that load on the sodium: special or signature mayonnaise-based sauces, bacon, olives, cheese, pickles, and salad dressings. Avoid or limit your consumption of these foods. ▶ Choose fresh rather than processed foods when you can. ▶ Don't use the salt shaker at the table.
3	*Guideline:* Reduce the intake of calories from solid fats. Consume less than 10% of calories from saturated fatty acids by replacing them with monounsaturated and polyunsaturated fatty acids. Keep trans fatty acid consumption as low as possible by limiting foods that contain synthetic sources [not natural such as in dairy and meats] of trans fats, such as partially hydrogenated oils, and by limiting other solid fats. Use oils to replace solid fats where possible. *Translation:* Based on research, there's now more focus on choosing to eat healthy fats vs. eating less total fat. Eat 25–35% of your calories as fat. Try to have most of your fat be from polyunsaturated and monounsaturated fats. Keep saturated fat and trans fat (a type of saturated fat) intake as low as possible to minimize the risk for cardiovascular disease.	▶ Use less fat—trim sour cream, cream cheese, mayonnaise, butter, and salad dressings from your diet to reduce both your total fat intake and intake of unhealthy fats. ▶ Opt for fat-free milk to reduce fat intake and limit unhealthy fats. ▶ Keep cheese (any form) to a minimum due to its total fat and saturated fat content. ▶ Ask about or observe what oil(s) the restaurants you eat in use. Commonly used liquid oils, such as soybean, corn, and canola oil, are low in saturated fat and contain no trans fats. ▶ Avoid fried foods due to the high total fat and calorie content. ▶ Dip bread in tiny amounts of olive oil (it's got more flavor than most vegetable oils) rather than using butter. ▶ Always order salad dressing on the side and use very little. Olive oil and vinegar is your best bet to keep the amount of saturated fat and sodium low. ▶ Order foods grilled, barbecued, roasted, steamed, or poached to limit fat.

Number	The Dietary Guideline*	Tips to Implement Healthy Eating Goals in Restaurants
4	*Guideline:* Consume less than 300 mg per day of dietary cholesterol. (The American Diabetes Association Nutrition Recommendations also recommend no more than 300 mg per day.) *Translation:* Limit your intake of cholesterol because of the link to a higher incidence of cardiovascular disease. Cholesterol is found in foods and ingredients that have an animal origin, such as cheese, full-fat dairy foods, meats, poultry, and seafood.	► Review the tips under Guideline #3. Reducing your total fat intake will help you limit the intake of animal fats that contain cholesterol. ► Opt for fat-free milk. ► Keep cheese to a minimum. ► Skip 3-egg omelets unless you'll be splitting or sharing them. ► Limit how often you order large portions of meats, poultry, and shellfish (shrimp, calamari, oysters). Enjoy some vegetarian meals or split portions of animal proteins to eat just 3–4 cooked ounces at a meal.
5	*Guideline:* Reduce the intake of calories from added sugars. *Translation:* Added sugars are a group of ingredients added to foods and beverages during processing to sweeten them. They all provide concentrated calories and have next to no nutritional value. Limit them as much as possible.	► The number-one source of added sugars is sugar-sweetened sodas and drinks. To quench your thirst at meals drink water, sparkling water, club soda, tea, or coffee. And don't be shy to order low-fat (or, better yet, fat-free) milk. Most restaurants have it on hand. ► Skip adding sugar to hot or cold beverages. One of the many low-calorie sweeteners available can help you sweeten foods and beverages without empty calories. ► Instead of pastries, Danishes, scones, and other breakfast sweets, opt for whole-grain bread, a roll, or half a bagel. ► If you want dessert and can afford to splurge, consider splitting it with two or more other people.

Number	The Dietary Guideline*	Tips to Implement Healthy Eating Goals in Restaurants
6	*Guideline:* Limit the consumption of foods that contain refined grains, especially refined grain foods that contain solid fats, added sugars, and sodium. Consume at least half of all grains as whole grains. Increase whole-grain intake by replacing refined grains with whole grains. *Translation:* Seek out and eat more whole grains and foods that contain whole-grain ingredients, such as whole-grain bread, crackers, and pasta, instead of those made with refined grains. This is a challenge in restaurants because they serve many refined grains and foods that contain them—from pizza crust to white-flour rolls and bread. Also limit grain-based foods which also contain solid fats, added sugars, and/or sodium, such as refined grain–based pastries and desserts and crunchy snack foods.	▶ Eat whole-grain bread or rolls. Have sandwiches made on these. ▶ Choose brown rice in Asian restaurants if it's an option. ▶ Skip the crunchy fried snack food. Opt for a side salad, side of cooked vegetable, or apple slices. ▶ Expand your palate and experiment with less familiar whole grains: barley, millet, quinoa, amaranth, and more (you'll find these being served more in upscale restaurants). ▶ Select whole-grain hot or cold cereals. ▶ Split and share desserts among many diners.
7	*Guideline:* Increase vegetable and fruit intake. Eat a variety of vegetables, especially dark-green, red, and orange vegetables and beans and peas.	▶ If you drink fruit juice, make it 100% fruit juice. But do watch the volume you drink. Restaurant portions, from a glass of orange juice at breakfast to a container purchased at a coffee or sandwich shop, tend to be large and often contain more than one serving. ▶ Make an entrée salad a meal. Or order a side salad in place of french fries or crunchy chips.

Number	The Dietary Guideline*	Tips to Implement Healthy Eating Goals in Restaurants
	Translation: Eat at least (within your calorie allotment) 2 1/2 cups of both fruit and vegetables each day. All fruits and vegetables that are prepared with no (or limited) added fats and sugars are excellent sources of nutrition.	▶ If a meal comes with a vegetable, ask for doubles and skip the serving of refined grains. ▶ Fit in beans and peas when you're able. Enjoy a cup or bowl of bean soup or chili made with beans. At a salad bar, include green peas, chickpeas, or kidney beans, if available.
8	*Guideline:* Increase intake of fat-free or low-fat milk and milk products, such as milk, yogurt, cheese, or fortified soy beverages. *Translation:* Americans, including children and young adults, only drink about one serving of milk a day when two 8-ounce servings per day are what we need. Fat-free milk is the optimal dairy food from which to get the calcium, vitamin D, and other important nutrients we need.	▶ Opt for fat-free milk when it's available. Otherwise try reduced-fat milk. ▶ Keep cheese to a minimum due to its saturated fat content. ▶ Yogurt, whether Greek or regular, has become more available in restaurants serving breakfast and in coffee shops. Unfortunately, it tends to be the type with fruit and added sugars. Plain, nonfat yogurt is ideal.
9	*Guideline:* Choose a variety of protein foods, which include seafood, lean meat and poultry, eggs, beans and peas, soy products, and unsalted nuts and seeds. Increase the amount and variety of seafood consumed by choosing seafood in place of some meat and poultry. Replace protein foods that are higher in solid fats with choices that are lower in solid fats and calories and/or are sources of oils.	▶ Poultry: Skip it fried. Order it grilled, sautéed, or stir-fried. If the skin is on, take it off prior to eating. ▶ Seafood: Skip it fried. Order it poached, boiled, steamed, or grilled with minimal butter or sauces. ▶ Red meats: Skip it fried. Order lean cuts. Order it grilled, barbecued, or broiled. Split and share large portions. ▶ Fit in beans and peas when you're able. Enjoy a cup or bowl of bean soup or chili made with beans. At a salad bar include green peas, chickpeas, or kidney beans, if available.

Number	The Dietary Guideline*	Tips to Implement Healthy Eating Goals in Restaurants
	Translation: Choose lean meats, prepare them with limited fat, and enjoy no more than 3–4 cooked ounces per meal. Take the skin off poultry before or after cooking. Enjoy seafood prepared with minimal fat. Try other healthy non–animal-based sources of protein like beans and peas, nuts and seeds, and soy-based foods.	► Opt for nuts and/or seeds for snacks.
10	*Guideline:* If alcohol is consumed, it should be consumed in moderation—up to one drink per day for women and two drinks per day for men—and only by adults of legal drinking age. *Translation:* Be moderate when it comes to alcohol. The calories add up. A moderate alcohol intake has minimal short- and long-term effects on glucose levels in people with type 1 or 2 diabetes. You should avoid drinking in excess because of the calories, the potential negative impact on glucose control, and the potential harm to yourself and others.	► Consider keeping your alcohol intake moderate by just drinking when you dine out. ► Choose beer, wine, or a simple mixed drink (such as a scotch and club soda or a rum and diet coke), rather than higher-calorie mixed drinks. ► Always have a noncaloric beverage by your side to sip rather than only sipping your alcoholic drink to quench your thirst. ► Read more about how to manage alcoholic beverages with diabetes in Chapters 5 and 9.

*Wording from U.S. Department of Agriculture and U.S. Department of Health and Human Services: Dietary Guidelines for Americans, 2010. Available at *http://www.health.gov/dietaryguidelines/dga2010/DietaryGuidelines2010.pdf*

As you make the effort to change your restaurant eating habits, keep these *Top 10 Healthy Eating How-Tos* in mind. And when you look at restaurant menus, ask yourself the following questions to help put these how-tos into action:

▶ How can I fit in more vegetables at this meal?

▶ Can I ask for olive oil to dip my bread in rather than butter? Better yet, to limit calories, can I skip the oil or butter? Or should I skip the bread or rolls altogether and send them back to the kitchen?

▶ Are there whole-grain breads I can have a sandwich made on or whole-grain side dishes available?

▶ Can I reduce my total fat grams by asking for an ingredient or two to be left out of my meal or replaced (e.g., replace mayonnaise with mustard on a sandwich)?

▶ Is it possible to split the portion of protein and take half home for tomorrow's lunch or dinner?

▶ Is there an appetizer, salad and/or cup of broth or bean-based soup that is healthy and can help me eat smaller portions of my main meal?

You get the picture: healthier restaurant eating is all about slowly changing your eating and ordering habits.

CHAPTER 3

The 10 Health and Nutrition Pitfalls of Restaurant Eating

L et's be clear: eating restaurant foods healthfully is downright challenging! That's true whether you're dining out for pleasure on upscale fusion cuisine that mixes ingredients and flavors from a cadre of cultures, blending business with lunch at a sit-down restaurant that serves typical American fare, or grabbing an on-the-run dinner from a fast-food restaurant along a highway or in a shopping mall food court. The next step on your journey is to raise your awareness of the 10 health and nutrition pitfalls of restaurant eating.

You need willpower (or "won't power") and perseverance to manage restaurant menu minefields and eat healthy. Challenges confront you when you have to pick and choose from a menu or menu board and cannot carefully control the ingredients or the portions of the meals you order. You can't march into restaurant kitchens and stop the chef or cook as they ladle butter, slather mayonnaise, or pour salt.

The pitfalls of restaurant eating range from huge portions to large quantities of fats, oils, sugar, and salt. But, please don't despair! These pitfalls aren't insurmountable and the more you raise your awareness, the better equipped you'll be to deal with them head on. You *can* learn to *choose*, or better stated, pick and choose, to eat healthfully in 99% of restaurants and not be trapped by these common pitfalls. (Chapter 4 on page 29 provides an in depth rundown of restaurant eating skills and strategies that will help.)

Sections 2 and 3 of *Eat Out, Eat Well* give you a head's up on the pitfalls you'll encounter with each type of restaurant fare or cuisine along with tips, tactics, and more.

The 10 Health and Nutrition Pitfalls of Restaurant Eating:

1 *Treating restaurant meals as special occasions:*
Back a few decades ago restaurant meals were reserved for special occasions. They celebrated unique events in a person's, couple's, or family's life, which took place once in a blue moon. Today people eat restaurants meals an average of five times a week. With this frequency of restaurant meals, you can't "afford"—when it comes to your weight, diabetes control, and health in general—to order with that old special occasion, splurge mindset every time you have a restaurant meal. Sure, you can still enjoy a splurge at celebrations. But to keep your waistline from expanding and to get and stay healthy, most people need to toe the nutrition line and make those frequent restaurant meals healthy.

2 *Not having direct access to the chef:*
Today your food is prepared either in a kitchen behind closed doors, in front of you in an open kitchen, or in assembly line fashion (think fast food chains and sub shops). In all cases, this goes on at least an arm's reach away. In fine dining restaurants, most dishes are prepared from scratch. These dishes start with basic ingredients, then sauces, seasonings, and more are added. These situations lend themselves to requesting simple changes to make your meal healthier; however, you need to have a willing chef or cook and a waitperson who will serve as your conduit.

In many restaurants (think fast-food burgers, sandwich shops, and large sit-down chains), foods come in the back door near-ready for their final preparation or assembly steps. Customizing items or orders isn't their specialty, though these types of restaurants are famous for telling you that you can "get it your way." In these situations you have less control, but you can still exert pressure to get foods as you need and want them. You'll learn to control these varied dining situations by asking questions and requesting changes. The good news is that restaurants need and want your business, and, with increased attention paid to health and nutrition, some restaurants are more open than ever to meeting your desires and customizing orders. Yes, a key to eating healthier is to get foods placed in front of you in the way and, importantly, in the amount you need them. Get ready to speak up and be assertive.

3 ***Fruits, vegetables, whole grains, legumes, and low-fat dairy options are few and far between:***
The very foods you should eat more of for good health are often limited or simply missing from restaurant menus. This includes fruits, vegetables, whole grains, legumes, and low-fat dairy foods.

Consider vegetables. You can find salads in fast-food restaurants. Side salads and entrée salads are present and accounted for in most sit-down American-style restaurants. But in fine dining establishments, vegetables, other than the occasional vegetarian entrée, are purely small side dishes used to fill out a plate with the protein source taking center stage. You'll have to work hard to satisfy that recommendation for 2 1/2 cups of vegetables a day.

Fruit is even less available than vegetables in most restaurants. You may find it camouflaged between two pieces of crust (fruit pie) or served in its liquid form as juice. To get the 2 1/2 cups a day you'll need to eat fruit as part of the meals you eat at home or bring it with you to enjoy during the day.

When it comes to whole grains, availability is improving. They're making their way onto the menus of more sandwich shops and better restaurants. You'll see whole-wheat or whole-grain breads and rolls available for sandwiches in sub and sandwich shops or in the bread baskets at nicer restaurants. You may—though this will still be tough—be able to order pizza made with a whole-grain crust or whole-wheat pasta. Brown rice may be available in Asian restaurants. But we've still got a ways to go before we can say that eating whole grains in restaurants is easy.

Low-fat dairy foods, such as milk or yogurt, can be challenging to find and incorporate into restaurant meals. Today, most fast food restaurants offer low-fat milk, which is lower in fat and calories than whole milk, but not as low in fat as fat-free milk. Low-fat milk is also available in most sit-down family-style restaurants. Don't count on milk being available in the majority of ethnic restaurants. Yogurt, particularly the healthier low-sugar plain yogurt, is not often found in restaurants. You'll find it served with Middle Eastern fare because it's an ingredient used to prepare some foods. Low-fat milk and lower-fat and lower-sugar yogurt are becoming more available in individual servings in supermarkets, convenience stores, and some sandwich shops.

4 Protein foods take center stage:

Protein foods often dominate the plate, particularly when it comes to American cuisines. (Protein includes but is not limited to red meats—beef, lamb, pork, and veal—as well as poultry and seafood.) When you look at a menu, is your focus usually on what will take center stage on the plate? Often that's the protein food. Healthy eating guidelines suggest that the portion of protein per meal should be no more than 3 ounces cooked for most adults. Unless you order an appetizer or mixed dish with vegetables and starch, such as stir-fry or pasta and clam sauce, you'll get served a portion of protein that's more in the realm of 6–8 ounces (cooked).

When you enjoy the food from some cuisines, such as Asian or Mexican, it's easier to eat a smaller portion of protein. In American and family-style restaurants you need to put the portion-control skills and strategies you'll learn in Chapter 4 (page 29) into action. For starters, consider how you can transition from thinking about a source of protein as the center of your main course to letting a hearty portion of a healthy side dish occupy your plate. Consider going meat-free, even for just one or two meals per week. When you do eat meat, it should only take up about one-quarter of the plate, whereas vegetables should take up one-half of the plate and the remaining quarter should contain a healthy starch.

5 Portions are HUGE:

It seems that a "value equals volume" mentality long ago invaded restaurant meals, especially in chain and fast-food restaurants. Portion sizes (and the plates to hold these massive portions) just keep getting larger. When you are served large portions, it's difficult to stop eating when there's still food on your plate. That's especially true if you were brought up holding membership in the clean plate club! One strategy you'll read about frequently in this book is to outwit large portions by controlling portions from the start—when you order,—by splitting and sharing menu items or ordering a 6-inch versus a foot-long sub, for example. Get less food placed in front of you and you'll eat less food during the meal. (You'll learn other strategies to combat large portions in Chapter 4.)

A word to the wise: limit all-you-can-eat restaurants and other settings that simply promote overeating, such as hotel breakfast buffets or salad or food bars. This is particularly wise if you don't have much willpower or if you like to "get your money's worth." However, if you feel these settings work well because they help you control portions, use them to your advantage.

6 Fats and oils are in, on, around, and through everything:

Fats and oils make foods taste good and stay moist for longer. That's just a fact about fats. It's a big reason why you see a wide variety of oils, fats, and high-fat ingredients used in restaurant foods from the start of the meal to the finishing touch. You may start a meal in a sit-down restaurant with bread and butter or olive oil. In a Mexican restaurant, it may be chips and salsa. Going Chinese, you may see fried noodles. The butter, chips, and fried noodles all contain a lot of fat, which means a hefty bunch of calories before you even take a bite of the food you've ordered.

In the kitchen, chefs use oil or butter to sauté or cook vegetables, grains, and starch dishes. Some even put pads of butter with herbs on a piece of beef to soak in when on the grill. Burgers and sandwiches often partner up with high-fat ingredients, such as cheese or bacon. Then a "special" or signature sauce may be added, which is usually mayonnaise-based and finishes off the dish with a flourish of extra calories.

Salad dressing gets tossed into salads and quickly raises the calories of a healthy fresh or cooked vegetable. Sour cream and butter get added to baked potatoes and cream and cheese sauces get added to meats, pastas, or sandwiches with the same disastrous results. Many foods, even healthy vegetables, are served fried, stuffed, and smothered, typically with high-fat ingredients that pack on the calories. Controlling the amount of fat in your restaurant foods is another BIG key to healthier restaurant eating. Stay tuned for plenty of tips and tactics on controlling fat in Chapter 4 (page 29).

7 *Unhealthy fats and oils abound:*
Not only is it important to not eat too much total fat, but research has shown it's even more important to eat more of the fats and oils that contain the healthier fatty acids—polyunsaturated and mono-unsaturated fat—and less saturated and trans fats. Diabetes and general nutrition guidelines encourage you to eat less saturated fat due to its negative effects on our circulatory system. Read more on trans and saturated fats in Chapter 2 (page 9).

When it comes to trans fat, you're advised to eat as little as possible, especially if you have diabetes. In 2006, the U.S. Food and Drug Administration (FDA) began requiring trans fat to be listed on the Nutrition Facts panel of packaged foods. The restaurant industry and the food manufacturers that supply the industry have been working to reduce the use of trans fats, also known as partially hydrogenated oils (PHOs), with some success. For example, cooking oils with zero trans fat are more commonly used today. But restaurant foods such as cinnamon rolls, pies (in the crust), cookies, pancakes and waffles, and non-dairy coffee creamers may still contain these PHOs. (We also eat a small amount of trans fat from animal-based foods, such as meat and dairy foods that contain fat.) As a result of these changes, our intake of trans fat has decreased, but not enough. In late 2013, the FDA announced further efforts to reduce trans-fat intake. This plan will likely take a few years to go into effect.

The cholesterol count from the foods you eat, though it is not fat per se, is another nutrition factor to consider. Limiting cholesterol from foods to less than the recommended 300 milligrams per day helps keep total cholesterol and LDL (bad) cholesterol levels down. Cholesterol is only found in animal-based foods, such as egg yolks, cheese, bacon and sausage, red meats, poultry, and seafood. Keeping portions of these foods small, and enjoying some of them only occasionally, helps reduce cholesterol intake.

8 *Sodium levels can skyrocket:*
When you consider the *Dietary Guidelines for Americans* recommendation of 2,300 milligrams of sodium per day (see page 14) and then observe the sodium counts of many restaurant meals, you'll understand why we eat way over the recommended sodium level.

Many restaurant meals can total 2,300 milligrams or higher on their own. Added salt in foods is not as much the sodium villain today as are processed and restaurant foods. While fine dining restaurants use mainly from-scratch ingredients, American, family, and fast-food restaurants use a number of processed foods. (Think cold cuts in sub sandwiches and chicken breasts in a grilled chicken sandwich.) These are often higher in sodium and add to the high sodium count of the meals. Sodium is used in excess because, just like fats and oils, it makes foods taste good. It's also used as a preservative to extend the shelf life of foods.

You'll learn to control the amount of sodium in your restaurants foods. For starters: limit known high-sodium foods, such as soup, cold cuts, and fast-food chicken products and french fries. Limit known high-sodium ingredients, such as anchovies, olives, and pickles. And limit high-sodium toppers, such as salad dressing, cheese sauce, or mayonnaise sauces. Limit servings of what the American Heart Association calls *The Salty Six* (see Chapter 2 on page 14). Don't shake the salt shaker. And keep in mind that if you eat fewer total calories, you'll also likely consume less sodium.

9 *Beverages (nonalcoholic) are big, bigger, biggest:* The selection of nonalcoholic beverages in most fast-food and sit-down family restaurants seems to focus on sugar-sweetened (usually made with high fructose corn syrup) drinks, such as soda, lemonade, sweetened ice tea, and fruit drinks. And the portions have become big, bigger, and biggest (even though they're called "small," "medium," and "large," or sometimes "jumbo," or "giant"). These giant portions of sugary drinks add a large amount of undesirable added sugars and hundreds of calories to your meal but have no nutritional value. In addition, the onslaught of hot and cold coffee beverages has upped our intake of added sugars and unhealthy fats (low-fat or whole milk, half and half, or whipped cream and non-dairy creamers). Explore options for healthier nonalcoholic beverages in Chapter 9 on page 87.

10 *Alcoholic beverages can run up calories and run down your resilience:*

Alcohol seems to go hand in hand with sit-down meals. You may enjoy a cocktail, one or more beers or glasses of wine, or perhaps an after-dinner drink when out for a business dinner or special celebration. When you total the calories from alcohol, the calorie count can easily be in the hundreds. Another downfall of consuming alcohol for some people is that it can weaken your resolve to eat healthfully. Learn the best ways to enjoy minimal amounts of alcoholic beverages in Chapter 9 on page 87.

Now on to Chapter 4: The 10 Skills and Strategies for Healthier Restaurant Eating, to begin to master the skills and strategies that will help you combat these 10 pitfalls.

The 10 Skills and Strategies for Healthier Restaurant Eating

At this point you may believe that the phrase "a healthy restaurant meal" is an oxymoron, or that finding a healthy restaurant meal is near to impossible. It's not impossible at all! With skills and strategies in hand, *you can choose* to eat healthier restaurant meals. "You can choose" are the operative words. As you put these skills and strategies into practice day after day and eventually reap health benefits, the job will get easier. Your new restaurant eating habits, the way you order, and the types of foods you eat will become second nature.

These skills and strategies range from the psychological—changing your mindset about restaurant meals—to the practical, such as when and how to put your knife and fork down and push your plate away or get up from the table.

Soak in these skills and strategies. (You'll also find cuisine-specific skills and strategies woven through the tips and tactics in the chapters of Sections 2 and 3.) You can apply these skills and strategies in just about any restaurant eating situation—whether you eat a meal in the restaurant or take out. In fact, these skills apply whenever you're faced with food choices outside of your home and beyond your control. Keep them in mind at your school or work cafeteria, at work celebrations or meetings when food is catered or brought in by co-workers, or when you eat a meal at a friend or loved one's home. Decisions, decisions!

The 10 Skills and Strategies for Healthier Restaurant Eating:

1 *Develop a healthy mindset and a can-do attitude:*
This is your crucial first step. Until you shift your mindset, you'll have a difficult time putting the other nine skills and strategies into action. Yes, this psychological shift is task number one.

Think about it: do you approach every restaurant meal as if it's a special occasion? Do you cast caution to the wind and choose whatever your taste buds and heart desire, eating until you are stuffed? Do you use frequent restaurant meals as opportunities to reward yourself, perhaps with a fat-drenched appetizer or a decadent dessert? Do you feel that, since you are paying for the meal, you might as well get your money's worth and eat all that's on your plate?

After you've given thought to and honestly owned up to your present attitudes, think about the small steps you can take to develop a healthier mindset about restaurant meals. Ask yourself what changes you need to make to find a balance between continuing to enjoy restaurant eating and ordering and eating healthier foods. Be kind to yourself. These changes will take some time, but you will build up a repertoire of positive experiences. You can do this!

2 *Examine your restaurant eating patterns (when, where, why, and what you eat):*
Take a look at how often you eat out. If your count verges on the excessive—at least once a day or more—then ask yourself why you eat out so frequently and how you can reduce this frequency. If you reduce the number of restaurant meals you eat and are willing to do some home food preparation, you'll have an easier time eating healthy.

The frequency with which you can "afford" a restaurant splurge really depends on a couple of factors. First, how often you eat restaurant meals. Second, your nutrition and diabetes goals. If you eat out quite frequently and need to keep your calories and fat grams pretty low, then you'll need to keep splurges to a minimum. Conversely, if you eat out pretty rarely, say even once a month, you might be able to take a few more liberties during a restaurant meal—perhaps with an alcoholic drink or a dessert. But then again, you may choose not to.

Get to know YOUR restaurant ordering and eating habits. Raise YOUR awareness about YOUR behaviors. Awareness is key to changing your behaviors. Answer the *Get to Know Yourself* questions at the end of this chapter (see page 42). What you learn about yourself will help you set some realistic goals to change your restaurant eating behaviors one step at a time.

3 Zero in on the right site:

Choose restaurants, when you can, that make it easier for you to eat healthfully. The reality is you can choose to eat healthfully in 99% of restaurants, but some restaurant menus definitely make it a bit easier than others. Steer clear of a few of your favorite restaurants in which you typically eat unhealthy meals or restaurants where the healthy pickings are slim, for example, a fried-chicken or fish-and-chips restaurant. One plus about large fast-food or chain restaurants that can make life easier is that you know the menu all too well. This can help you plan ahead, no matter which one of the chain's locations you pop into.

4 Set your game plan prior to your arrival:

"Think before you act" should be your modus operandi. If you're familiar with the menu offerings from a particular restaurant you frequent, take a minute on your walk or drive to think through what you might order before you cross the restaurant's threshold. If you know the menu well and are set on your order, don't even tempt your taste buds by looking at less healthy foods on the menu.

Be the first in your party to order. This strategy eliminates your time to ponder changes as you wait for your dining partners to place their orders. If you want to split and/or share menu items, ask who's willing to share as people peruse the menu. More often than not, people will be pleased you made the offer. This strategy has become increasingly acceptable in restaurants. The greater availability of small plates of food in better restaurants is another trend that makes portion control even easier. Yes, that's eating tapas style.

On a broader scope, think about your menu choices in the context of the whole day. Ask yourself these questions:

- ▶ Have I eaten enough servings of fruit and vegetables today?
- ▶ Will I be eating more protein at another meal?
- ▶ How much fat will I eat today?

A preplanning strategy that might help you is calorie and nutrient banking. Use this thought process for whatever you're trying to track—calories, fats, carbohydrate, fruits, and/or vegetables. "Calorie and nutrient banking" teaches you to think about your food intake more than one meal at a time and, if necessary, more than one day at a time. For example, if you plan to celebrate your anniversary at a swanky restaurant, you can "save" fat grams throughout the day or week to "spend" on a special sauce or a split of a favorite dessert.

When you practice banking strategies, don't fall into the trap of starving yourself prior to a restaurant meal. This practice is clearly a setup for overeating and, if you're at risk, possibly hypoglycemia. All in all, this plan usually backfires. For one thing, it makes you extremely hungry, which weakens your resistance to unhealthy foods and extras.

Another way to bank calories is through increased physical activity. Increase your activity and burn more calories before or after meals. Spend more time at the gym, take a longer walk or swim, or take a nice stroll after dinner. Be aware when you use this method of banking that you may require some adjustments in your glucose-lowering medications if you're at risk of developing hypoglycemia.

5 Be an avid fat detective:

Dodging the fats in restaurants is one of your a biggest challenges. Fat adds significant calories to your meal without adding any food volume (or "bites").

Here's a perfect example: Consider a medium baked potato, which contains about 100 calories and no fat. Add to that 1 teaspoon of regular butter or margarine at 50 calories and 2 tablespoons of regular sour cream at 50 calories and you've added another 100 calories of almost pure fat without adding any bites.

Fat is the most saturated form of calories, with 9 calories per gram. Carbohydrate and protein contain half the calories, at

4 calories per gram. Therefore, lowering fat intake, even just a little, can have a big impact on the number of calories you consume. Learn to be an avid fat detective. Consider the fats both on the menu and at the table when eating a restaurant meal.

Fats on the menu creep in as ingredients used in cooking and food preparation—butter, oil, cream, sour cream, mayonnaise—and as main ingredients used in dishes, such as sausage on pizza, prime rib, and pork spareribs. Certain preparation methods simply mean a food is drenched in fat, such as deep-fried, smothered, or covered with a cream-based sauce.

Particular menu items, by definition, are loaded with fat, such as pasta with Alfredo sauce or chimichangas, a fried burrito. Most of the chapters in Sections 2 and 3 contain lists of green- and red-flag words, which give the cuisine-specific ingredients, preparation methods, and menu descriptions that signal low-fat and healthy items (*Green-Flag Words*) or higher-fat and not-so-healthy items in each type of cuisine (*Red-Flag Words*). And don't be shy in restaurants. Ask questions about unfamiliar ingredients, preparations, and menu descriptions. Then you won't be unpleasantly surprised when your plate arrives.

Fat creeps in at the table in several ways. You might be greeted with rolls and butter, chips and salsa, Chinese noodles, or garlic bread. So, even before you order, the fat starts to tally up. Extra fats might be brought to the table in the form of sour cream, butter, margarine, mayonnaise, salad dressing, and cream for beverages. The best advice is to limit the fats at the table if this is agreeable with your dining partners. Perhaps keep the rolls but return the butter. Or return them both.

6 *Order with your diabetes and healthy eating goals top in mind:* You learned about the keys to healthy eating in Chapter 2. Go back to these on occasion. Keep them in mind as you select restaurant meals. More than likely you'll want to set these two goals: 1) eat more fruits and vegetables (because they're usually sparse or missing completely), and 2) lighten up on your portions of protein and fats (because they're often served in excess).

7 **Practice portion control from the start:**
Large portions tend to define restaurant meals. To cut portions down to a healthy size you'll need to "outsmart" the menu. One helpful strategy is to control portions from the start—when you place your order. The result? Less food will be in front of you and you'll eat less. This is the "out of sight, out of mind (or mouth)" technique. It's a lot more difficult to control the amount you eat if food is just a forkful or spoonful away. A few general tactics for controlling portions when you order:

- ► Steer clear of menu descriptions that mean large portions—"jumbo," "grande," "supreme," "extra large," "king size," "double," "triple," "feast," or "combo." (Unless you plan to split!)
- ► Go for the menu descriptions that mean small servings— "regular," "petite," "kiddie."
- ► Ask for and order half-, lunch-, or appetizer-size portions (if available).
- ► Choose from à la carte items and/or side offerings. Mix and match these to wind up with small servings of a few items.
- ► Split and share when you can or wrap part of your food up for another meal.

Throughout the book you'll learn ways to control portions in specific types of restaurants. You'll want to work toward eating smaller quantities of those restaurant foods you enjoy.

Portion control and guesstimating skills are particularly important for people with diabetes who are tightly managing their blood glucose levels and adjusting their mealtime blood glucose–lowering medications (usually insulin) based on the grams of carbohydrate they eat. With these skills fine-tuned, you can figure out a rough estimate of the amount of important nutrients in restaurant food. *Put Your Best Guesstimate Forward* (page 37) offers tips to improve your "guesstimating" skills.

8 **Practice menu creativity:**
To eat healthfully and to eat reasonable portions, you'll need to be creative with menus. Get started with these general creativity tips.

In Sections 2 and 3 you'll get cuisine- and menu-specific ways to practice menu creativity when eating restaurant fare.

▶ No rule says you must order an entrée. Mix and match items from the soups, salads, appetizers, and side dishes. There are countless ways to combine these to eat smaller portions.

▶ Order a cup of broth-based soup, such as chicken with rice or bean and barley, as a low-calorie filler, especially if your dining partners are partaking of high-fat appetizers. You can use a side salad in a similar way.

▶ Opt for a salad to start and then ask the waitperson to serve an appetizer of your choosing as a main course.

▶ Order two appetizers, one to eat as an appetizer and the other as your main course.

▶ Split portions with your restaurant eating partner(s). Go ahead, enjoy soup and a dessert with your entrée, but split everything down the middle. In better restaurants, you can ask the waitperson to split the items that can be split in the kitchen and serve them on two plates.

▶ Eat "family style." This is the eating style you'll find in some Asian restaurants, but it can be used in any type of restaurant— you can even split an order of french fries from fast-food restaurants. Order one or two fewer entrées than the number of people dining.

▶ Share nutritionally complementary dishes to eat more healthfully. For example, in an Italian restaurant, one person orders Pasta Primavera and the other orders Chicken Marsala. The chicken dish will be at least 6–8 ounces of chicken—that's enough protein for two. The pasta is also enough to provide starch servings for two. A salad will add a vegetable serving for two.

9 *Order foods as you need and want them:*
Special requests are key to being served dishes as you like (and want or need) them. A special request might mean asking for an ingredient to be left off, such as cheese, bacon, and/or sour cream. Or asking for a substitution: a baked potato rather than french

fries or potato chips or mustard rather than mayonnaise spread on a sandwich. Maybe you just want an ingredient, like salad dressing, butter, or guacamole, served on the side so you control the amount you eat. Perhaps your request is a cooking instruction, such as "broil my fish with a small amount of butter" or "use very little oil in the wok." Or maybe you have celiac disease as well as diabetes and special requests are critical to avoiding any gluten consumption (see Chapter 6, beginning on page 56, which is dedicated to people with gluten concerns). It's important to adopt the attitude that there's no harm in asking and the worst someone can say is no.

Special requests might make you feel like you are ruffling feathers or holding up other customers in line. However, there are ways to approach special requests that will put you at ease and won't make you or your eating partners sink into their seats or that won't delay others in a walk-up-and-order restaurant:

▶ Request simple changes or additions. For instance, request that salad dressing, sauce, or sour cream be served on the side or ask that french fries be replaced with a baked potato.

▶ Be reasonable and realistic. Don't try to remake a menu item by requesting that certain ingredients be left out and others added.

▶ Be pleasantly assertive. Let the waitperson know what you want by using non-threatening words and language. These phrases work:

▷ Do you think the chef will…?

▷ I'd really appreciate it if you could…?

▷ May I have … on the side?

▷ Would it be a problem to substitute … for…?

10 Know when to say "enough":

You already know that portion control is a key to healthier restaurant eating. Control portions from the start by ordering creatively. But if the portions are huge, request a take-home container and immediately set aside the portion to take home or back to work for a meal tomorrow or another day. If that feels uncomfortable in some situations, separate the portion you don't want to eat, place it on a small plate, and offer "tastes" to your dining companions or just move it to the side of your plate.

Be clear about your definition of fullness. Often, we respond to external rather than internal cues. An external cue is food left on your plate. An internal cue is a full stomach. Learn to listen to your internal signals: how does your stomach feel when you have had enough to eat? Begin to recognize this sensation as a message to stop eating and put down your knife and fork rather than waiting for that post–Thanksgiving-dinner stuffed-turkey feeling. Slow your pace of eating to give your stomach a chance to communicate with your brain that you are full. Put down your utensils regularly and sip a noncaloric beverage, like water. Lastly, take time to enjoy the taste of your food. Remember, you don't need to be a member of the clean plate club.

Enjoy the non–food-related pleasures of restaurant eating. Frequently, we focus just on the food due to time constraints, hunger, or other stresses. Doing this, you may miss enjoying the surrounding environment. Train yourself to enjoy all aspects of the restaurant experience, even if it's just a few minutes of relaxation or conversation with a friend. Think about how nice it is not to cook, put away leftovers, or do the dishes. Enjoying these pleasures makes it easier to limit portions and eat healthfully.

Put Your Best Guesstimate Forward

When you've got the Nutrition Facts label from a packaged food or nutrition information from a restaurant's website at your fingertips, it makes knowing the nutrients you're eating a snap. This book will also help you gather the nutrients in restaurant foods. Nearly every chapter in Sections 2 and 3 serves up the nutrition facts for a sampling of foods from the types of restaurants covered in that chapter. You'll find a list of foods in most of these chapters referred to as *Health Busters*. You can guess that these foods aren't strong contenders for healthy choices. Then you'll find a longer list of *Healthier Bets*. Yes, this represents a sampling of healthier foods in that type of cuisine. You'll also gain insight into the nutrition counts of various restaurant foods and meals in the *Menu Samplers* section of each cuisine-specific chapter in Sections 2 and 3. *Health Busters, Healthier Bets,* and *Menu Samplers* are further described in Chapter 10 (page

108). Need more nutrition information? Find the nutrition facts for thousands of restaurant foods in the *Eat Out, Eat Well* companion app.

Though more nutrition information for restaurant foods is available now than ever before, the nutrition facts for many restaurant items and/or specific nutrition information for carbohydrate, saturated fat, and other nutrients of concern to people with diabetes, are simply not available. This is particularly true for single-unit, independent restaurants that serve American or ethnic fare and just have one or a few locations. And, according to the National Restaurant Association, more than 7 in 10 restaurants have just one location. Learn more in Chapter 8 (page 78) about the availability of restaurant nutrition information.

If no nutrition information is available, then getting accurate nutrient counts presents a challenge. These tips will help you train your eyes to estimate portions and put your best guesstimate forward:

▶ Have measuring equipment at home and use it regularly. Have a set of measuring spoons, measuring cups, and an inexpensive (or, if you choose, a more expensive) food scale. Weigh and measure foods at home regularly to familiarize yourself with the portions you should eat. Eventually you'll be able to estimate portion sizes without a measuring tool. Then on occasion—say, once a month—weigh and measure foods, especially the starches, fruits, and proteins, to check your estimating abilities.

  Weighing and measuring foods regularly helps you keep portions in control at home. It also helps you more precisely estimate your portions and their nutrient content in restaurant meals. When you don't have your measuring tools, you always have your hands. Commit these "handy" portion guides to memory and use them to estimate restaurant food portions:

  ▷ Tip of the thumb (to first knuckle) = 1 teaspoon
  ▷ Whole thumb = 1 tablespoon
  ▷ Palm of your hand = 3 ounces (this is the portion size of cooked meat that most people need at a meal). Other 3-ounce portion guides: 3 ounces is about the size of a deck of regular-size playing cards or the size of a household bar of soap.
  ▷ Tight fist = 1/2 cup
  ▷ Loose fist or open handful = 1 cup

Note: These guidelines hold true for most women's hands, but some men's hands are much larger. Check the size of your hands out for yourself with real weighing and measuring equipment.

▶ Here's a rule of thumb to translate from raw to cooked portions of protein foods. It's reasonable to estimate you'll lose about one quarter of the weight in cooking. So 4 ounces of raw protein with no bones will serve up roughly 3 ounces cooked. To roughly estimate the weight of cooked protein with bone in it, say a T-bone steak or chicken legs, figure you'll lose another ounce. So, 4 ounces raw with bone, fat, and skin will result in 2 ounces cooked (with the bones and skin removed). These rules may vary based on several factors: the cut of protein, the amount of fat on the raw item and left on the cooked item, whether the cut contains bones or skin (for poultry), what cooking method you use (e.g., grilled versus braised), and the degree of doneness to which you cook it. For example, a 4-ounce raw portion of lean meat grilled to "rare" will weigh more after cooking than a steak with visible fat trim on it that is cooked to "well done."

One more tip for protein portions at restaurants: When you see an amount of protein described or named on restaurant menus or menu boards, it's typically referring to a raw weight, not the weight of the cooked food served to you. This is based on an industry standard, not a regulation. A hamburger described as a quarter-pound burger will be about 3 ounces by the time you bite into it and that 8-ounce filet will be about 6 ounces on your plate.

▶ Use the food scales in the produce aisle of the supermarket to educate yourself about the servings of foods you may be served in a restaurant, such as baked white or sweet potatoes, an ear of corn, a banana, or half of a grapefruit. Weigh individual pieces of these foods. Check out how many ounces an average potato or an ear of corn that you may be served in a restaurant is. You'll weigh these foods raw, but their weight doesn't change that much when they're served and eaten cooked. (This may sound silly or onerous, but it can really improve your guesstimating skills.)

▶ If there are no nutrition facts for a particular restaurant you frequent, use the information available for other similar restaurants as a guide.

Check out the nutrition facts in this book or the companion app. If you want to know the nutrient content of a food like french fries, a baked potato, stuffing, pizza, or a bagel, use the serving size and nutrition information for similar foods. Take a few examples and then do an average. For example: if you regularly eat two slices of cheese pizza at a local pizza shop (rather than a national chain) and they have no nutrition information available, look up the nutrition information for two slices of medium-size regular-crust cheese pizza from three other restaurants. Then calculate an average of each nutrient. This will come pretty close to the nutrition content of the two slices of cheese pizza you eat. It's way better than winging it.

▶ Use the nutrition information from the Nutrition Facts labels of foods in the supermarket to estimate what you might eat in a restaurant. You might find some similar foods in the frozen or packaged convenience food area. Again, take a couple of examples and then average them.

▶ If you regularly eat particular ethnic foods for which you can't find satisfactory nutrition information, look for recipes with nutrition information for similar dishes online. Look at a couple of similar recipes. Then get an average. This might work well for ethnic foods such as Indian, Japanese, or Thai, for which there's a scarcity of nutrition data.

▶ Build your own personal food and nutrition database. Most people regularly eat just 50–100 foods, including restaurant foods. People tend to frequent the same restaurants and order similar items. Is this true for you? Think about it. For this reason, it makes sense to spend a few hours gathering and estimating the nutrient content of your favorite restaurant items. Once you have this figured out, keep it somewhere that will always be accessible to you. Before you know it, you'll have the information for your regular restaurant meals committed to memory.

▶ And even when you have consulted the nutrition facts for restaurant menu items and have them in hand, practice defensive counting. Recognize that the nutrition information provided by restaurants is obtained from several samples of the foods prepared according to corporate specifications or based on the various ingredients. This is truer for large chain restaurants where quality and quantity control reign supreme. But, on any given day, the portions of foods and ingredients served may be slightly more or less than the samples on which the nutrition information is based. Even in fast-food hamburger chains, the same burger can include more or less ketchup, tomatoes, pickles, mayonnaise, or other ingredients. So, before you dig in, reassess your nutrition figures. Reflect on whether the nutrition numbers provided by the chain add up based on your nutrition knowledge. If not, revise your counts.

Get to Know Yourself

Taking time to assess the whens, whys, wheres, and whats of your restaurant meals is a key strategy to healthier restaurant eating, as discussed earlier in this chapter on page 30. Take a few minutes to answer the following questions. Be honest with yourself. Raising your awareness of your current restaurant eating habits and food choices is the first step to changing your behaviors.

With your current restaurant eating habits written down in black and white, you can set a few realistic, easy-to-accomplish goals to change your restaurant eating behaviors one step at a time. Experience some success with your first steps. Then make a few more changes. Come back to these questions on occasion to observe your successes and think about what you want to change next. Remember, slow and steady changes can last a lifetime and help you achieve your health goals.

1. What meals and snacks do you eat away from home?

2. How often during the course of a day, week, or month do you eat meals or snacks away from home? (Think about your weekdays and weekends and estimate the number of meals and snacks you eat away from home. Don't forget meals and snacks that you purchase at restaurants and eat somewhere else.)

3. Why do you eat meals and snacks away from home? (Check all that apply.)
    - ☐ Restaurant meals are convenient.
    - ☐ I do not like to cook.
    - ☐ I do not have/make time to cook.
    - ☐ I want to have someone serve me.
    - ☐ I enjoy various ethnic flavors that I cannot create in my kitchen.
    - ☐ I need a place and way to get together with friends, family, or for business.
    - ☐ I want to relax during lunch or at dinner after a long day.
    - ☐ I don't make time for breakfast.

4. What types of restaurants do you eat at or take food out from and how many times per day, week, and month?
    - ☐ Fast food (hamburger, chicken, or seafood chains)
    - ☐ Pizza
    - ☐ Sandwich shops
    - ☐ Coffee shops
    - ☐ American fare—family restaurant
    - ☐ Steak house
    - ☐ Fine dining
    - ☐ Ethnic fare (fast food)
    - ☐ Ethnic fare (table service)
    - ☐ Sweets/desserts/ice cream

5. Which foods do you order or eat in the restaurants listed above? In what amounts? Record what you usually order in the restaurants you frequent (make sure to include any nonalcoholic and alcoholic beverages you drink).

CHAPTER 5

Dealing with Diabetes Restaurant Eating Dilemmas

T oday many people who eat restaurant meals have concerns about their health and nutrition. It's become commonplace to ask questions and make special requests. However, as a person with diabetes or a diabetes caregiver, you'll deal with dilemmas and challenges in addition to unhealthy foods and ingredients, and large portions. This chapter offers guidance on three diabetes-specific dilemmas: delayed meals, alcohol consumption, and sweets and desserts.

Delayed Restaurant Meals

When it comes to restaurant meals, expect the unexpected. That's tough for people with diabetes, especially when it comes to the potential risk of hypoglycemia. But, it's the reality you've got to deal with. A restaurant might have lost your reservation or might not be able to seat you quickly, your meal-mate(s) might be late, the kitchen might be slow, there may be a mixup with your order, or your order might not come out right. And, as you know, the list of possible issues goes on. Your modus operandi should be, "better to be safe than sorry."

A big challenge, if you take one or more blood glucose–lowering medication that can cause hypoglycemia, is how to manage delayed meals. For example, if you usually eat lunch between noon and 12:30 pm, and you take a mixture of intermediate-acting and rapid-acting insulin before breakfast, what steps can you take to safely delay your meal until 1:00 or 1:30 pm when your friends or business associates want to eat? Or what should you do if you want to dine at 8:00 pm on a Saturday night, when your usual dinner time during the week is 6:30 pm?

Blood Glucose–Lowering Medications and Delayed Meals

All types of insulin can cause hypoglycemia, as can a couple of categories of oral medications (see Table 5.1 on page 54). If you take one or more of these medications, you'll need to put a game plan in place to deal with delayed meals.

- ▶ Insulin: Everyone with type 1 diabetes takes insulin, as do millions of people with type 2 diabetes. These days, people typically take two types of insulin, either separately or in combination.
  - ▷ Long-acting and rapid-acting insulin: Many people take one of the two currently available longer-acting insulins, such as detemir (Levimer) or glargine (Lantus), once or twice a day, either in the morning or before bed or at both times. Then they take one of the three rapid-acting insulins prior to eating. The rapid-acting insulins are: lispro (Humalog), aspart (Novolog), and glulisine (Apidra). These must be given as separate shots because the insulins can't be mixed. These insulins can be taken using a pen, a patch (these are newer devices, such as V-Go or PaQ), or, the old-fashioned way, with vial of insulin and a syringe. People who use an insulin pump use only one type of insulin. Most often that's rapid-acting insulin, but sometimes slower-acting U500 insulin is used. If you use rapid-acting insulin to manage the rise of glucose from meals (food), you can delay taking a dose until about 15 minutes before you eat your delayed meal (but follow what you know best keeps you safe). For pointers on using rapid-acting insulin with restaurant meals read the practical tips in this chapter on page 47.
  - ▷ Pre-mixed insulin combinations: Some people take pre-mixed combinations of two types of insulin. These come in various ratios. Typically it's a mixture of an intermediate-acting insulin (NPH) with a rapid-acting or short-acting insulin (Regular). The ratios for pre-mixed insulins range from 50% of each insulin to 70–75% of intermediate-acting insulin and the remainder (30–25%) of the rapid-acting or short-acting insulin. Typically people take two shots a day; one in the morning and one before dinner. A

disadvantage of these insulin regimens is that they do not allow much adjustment of dose or flexibility in meal times. If you use one of the pre-mixed combinations, you'll need to have a game plan to avoid hypoglycemia with delayed meals. If you find you regularly need more flexibility in your schedule, talk to your health-care providers about getting on a more flexible insulin regimen than pre-mixed dosing.

▶ Oral medications: Medications in the sulfonylureas category and the pills Prandin (repaglinide) and Starlix (nateglinide) can cause hypoglycemia (see Table 5.1 on page 54). These pills work by making the pancreas put out more insulin. The sulfonylureas, which are taken once or twice a day, lower glucose more slowly than Prandin and Starlix. If you take a sulfonylurea, you'll need to pay attention to your meal times and possibly put an action plan in place for delayed meals.

One positive aspect of the management of diabetes today is the availability of a slew of new oral blood glucose–lowering medicines (pills) and new types of insulin and other injectable medications that better mesh with the realities of life in the 21st century. Another big plus, as you'll see in Table 5.2 on page 54, is that many of these newer medications aren't likely to cause hypoglycemia, even if you delay a meal. This can allow you the flexibility to manage your diabetes in the manner that best suits your needs and lifestyle. If your current blood glucose–lowering medication regimen is not in sync with your life schedule or style, speak up. Do the same if you aren't meeting your glucose and A1C goals (see the table on page 10 in Chapter 2). Learn about other glucose-lowering medications. Then talk with your health-care providers about your lifestyle and medication options. Don't wait for them to ask you.

Have an Action Plan to Prevent Hypoglycemia

If you need to delay a meal and you take a glucose-lowering medication or a type of insulin that has the potential to cause your blood glucose to get too low, put a preventive action plan in place using the following guidelines:.

▶ Check your blood glucose at the usual time of your meal.
  ▷ If your blood glucose is high (>130 mg/dl), you can wait a short time before you eat without concern. But do check again if you develop symptoms of low blood glucose before your meal.

▷ If your blood glucose is around your premeal goal (70–130 mg/dl is the American Diabetes Association goal) and you feel it will fall too low before you get to eat, eat some carbohydrate (start with 15 grams) to make sure your blood glucose doesn't go too low before your meal.

▷ If your blood glucose is lower than 70 mg/dl and/or you feel the symptoms of low blood glucose, then you can use 15 grams of some source of carbohydrate that you carry or is accessible to you, such as glucose tabs, gels, sugar-sweetened soda, or juice, to treat your hypoglycemia. Try to eat your meal soon after.

► If you delay your meal more than one hour and your blood glucose is around your premeal goal, you may need to eat more than 15 grams of carbohydrate to keep it from going too low before your meal. Then you may want to eat fewer grams of carbohydrate at the meal when you finally eat.

► Keep easy-to-carry and quick-to-eat foods that contain carbohydrate or a source of glucose, like tablets, gels, or liquid, in places such as your desk, briefcase, purse, locker, glove compartment, night stand, and any other places you may need it. These can come in handy with delayed meals or any time your glucose may be getting too low. A few suggestions for nonperishable foods to carry are: dried fruit, cans of juice, pretzels, lifesavers, gumdrops, gummy bears, or snack crackers. Try out a few items and learn what works best for you in a variety of situations. Check the Nutrition Facts label on the food to determine the serving size equivalent to 15 grams of carbohydrate.

These suggestions offer you general rules of thumb. Check with your health-care providers to learn the best alternatives for you based on your diabetes goals and the types of medication you take.

Practical Tips for Using Rapid-Acting Insulin with Restaurant Meals

Rapid-acting insulin came on the market in the mid-1990s. Prior to its availability, Regular (short-acting) insulin was the quickest acting insulin available. Though it's called "rapid-acting" insulin and health-care providers initially encouraged people to take it right before eating (the advertisements still advise this for regulatory reasons), for most people it doesn't get absorbed or lower blood glucose as quickly as you'd like it to. Today, diabetes experts agree that rapid-acting insulin doesn't really start lowering glucose for a good 15–30 minutes after taking it. The maximum blood glucose–lowering effect of rapid-acting insulin occurs more often in the range of 90–120 minutes after it's injected rather than around an hour after injection. People who wear a continuous glucose monitor (CGM) have made these observations as well.

Taking rapid-acting insulin 10–15 minutes before you eat and carefully calculating your dose according to the grams of carbohydrate you'll eat is ideal for blood glucose control. However, this isn't always possible and restaurant meals present a common challenge with dosing rapid-acting insulin. If you take rapid-acting insulin when you start to eat, or perhaps during or after eating, and find that your glucose rises quickly after you eat, then you may want to try to take at least some portion of your premeal insulin dose about 10–15 minutes before you eat and then take the rest of the dose once you know how much you'll eat. In general, the best thing to do is test out what works best for you in various situations, with the goal of preventing hypoglycemia.

These practical tips can help you achieve better glucose control after eating a restaurant meal. Several of these suggestions are easier to implement if you wear an insulin patch or pump because, with these devices, no additional injections are necessary. Discuss these suggestions with your health-care provider. Your safety is top priority!

▶ High blood glucose before a meal: If you have high blood glucose prior to your meal, take some rapid-acting insulin about a half hour before your meal to give the insulin time to get your glucose coming back down. It might take longer than the time you have before you eat to come down, but at least it will be on the downswing.

▶ Uncertain carbohydrate intake: If you don't know how much carbohydrate you will eat at a meal or you don't quite know how fast the restaurant meal will be delivered, consider splitting your rapid-acting insulin dose. Take enough insulin 15 minutes before the meal to cover the minimum amount of carbohydrate that you know you will eat (say 30–45 grams) and to keep your glucose from rising high. Then, as the meal goes on and you know how much more carbohydrate you will eat, take the remaining amount of insulin you need to cover the carbohydrate.

▶ Long, lingering meals or food events: Pump users who plan to have a long, lingering meal (say at a cocktail party or celebratory event) or are eating a meal that is high in fat may want to use the bolus delivery tool that allows you to extend a bolus dose over an hour or more.

Most importantly, learn from your experiences. There is a large variation in individual blood glucose responses to food and insulin among people with diabetes. The more you check your glucose after eating and observe changes, the more you will learn and be able to fine-tune your control. Keep notes of your responses to various foods and activities. Everyone is unique. Create your history based on your unique experiences.

Alcohol—When, What, and How to Drink Safely

Restaurant meals are a common time to consume alcohol. Drinking alcohol can present a couple of dilemmas for people with diabetes. The number-one dilemma is the risk of hypoglycemia with excess alcohol consumption, especially if you take a blood glucose–lowering medication that can cause hypoglycemia, like insulin or a sulfonylurea (see Table 5.1 on page 54). Dilemma number two is the challenge of excess calories from alcohol. All things considered, moderate consumption of alcohol, believe it or not, has health benefits. But excessive alcohol consumption can derail your eating plan and even endanger your health. Learn more about alcohol's health benefits and pitfalls, the calorie and nutrition profile of alcoholic beverages, and tips to limit excess calories in Chapter 9 (page 87).

Alcohol and Hypoglycemia: Preventive Steps

For people with diabetes who take insulin and/or a glucose-lowering medication that can cause hypoglycemia, excess alcohol intake can cause hypoglycemia up to 24 hours after it is consumed. For example, if someone has several alcoholic beverages at a special celebration one evening, hypoglycemia can occur shortly after drinking or in the wee hours of the night. Practice hypoglycemia prevention with these steps:

1) Limit excess alcohol intake.
2) Check glucose levels often when drinking alcohol, especially before going to sleep. If necessary, consume some carbohydrate-containing food before going to sleep.

3) Consume some source of carbohydrate, in the form of snacks or as part of a meal, along with the alcoholic beverages to keep your glucose from becoming too low. Never drink on an empty stomach.

How to Count Alcoholic Beverages in Your Eating Plan

Over the years the answer to the question, "How should I factor alcohol into my eating plan to account for the calories?" has changed. Today, the answer, according to the American Diabetes Association, is that you can drink a moderate amount of alcohol without making changes to your eating plan. You don't need to omit foods to account for the alcohol. However, if you drink a moderate amount of alcohol daily and your weight is a concern or you want to lose weight, you'll need to determine how many calories you can allot for alcohol. If any of your alcoholic beverages contain grams of carbohydrate from calorie-containing mixers, you need to count them.

Tips to Drink Alcohol Safely with Diabetes

► Check your blood glucose to help you decide whether you should drink and when you need to eat something.
► Don't drink when your blood glucose is below 70 mg/dl and/or you have symptoms of hypoglycemia.
► Remember that alcohol can cause low blood glucose hours after you consume alcohol (see *Alcohol and Hypoglycemia: Preventive Steps* above).
► Wear (preferably) or carry identification that states you have diabetes. Keep in mind that signs of hypoglycemia can be mistaken for being drunk.
► Don't drink on an empty stomach. Munch on a carbohydrate source (popcorn or pretzels) as you drink or wait to drink until you get your meal.
► Do not drive for several hours after you drink alcohol. Never drink and drive.

Sweets and Desserts

Nearly everyone has a sweet tooth or two! We're born with an innate desire for sweets. You don't all of a sudden lose your desire for sweets when you're diagnosed with diabetes. Granted, some people like (some would even say "need") sweets more than others. The advice for people with diabetes, historically, was no sweets or sugary foods. That is no longer the recommendation from the American Diabetes Association; in fact, that hasn't been the advice about sweets for people with diabetes for a couple of decades.

The current *Nutrition Therapy Recommendations for the Management of Adults With Diabetes* from the American Diabetes Association suggest that if you want to integrate a small amount of sweets into your healthy eating plan, you should substitute these for other foods that contain carbohydrate. In small amounts and only eaten on special occasions, sweets won't affect glucose or blood fat (lipid) levels. The amounts of sweets you choose to fit into your eating plan and how frequently you indulge will need to depend on your weight status and your glucose and lipid levels. It also depends on whether or not you use a blood glucose–lowering medication, like rapid-acting insulin, that you can take more of to compensate for the extra carbohydrate load from desserts. But do be careful of excess calories and weight gain. Talk to your health-care provider about how to fit sweets into your meal plan.

Sweets and desserts certainly make their appearance on all types of restaurant menus, from fast food to fine dining. It may be a fried apple pie, a brownie, or cookies the size of your face. At coffee shops there are breakfast pastries, donuts, and more. Most ethnic restaurants serve up the favorite sweet treats of their cuisine—think baklava in Middle Eastern restaurants and cannoli in Italian restaurants. You'll see that dessert draws little attention in some cuisines, like Japanese and Chinese. Then there are fine dining restaurants where an award-winning pastry chef may be on staff to whip up delectable desserts. Sugary foods that aren't desserts show up on menus as well, from a long list of sugar-sweetened beverages, to those more-prevalent-than-ever smoothies and sugar-laden sauces and syrups, such as maple syrup, barbecue sauce, and ketchup, to name a few. You'll find information and guidance about desserts in the chapters in Sections 2 and 3.

When it comes to choosing the sweets you eat, here are two essential bits of advice. One, eat them in small portions. Two, make sure each and every morsel quenches your sweet tooth to the max. The more satisfied you are from a small amount of sweets, the easier time you'll have following a healthy eating plan. Here are some other healthy eating tips and tactics for sweets and desserts:

► Prioritize your personal diabetes and nutrition goals. Which are most important to you and your health: blood glucose control, blood lipid control, and/or weight loss or maintenance? Your priorities should dictate how you strike a balance with sugars and sweets.

▶ Think about a few of your very favorite desserts, those that are mouth-watering to you! Think about where and when you eat these (perhaps you prepare and serve them at home or eat them on a special occasion or holiday). Decide how often you can eat them and how you can fit them into your healthy eating plan.

▶ It may be best for you to keep sweets and desserts out of your home (if possible, based on who else you're living with) and just plan to enjoy them at an occasional and special restaurant meal.

▶ In ice cream and yogurt shops, don't think kiddie- or junior-size servings are just for kids. Think of them as portion-controlled sizes for calorie and carbohydrate counters too.

▶ If you want a topping for your small serving of ice cream or frozen yogurt, go for nuts, fresh fruit, raisins, or granola. Steer clear of the toppings made from chopped-up candy.

▶ Order one dessert and two (or more, depending on the number of diners) spoons or forks. Quite often just a few bites of a fantastic dessert will quench your sweet tooth.

▶ Can't find anyone to share with? Split it! Eat a portion of your dessert and take home the rest. But practice that "out of sight, out of mouth" tactic. Set aside the portion you'll take home before you dig into the rest.

▶ Looking for the nutrition information for desserts, particularly calories and carbohydrate, total fat, and saturated fat grams? In Sections 2 and 3, at the end of most of the chapters, you'll find the nutrition information for some sweet treats in the *Health Busters* and *Healthier Bets* tables. If you're determined to find the nutrition information for desserts from your favorite ethnic and fine dining restaurants, do some extrapolating from websites and online recipes or recipe books loaded with nutrition information. Then put your guesstimating skills into action.

▶ When you do eat sweets, check your blood glucose 1–2 hours later to observe your body's response. Do this repeatedly because different sweets will impact your glucose differently at different times.

▶ Keep an eye on your A1C (your average glucose measure over the past 2–3 months) and your blood fat (lipid) levels to see whether eating more sweets affects these numbers.

▶ Keep an eye on that scale. Excess sweets and desserts can make holding the line on your weight or losing weight more challenging.

Blood Glucose–Lowering Medications

Many people with diabetes, type 1 or 2, take several types of medications. One or more of these medications may be used to lower blood glucose. Others may reduce the risks of heart disease by lowering bad cholesterol or treating high blood pressure. Prior to 1995, there were only two categories of glucose-lowering medications to treat type 2 diabetes—sulfonylureas, like glyburide and glipizide, and various types of insulins. Much has changed since then! During the last couple of decades a number of new categories of these medications have been approved and added to the choices your health-care providers have to help you keep your glucose levels in control.

What's particularly good news about these newer blood glucose–lowering medications is that most of them are unlikely to cause hypoglycemia, due to the way they work (unless they are taken with other medications that can cause hypoglycemia). It is common for people with type 2 diabetes to take more than one medication to lower blood glucose. This may mean two different pills or taking one pill that combines two categories of blood glucose–lowering medicine. Or you may take one or more pills and/or an injectable medicine, like insulin or a GLP-analog. It may be that one of the medications you take can cause hypoglycemia and another is unlikely to do so. Or it may be that none of the blood glucose–lowering medications you take may cause hypoglycemia. Learn the actions of the medications you take from your health-care providers, including your primary care provider, diabetes educators, or pharmacists and determine whether any of them put you at risks for hypoglycemia.

Several of the diabetes restaurant eating dilemmas detailed in this chapter revolve around how to stay safe. This mainly involves how to prevent or, if you experience it, treat hypoglycemia. It's important to know which glucose-lowering medication(s) you take and whether or not any of them put you at risk of hypoglycemia. Tables 5.1 and 5.2 on the next page list the blood glucose–lowering medications currently approved by the U.S. Food and Drug Administration and available on the U.S. market. Keep in mind, these days, this is changing rather frequently.

Table 5.1	Medications That May Cause Hypoglycemia	
ORAL MEDICATIONS		
Category Name	**Generic Names**	**Brand Names (in U.S.)**
Sulfonylureas	glimepiride	Amaryl
	glipizide	Glucotrol, Glucatrol XL
	glyburide	Diabeta, Micronase, Glynase (micronized glyburide)
D-Phenylalanine Derivative	nateglinide	Starlix
Meglitinide	repaglinide	Prandin
INSULINS		
Insulin	all	all

Table 5.2	Medications Unlikely to Cause Hypoglycemia	
ORAL MEDICATIONS		
Category Name	**Generic Names**	**Brand Names (in U.S.)**
Biguanides	metformin (most metformin prescribed now is generic)	Glucophage Extended release: Glucophage XR, Glumetza, Fortamet Liquid: Riomet
Glitazones (TZDs)	pioglitazone	Actos
	rosiglitazone	Avandia
Alpha-glucosidase inhibitor	acarbose	Precose
	miglitol	Glyset
DPP-4 inhibitor	sitagliptin	Januvia
	saxagliptin	Onglyza
	linagliptin	Tradjenta
	alogliptin	Nesina

(table continues on next page)

Table 5.2   Medications Unlikely to Cause Hypoglycemia
(continued)

ORAL MEDICATIONS

Category Name	Generic Names	Brand Names (in U.S.)
Bile sequestering agent (removes glucose and LDL-cholesterol from the body)	colesevelam	Welchol
Dopamine agonist	bromocriptine	Cycloset
Sodium-glucose co-transporter 2 (SGLT2) inhibitors	canagliflozin	Ivokana
	dapagliflozin	Farxiga
	empagliflozin	Jardiance

INJECTABLE MEDICATIONS

GLP-1 analog/incretin mimetic	exenatide (twice daily)	Byetta
	liraglutide (once daily)	Victoza
	extenatide extended release (once weekly)	Bydureon
	dulaglutide (once weekly)	Trulicity
Amylin analog	pramlintide	Symlin

CHAPTER 6

Healthy and Safe Restaurant Eating with Celiac Disease or Gluten Sensitivity

by Carol Brunzell, RD, LD, CDE

Carol Brunzell is a registered dietitian and certified diabetes educator who has worked at the University of Minnesota Medical Center, Fairview, for the past 27 years. She specializes in counseling people with diabetes, cystic fibrosis–related diabetes, and celiac disease and diabetes. She is considered by many to be the go-to dietitian on living with diabetes and celiac disease. Due to her expertise, the author of this book requested that Brunzell contribute this chapter and the Tips and Tactics for Gluten-Free Eating you'll find in the chapters in Sections 2 and 3.

E ating restaurant foods and meals, whether you eat them in the restaurant or take them out, when you have diabetes and celiac disease can be VERY challenging. There are many questions to consider. How can I be sure this or that food or meal is gluten-free? Having diabetes by itself is stressful, but adding celiac disease takes managing diabetes to a whole different level. More restaurants are aware of the importance of serving safe, gluten-free healthy foods and want to make sure your experience in their restaurant is pleasurable. It is important that you know how to find restaurants that are safe to eat in and know the critical questions to ask in order to keep your foods and meals gluten-free.

This chapter reviews the signs and symptoms of celiac disease and non-celiac gluten sensitivity, how these conditions are diagnosed, the basics of eating gluten-free, the gluten-free food labeling law and its impact on restaurant foods, and strategies to eat safely in restaurants. References are provided at the end of the chapter with lists of certified training programs for restaurants, support groups, gluten-free dining resources, and other celiac resources.

What Is Celiac Disease?

Celiac disease is an autoimmune disorder (just like type 1 diabetes) that occurs more often in people with type 1 diabetes. It has been estimated by the American Diabetes Association that about 10% of people with type 1 diabetes also have celiac disease, compared with about 1% of people in the general population (about 1 in 133 people). Having one autoimmune disorder increases your chances of having another autoimmune disorder, hence the link. The incidence of celiac disease in people with type 2 diabetes is not known, but has been estimated to be similar to the incidence rate in the general population.

In people with celiac disease, eating foods with gluten injures the lining in the small intestines. Gluten is a protein made up of gliadin and glutenin. It's found in wheat and other grains. This causes the body to not absorb nutrients from food normally, which can result in a wide variety of health problems if not diagnosed or treated. The only treatment for celiac disease at this point is following a strict, lifelong gluten-free diet.

Signs and Symptoms

Celiac disease can be difficult to diagnose as symptoms are variable and may often be subtle. Symptoms vary because when individual nutrients are not being absorbed normally by the body, it can lead to all kinds of different health problems. Some symptoms of undiagnosed or untreated celiac disease include diarrhea, unintentional weight loss or poor weight gain, growth failure, abdominal pain, bloating, fatigue, constipation, vomiting, and malnutrition due to malabsorption of food nutrients. Some people who have celiac disease have a higher incidence of being diagnosed with bone diseases, such as osteoporosis, because they are not absorbing adequate calcium and vitamin D. Other people may develop anemia because they aren't absorbing iron properly. People with diabetes and celiac disease may have unexplained hypoglycemia or blood glucose levels that are difficult to control for no apparent reason. Some people can develop neurological conditions like peripheral neuropathy or ataxia (the loss of full control of body movements) due to malabsorption of certain B vitamins. One manifestation of celiac disease that affects the skin is dermatitis herpetiformis, which occurs in about 15–25% of people with celiac disease. Dermatitis herpetiformis causes an itchy, blistering rash which mostly affects the knees, elbows, butt, scalp, and back in a symmetrical pattern (on both sides of the body). If these signs and symptoms sound familiar to you, mention them to your health-care provider.

Testing Recommendations for Celiac Disease

No one should begin following a gluten-free diet until they get a firm diagnosis from a health-care provider. Testing for celiac disease starts with a simple blood test that looks for certain antibodies. If this test is positive, then your health-care provider should order a biopsy of the small intestine. This test is considered the gold standard for diagnosing celiac disease. To ensure an accurate diagnosis, these tests must be done while the patient is still eating gluten.

Why Omit Gluten?

The gluten-free diet is currently the only treatment for celiac disease. To learn the ins and outs of following a gluten-free diet, it's important to meet with a registered dietitian who is familiar with diabetes and celiac disease. Refer to the resource list at the end of this chapter to find a registered dietitian with this expertise. Following a gluten-free eating plan may seem overwhelming at first, especially since you are already dealing with your diabetes, so plan to meet with a dietitian more than once. There is a lot of information to learn, but you will get used to it with time. More importantly, once you eliminate gluten you will feel much better and your health will improve. There are many national and local celiac organizations that provide updated information and research, as well as help and support, for people with celiac disease. See the resource list on page 69 for more information.

Fortunately, gluten-free foods are more plentiful and taste much better today than they used to. However, just because a food or menu item is called gluten-free, does not necessarily mean it is healthy. Many processed gluten-free foods are made from refined gluten-free flours and starches. They may be high in fat and calories and low in fiber, vitamin B, and iron. So just like you pay attention to your food choices for diabetes, it is important to choose healthy gluten-free food by reading food labels. Try to limit excess carbohydrate, fat, and sodium.

Once you remove gluten from your food choices, the intestinal damage can heal. The amount of time this takes varies from 6 months to 2 years. If you have celiac disease, it's important to understand that if you eat gluten, injury to your intestinal lining may still be occurring even if you do not have noticeable symptoms of celiac disease. So to protect your health, carefully follow a gluten-free eating plan.

Non-Celiac Gluten Sensitivity vs. Celiac Disease

Gluten sensitivity or non-celiac gluten sensitivity is not the same as celiac disease. It is not an autoimmune disorder. It is considered a nonallergic, non-autoimmune reaction to gluten. It is typically diagnosed after all other possible digestive diseases causing celiac disease–like symptoms have been ruled out. People who have non-celiac gluten sensitivity feel much better when they eliminate gluten from their diets, but they don't have the same health risks as people with celiac disease if they eat gluten. There is a lot we don't know about this condition.

Basics of Eating Gluten-Free

People with celiac disease are advised to choose a well-balanced, healthy, gluten-free eating plan. Focus on the many foods you *can* eat, not the foods you need to avoid. Choose more whole or enriched gluten-free grains and products such as brown rice, wild rice, buckwheat, quinoa, amaranth, millet, sorghum, and teff (make sure they are labeled "gluten-free" because cross-contamination from equipment in processing plants can be a problem).

All fresh fruits and vegetables, fresh milk and yogurt, unprocessed lean meats, poultry, fish, eggs, peas, beans and legumes, unflavored nuts and seeds, and oils are naturally gluten-free. Do keep in mind that grains, legumes, and seeds can potentially have cross-contact issues. Check out the lists of gluten-free foods below to help you make healthy food choices.

Gluten-Free Grains and Flours:

- ▶ Amaranth
- ▶ Arrowroot
- ▶ Buckwheat
- ▶ Corn, cornstarch, corn bran, natural popcorn
- ▶ Flax
- ▶ Millet
- ▶ Montina® (Indian rice grass flour)
- ▶ Oats (labeled gluten-free)
- ▶ Quinoa
- ▶ Rice: brown, white, wild, rice bran, rice flour
- ▶ Sago
- ▶ Sorghum
- ▶ Soy
- ▶ Teff
- ▶ Whole beans/legumes and flours (garbanzo, lentil, pea, kidney, black, red, pinto, white, etc.)
- ▶ Nut and seed flours (almond, hazelnut, pecan, sesame)
- ▶ Tapioca (also called cassava or manioc)
- ▶ Potato, sweet potato, yam, potato flour, potato starch

Other Non–Grain-Based Gluten-Free Foods:

- ▶ Fresh, frozen, or canned unprocessed fruits and vegetables
- ▶ Fresh meats, poultry, seafood, fish, wild game, eggs, some processed meats with gluten-free ingredients
- ▶ Dried peas, beans and lentils, tofu
- ▶ Milk, yogurt, and aged natural cheese made with gluten-free ingredients
- ▶ Oils, tree nuts, seeds, natural peanut butter, and salad dressings and spreads with gluten-free ingredients
- ▶ Sugar substitutes, sugar alcohols, honey, sugar, pure maple syrup, corn syrup, jams, jellies, candy and ice cream with gluten-free ingredients
- ▶ Pure spices and herbs, salt, soy or tamari sauce made without wheat, cider, and distilled and non-malt vinegars
- ▶ Coffee ground from whole beans, brewed tea
- ▶ Distilled alcoholic beverages (gin, vodka, whiskey, etc.) and wine

Reading Food Labels for Gluten

All foods sold in the U.S. are regulated by the U.S. Food and Drug Administration (FDA) and the U.S. Department of Agriculture (USDA). Most foods are under FDA jurisdiction. The following lists will give you an idea of the kind of foods and ingredients you need to avoid if you are eating gluten-free.

FDA Regulated Foods

When reading the labels for foods regulated by the FDA, look out for the following words/ingredients, which indicate that the food contains gluten:

- ▶ Wheat
- ▶ Rye
- ▶ Barley
- ▶ Malt and malt flavorings (e.g., malt vinegar, malt extract, malt flavor)
- ▶ Oats (which have not been labeled gluten-free)
- ▶ Brewer's yeast

USDA Regulated Foods

Meats, poultry, eggs, and most packaged products prepared with meat, poultry, and/or eggs are regulated by the USDA. In addition, the USDA also regulates mixed foods, like tuna noodle casserole, which contain a percentage of meat or poultry. When reading the labels of these foods, watch out for the same ingredients in the list above (FDA regulated foods) and also look for these additional ingredients, which may be derived from wheat:

- ▶ Starch
- ▶ Modified food starch
- ▶ Dextrin

If you are not sure whether or not a food contains gluten, and the food is something you'd like to eat regularly, consider calling the food manufacturer. Food must contain the manufacturer's phone number on the packaging of the product. Today many products also have the manufacturer's website, which may contain the ingredient lists of their foods.

Gluten-Containing Grains and Grain Products:

- ► Atta (chapatti flour)
- ► Barley
- ► Bran
- ► Bulgur
- ► Communion wafers
- ► Couscous
- ► Cracked wheat/tabbouleh
- ► Durum flour
- ► Einkorn
- ► Emmer
- ► Farina
- ► Farro or Faro
- ► Graham flour
- ► Kamut
- ► Malt, malt extract, malt flavoring, malt syrup, malt beverages, malted milk, malt vinegar, matzo
- ► Modified wheat starch (it might just say "wheat starch" on the food label)
- ► Oatmeal, oat bran, oat flour, whole oats (that are not labeled gluten-free). Commercial oats have been found to be highly contaminated with wheat flour. They may also be contaminated with barley or rye grain. Oats that are labeled gluten-free are not contaminated and are safe to eat.
- ► Pasta, ravioli, gnocchi, lasagna, ramen, udon, soba, egg noodles, chow mein noodles, and dumplings
- ► Rye
- ► Semolina
- ► Spelt (dinkel is another name for spelt)
- ► Triticale
- ► Wheat, wheat bran, wheat germ, wheat berries, bread, croissants, pita, naan, bagels, flatbreads, cornbread, potato bread, muffins, donuts, rolls, or any unidentifiable grain or flour product

Other Foods That May Contain Gluten:

- ► Fruits and vegetables with sauces, breading, or thickeners
- ► Breakfast cereals with gluten-free grains but that contain malt flavoring or granola with regular (not gluten-free) oats

- Pancakes, waffles, French toast, crepes, muffins, and biscuits
- Flavored milk, flavored yogurt, processed cheese, and spreads made with gluten-containing ingredients
- Canned soups, soup mixes, bouillon, broth and soup bases, miso
- French fries fried in oil along with gluten-containing foods
- Processed meats and luncheon meats containing hydrolyzed vegetable or plant protein (HVP and HPP)—the protein source must now be mentioned on the ingredient list—breaded and battered meats, meats with sauce or gravy, seitan (made from wheat gluten, often referred to as Mock Duck), vegetarian burgers, vegetarian sausage, casseroles, or other mixed dishes made with gluten-containing grains
- Ground spices and spice mixes, seasonings, condiments, and soy sauce made with gluten-containing ingredients
- Salad dressings and dips with gluten containing ingredients
- Candy and desserts such as cake, cookies, pie, brownies, bars, frozen yogurt, and ice cream with gluten-containing ingredients (like candy).
- Snack foods, crackers, pretzels, granola bars, energy bars, chips with gluten-containing ingredients
- Instant coffee, instant tea, instant cocoa mixes, with gluten-containing ingredients
- Fermented beverages including beer, ale, lager, porter, pilsner, and stout

Commonly Overlooked Sources of Gluten:

- Breading, bread stuffing, dressing, panko breadcrumbs
- Breadcrumbs added to meats such as meatballs or crab cakes
- Broth/bouillon
- Coating mixes
- Communion wafers
- Croutons
- Imitation bacon
- Imitation seafood
- Marinades
- Modified plant and vegetable protein (the protein source must now be mentioned on the ingredient list)

- ▶ Some salad dressings
- ▶ Processed meats
- ▶ Roux (flour and water mixture to thicken dishes)
- ▶ Sauces/gravies
- ▶ Seasonings
- ▶ Self-basting poultry purchased uncooked (injected with broth)
- ▶ Smoke flavoring
- ▶ Soup bases and cream-based soups
- ▶ Soy sauce, teriyaki sauce (check the label, some may contain small amounts of gluten and may not be gluten-free)
- ▶ Thickeners

FDA Regulations for Gluten-Free Foods in Supermarkets and Restaurants

In late 2013, the FDA issued new rules for foods that are labeled "gluten-free." This ruling was several years in the making because it was necessary to first determine the threshold of safety for gluten in foods for people with celiac disease and to determine the most reliable testing method to detect gluten in foods. The FDA's new rule became effective in 2014. This rule requires that a food labeled gluten-free:

- ▶ Cannot contain wheat, barley, rye or a crossbred hybrid of these grains.
- ▶ Cannot contain an ingredient derived from wheat, barley, rye, or a crossbred hybrid of these grains that has not been processed to remove gluten.
- ▶ Can contain an ingredient derived from wheat, barley, rye, or a crossbred hybrid of these grains that has been processed to remove gluten, but with final product containing less than 20 parts per million gluten.
- ▶ Must contain less than 20 parts per million gluten, whether gluten comes from an ingredient or is in the food unintentionally due to cross contact.

The FDA states that any use of an FDA-defined food labeling claim on a restaurant food, including "gluten-free," should be consistent with the same regulatory definition used on supermarket foods.

Skills and Strategies for Safe Restaurant Eating with Celiac Disease

First and foremost, it's important to be very familiar with the gluten-free eating plan and the potential for cross-contact or cross-contamination with gluten-containing foods. Cross-contact or -contamination means that the gluten-free food has been cooked with or has touched one or more gluten-containing foods during preparation and is no longer considered gluten-free.

Whenever possible, go to restaurants that have a gluten-free menu and have training or certification though one of the celiac disease organizations. To find these restaurants, see the links under *Restaurants with Certified Gluten-Free Training or Accreditation* (page 69). This will help you to trust that the restaurant is knowledgeable about gluten-free dining and the importance of using gluten-free ingredients and preparations that are free of cross-contamination. Many national chain restaurants and smaller local restaurants are certified.

Regardless of whether or not a restaurant is certified, it is still important to ask questions before you eat there. Here are a few steps to take to make sure that the food you order will be gluten-free:

1. Check out the restaurant's menu ahead of time. The restaurant's menu will likely be posted on their website (if they have one). If you eat in certain chain restaurants frequently, contact the corporate office to inquire if they have a gluten-free menu or check out their website.
2. If this is a special occasion or an unusual situation, call the restaurant ahead of time, preferably when they are not busy, and speak with the owner, manager, and/or chef. Tell them about your gluten-free diet needs and, if possible, make a reservation ahead of time so they know you are coming. Ask them if they have a gluten-free menu and if they'll be willing and able to meet your needs.
3. Ask what precautions the restaurant takes to ensure that the food is not cross-contaminated with gluten-containing ingredients or products, with these questions:
   ► Do they understand the need to keep your food free from cross-contact/cross-contamination with gluten-containing foods?

▶ Do they have a separate storage and preparation area for gluten-free menu items?

▶ Do they know what ingredients to look for on food labels to detect gluten?

▶ Do they use separate cleaned utensils, cooking pots, pans, and strainers for the gluten-free food?

▶ Do they clean the grill before gluten-free foods are made?

▶ Do they have a dedicated fryer for gluten-free foods?

Once you get to the restaurant, don't assume that just because you called ahead, you do not need to continue to ask additional questions. Here are a few more strategies to help you order gluten-free once you get to the restaurant:

1. Introduce yourself to your server and tell them you have to follow a gluten-free eating plan. Note that you can't eat anything with wheat, barley, rye, or oats (unless the oats are gluten-free). Ask for a gluten-free menu if it's available.

2. In the resources at the end of this chapter (page 69), you'll see a listing of gluten-free dining card resources. Having a dining card in hand to give to your waitperson can help you explain your needs.

3. Don't be hesitant to ask questions. Even if the restaurant has a gluten-free menu, it is important that you still ask your server the right questions to avoid potential mistakes. Talk with your waitperson, the manager, or chef (if possible) about your gluten-free needs.

4. Most restaurants, especially sit-down restaurants that prepare food from scratch, do take special requests. Don't be intimidated, they want you to have a pleasant dining experience and come back. If there is no gluten-free option available, tell the server *exactly* what you want and how it should be prepared. To minimize challenges, you can usually put together restaurant meals that combine naturally gluten-free foods, such as lean meats, poultry, seafood, vegetables, and fruits, without breading, sauces, or toppings. Ask the server to show you food labels if you are not convinced that an ingredient or food is gluten-free. As a last resort, bring some of your own foods such as gluten-free sauces or salad dressing, bread or crackers, or gluten-free pasta and ask the chef to prepare it in a clean pot and use a clean strainer.

5. Understand that, realistically, there is no way any restaurant can completely guarantee that the food will be 100% gluten-free. The gluten-free diet is complicated, so it is not realistic to expect that employees will know as much as you do. Be cautious, courteous, and diligent when you eat out.

6. When your food arrives, double check with the server that your meal is gluten-free. Ask again about sides, topping, and sauces to ensure that nothing was added to your food. If you are not confident that the food is gluten-free, either send it back or go without. It is better to not eat rather than risk eating food that can make you sick. If you take insulin to cover the rise of glucose for meals, don't take it until you are confident that the food is safe to eat. (Read more in Chapter 5 on page 44 about delayed meals.)

7. Unless you are dining with another person who also has celiac disease or non-celiac gluten intolerance, do not split or share food with others. Portion sizes may be too large, so gauge how much you want to eat before you start. If the portion served is too much, ask the server for a to-go container right away, pack half of it up before you start eating, and put it aside. This way you'll already have a future lunch or dinner!

8. Thank the restaurant personnel when you have had a good experience. Leave a good tip for the extra work they did to assist you. They will remember you and appreciate your feedback and hopefully your continued patronage and that of others who must eat gluten-free!

Pitfalls of Healthy Restaurant Eating with Celiac Disease

Healthy eating and a gluten-free diet are not always compatible. A gluten-free diet does not automatically equal a healthy eating plan. Many gluten-free foods can be just as high in fat and sodium as their gluten-containing counterparts and they may be high in refined flour or starch. For example, a slice of gluten-free bread may contain more carbohydrate than a slice of wheat bread. As always, it's important to pay attention to what you order and how it is prepared. Additionally, you want to look for hidden sources of gluten in restaurant foods. Keep the following pitfalls in mind when eating to manage celiac disease and diabetes at a restaurant.

1. Many restaurants offer refined grains such as white rice. Try to order gluten-free whole grains whenever possible, such as brown rice, wild rice, quinoa, or others (see the list above). Risotto or polenta are also options. Ask if the grain is cooked in water rather than a stock that may contain gluten. Other gluten-free starch alternatives are baked potatoes or baked sweet potatoes, or beans such as kidney, garbanzo, black beans, split peas, or lentils. Mashed potatoes may be made from a mix that contains gluten and hash browns may also contain gluten, so if you want these, ask how they are prepared.

2. Meats, poultry, fish, and seafood in restaurants are frequently served fried or battered or with sauces, gravies, or breading. Not only are these dishes high in fat but they typically contain gluten. Egg dishes may contain wheat flour. Request that egg or meat dishes be grilled, roasted, broiled, baked, or lightly sautéed with olive oil on a cleaned surface with fresh herbs or spices and lemon.

3. Most soups are high in sodium and also contain gluten (flour, soup base, bouillon cubes, noodles, barley) unless otherwise noted. If the restaurant prepares their soup from scratch, ask what the ingredients are. If there are no gluten-containing ingredients, broth-based soups are a better choice than cream-based soups, as they are lower in total and saturated fat.

4. Plain steamed vegetables are always a good bet, or you can order them lightly sautéed in olive oil and garlic in a clean pan. If you order a salad, be sure to tell the server you cannot have any croutons or other toppings that may contain gluten. Olive oil and balsamic vinegar (or another non-malt vinegar) is a healthy dressing for salads. Make sure your salad is prepared separately from other salad-making ingredients that may contain gluten.

5. Desserts in restaurants are typically very high in sugar and fat and typically have one or more gluten-containing ingredients. You can always be safe with fresh fruit.

6. Wine and hard liquor are gluten-free. All beers, ales, stouts, and porters contain gluten. However, there are a variety of gluten-free beers available. Make sure the beer is "gluten-free" and not "low-gluten."

Eating out with diabetes and celiac disease can be challenging, but it's easier than it used to be. Be prepared, call ahead of time, ask the right questions, and over time you will become more confident communicating your needs clearly to restaurant staff. They want you to have an excellent dining experience just as much as you do! Get specific advice about eating gluten-free in different types of restaurants in the chapters in Sections 2 and 3 under *Tips and Tactics for Gluten-Free Eating.*

Resources

Restaurants with Certified Gluten-Free Training or Accreditation

- ▶ Gluten Intolerance Group: http://www.glutenfreerestaurants.org/
- ▶ National Foundation for Celiac Awareness: http://www.celiaccentral.org/great-gluten-free-foodservice-training/
- ▶ Celiac Sprue Association: http://www.csaceliacs.info/gluten_free_restaurants.jsp

Gluten-Free Dining Cards and Celiac-Friendly Restaurants

- ▶ Triumph Dining: http://www.triumphdining.com/products/gluten-free-dining-cards
- ▶ Celiac Support (Sprue) Association: http://www.csaceliacs.info/shop.jsp
- ▶ Gluten Intolerance Group: http://www.glutenfreerestaurants.org/
- ▶ National Foundation for Celiac Awareness: http://www.celiaccentral.org/great/gluten-free-dining-card-tips-887/rev—2/
- ▶ Gluten Free Passport: www.glutenfreepassport.com
- ▶ Celiac Travel.com: http://www.celiactravel.com/cards/
- ▶ Gluten Free Registry: http://www.glutenfreeregistry.com/
- ▶ Find Me Gluten Free.com: http://www.findmeglutenfree.com/
- ▶ Food Allergy Research & Education: http://www.foodallergy.org/related-conditions#celiac

Apps for Restaurant Eating

- Allergy Eats: http://www.allergyeats.com/
- Gluten Free Registry: http://www.glutenfreeregistry.com/
- Find Me Gluten Free: http://www.findmeglutenfree.com/
- Gluten Free Passport: http://glutenfreepassport.com/
- Triumph Dining: http://www.triumphdining.com/glutenfree/shop.php
- Dine Gluten Free: http://glutenfreetravelsite.com/mobileresources.php
- Glutenfree Roads: http://www.glutenfreeroads.com/en/app/

National Celiac Disease Support Groups

- Celiac Disease Foundation: www.celiac.org
- Gluten Intolerance Group: www.gluten.net
- Celiac Support (Sprue) Association: www.csaceliacs.org
- National Foundation for Celiac Awareness: www.celiaccentral.org

Medical Centers

- University of Chicago Celiac Disease Center: www.celiacdisease.net
- Center for Celiac Research and Treatment at Massachusetts General Hospital for Children: www.celiaccenter.org
- Celiac Disease Center at Columbia University Medical Center: www.celiacdiseasecenter.columbia.edu
- Celiac Center at Beth Israel Deaconess Medical Center: www.celiacnow.org

Magazines

- Gluten-Free Living: www.glutenfreeliving.com
- Delight Gluten Free Magazine: www.delightglutenfree.com
- Living Without's Gluten Free & More: www.livingwithout.com

Books

- Triumph Dining: *The Essential Gluten-Free Restaurant Guide.* 6th ed. Burlingame, CA, Triumph Dining, 2013

Other Resources

- ► FDA gluten-free labeling law: http://www.fda.gov/Food/Guidance Regulation/GuidanceDocumentsRegulatoryInformation/Allergens/ ucm362880.htm
- ► Dietitians with resources on gluten-free eating:
  - ▷ Tricia Thompson, MS, RD: http://www.glutenfreedietitian.com/
  - ▷ Suzanne Simpson, RD, LD: http://celiac.org/provider/ suzanne-simpson-rd/
  - ▷ Marlisa Brown, MS, RD, CDE, CDN: http://www.twellness.net/
  - ▷ Shelly Case, RD: http://glutenfreediet.ca/bio.php
  - ▷ Melissa Dennis, MS, RD, LDN: http://www.bidmc.org/ CentersandDepartments/Departments/DigestiveDiseaseCenter/ CeliacCenter/OurCeliacCenterTeam/OurDietitiansandStaff.aspx
- ► Academy of Nutrition and Dietetics: www.eatright.org

CHAPTER 7

Healthy Restaurant Eating with Kids and Teens with Diabetes

C hildren and teens growing up today will likely eat restaurant meals more frequently during their lives than any generation before, for many of the same reasons that we enjoy restaurant meals today. They are quick, convenient, and available 24/7 to fit our fast-paced lifestyles. With the digital age exploding and impacting restaurant eating as well as many other aspects of life, the easy access to and availability of restaurant foods will only become more prevalent in the coming years. So yes, today's youth will need a set of skills and strategies for eating healthy restaurant meals even more than adults do now. This is particularly true for children and teens who have diabetes and/or are overweight or at risk of becoming overweight.

While not typically true for children with type 1 diabetes, too many kids and teens today are overweight or obese. Many of these children either have, or are at risk for developing, type 2 diabetes and other diseases related to being overweight. Prior to the last decade, prediabetes and type 2 diabetes were a rarity in children; so was excess weight. Today, about one in three American children and teens is overweight or obese. This is nearly triple the rate in 1963. Overweight and obesity for children and younger teens are defined, using the CDC growth charts from the year 2000, as age- and sex-specific BMIs between the 85th and 95th percentile, and at the 95th percentile or above, respectively.

Frequent restaurant meals have been shown through research to contribute to obesity-related health problems. Restaurant meals for kids and teens are often eaten in or taken out from fast-food chains, sandwich shops, or pizza joints. Ah, yes, pizza, the seemingly ubiquitous food for children and family events. Research shows that kids eat more calories, total fat, and saturated fat during restaurant meals than from home-cooked meals. And, as you might guess, they eat fewer servings of fruits, vegetables, and milk when they eat out.

Whether you are a parent, grandparent, or caregiver of a child or teen who has or is at risk for diabetes, take on the responsibility to train the younger generation in the ways of healthy restaurant eating. The reality is, food choices and eating habits become ingrained early in life. So it's never too early to make healthy eating practices part of your normal family life. The sooner the better! Don't single out the child with diabetes. Make healthy eating for diabetes management and beyond a family affair.

Those Darn Kids' Meals and Menus

Yes, there are hurdles and high jumps in your way when it comes to teaching kids about healthy restaurant eating—kids' meals, kids' menus, and kids-eat-free special offers, to name a few.

Kids' meals and menus are those listings of supposedly kid-friendly and kid-favorite foods posted in a special section of the menu board at fast-food restaurants or on a laminated card you're often handed, whether you want it or not, at sit-down restaurants. These kid-friendly meals are most often a narrow list of foods that don't score well when graded for healthfulness. When it comes to kids' meals at American or family-fare restaurants, you can name the offerings on kids' menus in your sleep: the sandwiches are hamburger, cheeseburger, hot dog, or grilled cheese, all served with french fries or chips. The entrées are macaroni and cheese, pizza, pasta and tomato sauce, and fried chicken fingers (or fried fish, in seafood spots). And all of these meals are most often served with sugar-sweetened beverages. One positive aspect of kids' meals at fast-food restaurants is their smaller portions, which can be a benefit for adults who want to eat smaller fast-food portions. Fast-food restaurants won't stop adults from ordering kids' meals, but sit-down restaurants will. But, whether young or older, you'll need to pick and choose to eat healthier fast-food meals.

Repeatedly feeding children these kid-favorite (but less-than-healthy) restaurant foods from a young age can result in several problems. The first is that children develop a taste for these high-fat foods rather than healthy ones. Another issue is that the scope of foods that children get exposed to narrows rather than widens. If kids are served the same short list of foods at home, at school, at family gatherings, and at restaurants, then those foods are all they'll want and expect to eat. Let's widen, not narrow, our kids' palates. You'll find plenty of ways in the pages ahead to expose children and teens to a wide range of restaurant cuisines, foods, and flavors.

Where are the vegetables, whole grains, fruits, and low-fat (or, better yet, fat-free) milk options? They're still not plentiful on most kids' menus, but due to the overweight and obesity epidemic in our younger generation, the pressure from many avenues is finally on large restaurant chains to take some responsibility and provide healthy offerings for kids. And they are beginning to make positive changes! Today, and this is expected to continue, fast-food burger-and-fries meals can be ordered with healthy kid-friendly sides—mini carrots, apple slices, applesauce, or fruit cup. Oh yes, there are still plenty of french fries, but the portion size is child appropriate, at least at some venues. To drink? Reduced-fat or fat-free white or chocolate milk and 100% orange or apple juice have become more readily available. Changes are also afoot in sit-down chains. Read about the National Restaurant Association's Kids LiveWell program initiated in 2012. It's catching on! This is all good news and can make parents' efforts towards healthier eating just a bit easier to accomplish.

Kids LiveWell Program

In response to the pressure of childhood obesity advocates and in an attempt to do the right thing, the National Restaurant Association (NRA) has partnered with Healthy Dining Finder, an online resource to help find restaurants serving healthy options, to develop the Kids LiveWell program. It's a voluntary program that restaurant chains of varying sizes can sign onto to endorse and put into practice in their restaurants. By early 2014, the program was being delivered by over 40,000 restaurants, many of which are part of restaurant chains.

The goal of the program is to help parents and children select healthier restaurant menu options. The program's big push is to make it easier for kids to eat more fruit and vegetables, lean protein, whole grains, and low-fat dairy foods in restaurants. Another goal of the program is to limit unhealthy saturated fats, added sugars, and sodium in restaurant foods. Restaurant chains that participate can tout their involvement in the program and can promote the meals they serve that meet the specified nutrition guidelines. The nutrition guidelines and criteria for the program are in sync with the healthy eating guidelines in the *Dietary Guidelines for Americans* and with other leading health associations. These match well with the American Diabetes Association's *Nutrition Therapy Recommendations for the Management of Adults With Diabetes.*

Kids LiveWell Nutrition Criteria

▶ Offer at least one full children's meal (an entrée, side, and beverage) that is 600 calories or less; contains two or more servings of fruit, vegetables, whole grains, lean protein, and/or low-fat dairy; and limits sodium, fats, and sugar.

▶ Offer at least one other individual item that has 200 calories or less, with limits on fats, sugars, and sodium, and contains a serving of fruit, vegetables, whole grains, lean protein, or low-fat dairy.

Gather more details about the nutrition criteria at http://www.restaurant.org/Industry-Impact/Food-Healthy-Living/Kids-LiveWell/About. Learn more about Kids LiveWell at: http://www.restaurant.org/Industry-Impact/Food-Healthy-Living/Kids-LiveWell-Program. You can see what kind of healthy kids' meals are available at each participating restaurant and find the exact nutrition information for these meals on the program's website.

Tips and Tactics to Help Kids Eat Healthy

Here are a slew of general tips and tactics to help children and teens make healthy restaurant choices. Find cuisine-specific tips and tactics to help kids eat healthy in the chapters in Sections 2 and 3.

▶ Make healthy eating in restaurants a family affair. If you eat out frequently (a couple of times a week or more), it's important to not think of or portray restaurant meals as special occasions. Rather, continue to practice the healthy eating habits you practice at home. Make this your modus operandi right off the bat. There's no need to wait until kids are a certain age or have a health issue to make healthy eating a priority.

▶ Develop family guiding principles for restaurant eating. Then get buy-in from everyone. Say, for example, that everyone needs to try at least a few bites of each vegetable.

▶ Be a role model. As the saying goes, "Monkey see, monkey do." Another expression that echoes the same sentiments is, "Actions speak louder than words." If your children see you ordering healthy foods and not overeating, they are likely to follow suit without you even whispering a word. Be a constant and consistent role model. Over time, they will begin to practice healthy eating habits.

▶ Limit the use of kids' menus unless they will help your children eat smaller portions or healthier foods and/or fit in some healthier fruits and vegetables.

▶ Take advantage of fast-food kids' meals. They're getting healthier, with the inclusion of fruit, juice, and/or low-fat or fat-free milk. Also the portions sizes (and thus calories and carbohydrate) are more appropriate for children. They could still use more vegetables, but we can hope this will come with time. In the meantime, include a side salad, if possible.

▶ Expose your children to a wide variety of cuisines, foods, and flavors. Widen the scope of foods they enjoy rather than narrowing their list to what adults believe are kids' foods. Take them to ethnic restaurants— the common ones include Mexican, Chinese, and Italian; less common options are Thai, Middle Eastern, or Indian. Expose them to foods and people from around the globe. Beyond widening their palate, these ventures can help them increase their perspective of the vastness of the world and the myriad cultures.

▶ Order from the main menu and eat family style. Order fewer entrées than people at the table. Put the entrées in the middle of the table and request empty plates for everyone. Then split and share the entrées. Remember you are modeling healthier eating behaviors.

▶ Help your kids eat small portions by encouraging them to choose from the soups, salads, appetizers, and side dishes. Mix and match for a healthy and palate-pleasing meal that is kid sized. This may be easier in ethnic restaurants.

▶ Practice portion control when ordering in fast-food or sandwich shops. When dining on fast-food burgers and fries, split a larger order (medium or large size) of fries between several or all of the family members. Or order one sandwich and split it. Then split the sides as well. That's often enough for you and one child.

▶ Fit in fruit as snacks if kids miss fruit at restaurant meals. Kids, as a group, are not eating enough fruit for good health.

▶ Divide up dessert. Kids love sweets, and teaching children with diabetes how to enjoy a small amount of sweets and control their glucose levels is an important lesson. A few sweet bites for each family member is enough, plus it teaches kids healthy behavior. Read more about managing sugary foods and sweets with diabetes in Chapter 5 on page 50.

▶ Encourage the selection of healthier, nutrient-dense beverages or choose those with no calories. Lay low on sugar-sweetened beverages such as soda, fruit drinks, lemonade, and the like, unless they are sweetened with no-calorie sweeteners (or you are treating hypoglycemia). Most restaurants offer low-fat or fat-free milk. Make milk the number-one choice whether at home or eating out. Kids need their milk for calcium, vitamin D, and other essential nutrients—unless, of course, your child is lactose intolerant and needs to drink a lactose-free beverage. To keep calorie, carbohydrate, and sugar consumption low, water, sparkling water, club soda, and iced tea are good options depending on the child's age. A splash of fruit juice may dress up these drinks. Fruit juice, as long as it is 100% fruit juice, is another option if your child has room for a fruit serving and the portion size is appropriate.

Find more *Tips and Tactics to Help Kids Eat Healthy* in the chapters in Sections 2 and 3. And thumb through Chapter 5 to get some assistance dealing with the diabetes-specific dilemmas of delayed meals and fitting in sugary foods and sweets. These tips may offer you guidance that extends beyond just restaurant meals.

As a parent or grandparent charged with fostering the healthy development of children (with or without diabetes), you have an opportunity to help them learn healthy restaurant eating habits from the start. Don't give them a chance to learn unhealthy habits that they'll need to unlearn. Unlearning bad habits is much tougher than learning good habits from the start. Help children and teens discover how to select healthier menu items in restaurants and put healthy eating skills and strategies into action. These habits will serve them well through their life. Though you may get screams, tugs, and pushback along the way, remember what's best for the kids. Apply grit and determination. It may take a couple of decades, but they'll thank you eventually.

CHAPTER 8

Restaurant Nutrition and Ingredient Facts

W hat a difference a decade or so makes when it comes to access to and availability of restaurant nutrition and ingredient information! The Internet offers access to a website for nearly every restaurant, whether they boast of one location or thousands. Many, but not all, restaurants are open books (or rather web pages), when it comes to their menu, nutrition facts, ingredients, and even allergen information (if they have them). Plus we've got access to food and nutrition databases galore, which we can access through the internet or a mobile app. That includes the companion app to this book.

In recent years, the push for healthier restaurant foods and nutrition and ingredient information has escalated—for reasons including widespread concern about health and food allergies—to the level of having city, state, and even federal regulations passed. This drumbeat for healthier foods and a tell-all approach to nutrition facts and ingredients will continue to mount as people increasingly rely on restaurant meals to get the job of eating done. This chapter provides a quick look back at the history of nutrition facts, and then focuses on the recent federal regulations on restaurant nutrition and ingredients. Let's explore what types of nutrition information you can expect to find both at restaurants and at your fingertips when you use your device of choice to search the particulars.

A Bit of History on Nutrition Facts

When the first edition of this book, originally titled *Guide to Healthy Restaurant Eating,* was published in 1999, the Internet was in its infancy. Restaurants generally did not have websites—even most of the large chain walk-up-and-order types. The minimal nutrition information that *was* accessible was in a brochure, which may or may not have been available at each restaurant location. While nutrition facts have long been available on packaged foods in supermarkets, restaurants weren't, until recently, required to serve up this information.

Slowly over the early 2000s, as the Internet infiltrated our lives and as consumer demand for nutrition information increased, fast-food and walk-up-and-order type restaurants began divulging their facts both online and in each restaurant location. In both the previous and current decades, there has been an explosion in the availability of nutrition and ingredient information for restaurant foods. Also during this timeframe several cities (including New York, Philadelphia, and Seattle) and the state of California passed regulations that required larger chain restaurants serving the same menu in each location to provide their nutrition facts in the restaurants.

At this point it continues to be difficult to find nutrition information for single-unit, independent restaurants no matter what kind of cuisine they serve, from pizza joints to fine dining establishments to ethnic restaurants. There are a couple of reasons why. First, it can be expensive to obtain nutritional analyses for menu items. Some single-location restaurants can't afford to do this. Second, these restaurants tend to change their menus more frequently than larger chains, which makes keeping the information up to date a challenge. As you'll see, this book contains nutrition information on some of the best and some less than healthy food options—in sections called *Health Busters* and *Healthier Bets*—in most of the cuisine-specific chapters of Sections 2 and 3. However, there are no *Health Busters* or *Healthier Bets* for Chapter 16: Fine Dining or Chapter 24: Indian. There's simply not enough nutrition information available for these types of restaurants to make the sharing of that info in this book educationally valuable.

Your ability to decipher the nutrition facts of restaurant foods can help you fit these foods into your diabetes eating plan. But this requires know-how and, oh yes, definitely effort. Read *Put Your Best Guesstimate Forward* (page 37) in Chapter 4 and learn to fine-tune your guesstimating skills; they're essential when eating restaurant foods. Also, make your job of searching for the nutrition facts of the restaurant meals you regularly eat a bit easier by building your own personal food and nutrition database.

Federal Regulations Put Nutrition Facts Front and Center

Fast forward to the present. You can now access nutrition information and ingredients for the vast majority of large national and regional chain restaurants and even some smaller chains. Until recently, much of this information was provided voluntarily. Around 2008, with the concerns about obesity and the closely related epidemics of prediabetes and type 2 diabetes mounting, several cities and states passed legislation to require some restaurants to disclose certain nutrition facts. With these efforts snowballing around the country, food and nutrition activists, the National Restaurant Association (NRA), and other interested parties began pushing for federal restaurant menu labeling. Did NRA and restaurant chains *really* want these regulations? Well, not really, but they definitely preferred having one set of federal regulations over a myriad of city and state regulations.

In early 2010, as part of the Patient Protection and Affordable Care Act (aka Obamacare), Section 4205 of the law amended (revised) the Food, Drug, and Cosmetic Act to require chain restaurants, retail food establishments, and vending machines with 20 or more outlets in the U.S., doing business under the same name, and offering for sale substantially the same menu items to provide specific nutrition information. Restaurants and similar retail food establishments that are not covered under the regulation can choose to "opt in" to the federal menu labeling requirements by registering with the FDA every other year. For example, a chain with fewer than 20 locations may choose to do this.

The focus of this regulation is on calories, not so much on nutrients, like carbohydrate or saturated fat, that may be of interest to people with diabetes. The number of calories, with the word "Calories" (or "Cal" for short), for standard menu items must be listed adjacent to the name of the menu item. (Think about the menu board in a fast-food burger chain or a coffee shop.) Calories must be disclosed prominently on all menus and menu boards, including menu boards at drive-through locations. The calories for variable menu items, such as combination meals, should be displayed in ranges. (A combination meal could be a choice of a sandwich, side dish, and beverage.) If foods are on display, calories must be listed per item or per serving on a sign next to the food. For self-service foods, such as a salad bar in a restaurant, calories also should be listed per serving or per item on a sign next to the food.

This is important for people with diabetes: In addition to calorie information, a clear and prominent statement must be posted on menus and menu boards stating that additional nutrition information for standard menu items is available to consumers on request. The restaurant must have the ability to provide you with the information on site. This additional information includes: total calories, calories from fat, total fat, saturated fat, cholesterol, trans fat, sodium, total carbohydrate, sugars (this includes both total added and naturally occurring sugars), dietary fiber, and protein. As a person with diabetes or a caregiver, don't be shy to ask about carbohydrate or fat grams, sodium counts, or other nutrients of interest on the list. As you know, the calories are really just the tip of the iceberg of the information you, as a person with diabetes, need. The overarching goal of this federal regulation is to ensure that consumers have adequate nutrition information to make healthier food choices away from home, just like we've become accustomed to having in the supermarket and other places where labeled food is purchased, such as convenience stores.

A stipulation of this regulation is that it supersedes (replaces) the existing city and state laws already on the books. State and local governments are not allowed to impose any different or additional nutrition labeling requirements on foods sold in restaurants or similar retail food establishments covered by the federal requirements. However, they can establish nutrition labeling requirements for food-serving establishments that aren't covered by the new law or regulations.

Non-Government Restaurant Nutrition Labeling Programs

Other restaurant nutrition labeling programs have come and gone over the years, always making an effort to help people eat healthier and, of course, generate interest in (and in some cases income for) the organization promoting the program. One program was started in San Diego, California, in 1991 by Anita Jones-Mueller, MPH. Anita was the mother of a child with type 1 diabetes and had a need for restaurant nutrition information. She developed

Healthy Dining Finder and today serves as the president and founder of the program. Healthy Dining Finder has evolved to be Internet and app-based. It's a great resource! Check it out at: http://www.healthydiningfinder.com/. Healthy Dining Finder has also partnered with the National Restaurant Association to bring us the Kids LiveWell program, which focuses on offering nutritional restaurant meals for children. Learn more about this program in Chapter 7 on page 74.

The American Heart Association has teamed up with some restaurants that use their Heart-Check Meal Certification Program. Learn more about this program on the American Heart Association website: http://www.heart.org/HEARTORG/GettingHealthy/NutritionCenter/DiningOut/Heart-Check-Meal-Certification-Program-Foodservice_UCM_441027_Article.jsp.

Nutrition Facts in This Book (and App)

This book contains a sampling of nutrition information for popular restaurant foods, mainly for the purpose of raising your awareness about what's in restaurant foods—both the healthy and not-so-healthy options.

A note of caution about the accuracy of the restaurant nutrition facts in some online resources and apps: While much of the content in these databases is based on USDA data and some is from major national chains and food manufacturers, some of these resources allow what's called crowdsourcing. Crowdsourcing allows people who access the database to add information they've collected. Crowdsourced information may or may not be reliably accurate. So, if data for a food looks fishy to you, revise your estimate based on your own knowledge base or go directly to the restaurant's nutrition information, if available.

Can Having the Facts Help You Eat Healthier?

You'd think that if people have access to the calories and other nutrition facts for restaurant foods, whether they are provided by restaurants or accessible online, it would be hard for them *not* to change their restaurant food choices and eat healthier. Well, think again! A few handfuls of studies conducted over the last decade or so delve into this question. The research does not conclude hands down that having access to the nutrition facts always leads people to make healthier decisions. The results are mixed and depend on the population of people and the types of restaurants studied. The research does find that if people use the nutrition information, it can save a few calories here and there. The bottom line for people with diabetes should be that the nutrition information for restaurant foods is becoming increasingly available and that you have access to it to help you make healthier, more nutrition-conscious decisions about what you eat. Please, use it to benefit your glucose control and overall health.

One plus of getting the nutrition facts front and center is that it may lead to more restaurants offering a few more healthy and nutrition-conscious choices or changing the formulations of some menu items to lighten their fat, calorie, or sodium load. But, not to worry, you'll still have to navigate your way through plenty of less-than-healthy options in most restaurants for years to come.

How Well Do People Estimate Calories?

It's well known that people underestimate the calories they eat and overestimate the calories they burn. Surprised? Perhaps it's simply human nature! A few studies show that people respond similarly when it comes to estimating calories in their restaurant foods. One study showed that teens eating in fast-food restaurants underestimated the calories in their meals by nearly 35%. In another study among more than 500 adults, only 11% could identify the restaurant choice that was highest in calories. Another study determined an underestimation of more than 600 calories in less-healthy restaurant items by 9 out of 10 people studied. And last, but not least, one study showed that even health professionals underestimated the number of calories in restaurant food by 200–600 calories! So, rather than relying on your estimating skills, which may have room for improvement, use the restaurant nutrition facts where and when you can. And always put your guesstimating training and skills into action. (Check these out the guesstimating tips in Chapter 4 on page 37.)

Restaurants' Use of Nutrition and Health Claims

Restaurant menu labeling regulations also include guidelines about restaurants' use of nutrition and health claims. Some examples of nutrition claims are "low fat," "low sodium," and "healthy." Nutrition claims like these were originally defined in the 1994 regulations that implemented the Nutrition Labeling and Education Act. Table 8.1 on page 86 provides you with the definitions of some common nutrition claims used on packaged foods and by restaurants. Health claims (there are a few different types) are scientific statements approved by FDA and used to explain the relationship between one or more categories of foods and the reduction of a particular disease— for example, the claim that eating more fruits and vegetables or dietary fiber is linked to the reduction of cancer or heart disease risks. Learn more about FDA-approved health claims at www.fda.gov.

The restaurant menu labeling regulations enacted within the Affordable Care Act (see page 80), permit restaurants to make specific nutrition claims about a menu item's nutritional content and require the use of terms to be consistent with the respective regulatory definitions used on packaged foods. If a nutrition claim is used, the restaurant must be able to provide you with the nutrition information to back up their use of the claim. The claim can be substantiated by a nutrition database, nutrition information in the cookbook from which the recipe was made, or another source that provides nutrition information. Regarding health claims, the FDA criteria to make the health claim must be met and the information used to support this claim must be made available to you upon request. At present there's minimal use of health claims for restaurant foods. Nutrition claims, while also minimally used, are used a bit more often than health claims.

Food and Ingredient Allergen Labeling in Restaurants

Today, there's greater awareness of and attention paid to food allergies of all kinds, including shellfish allergies, nut allergies, and gluten intolerance. As restaurant foods represent an increasing percentage of our food choices, ingredient and allergen labeling has increased in importance. Activists in this area have also pushed for local and federal regulations.

The big question on this topic is: how do federal regulations impact the allergen labeling of restaurant foods? Food and ingredient allergen information became more plentiful in 2006. This was due to the federal Food Allergen Labeling and Consumer Protection Act of 2004 (abbreviated as FALCPA), an amendment to the Federal Food, Drug, and Cosmetic Act. The FALCPA requires that the label of a packaged food that contains an ingredient that is, or that contains, a "major food allergen" declares the presence of the allergen. There are eight major food allergens: wheat, crustaceans (e.g., shrimp, crab, lobster), eggs, fish, peanuts, milk, tree nuts (e.g., almonds, pecans, walnuts), and soybeans. The FALCPA regulation only applies to packaged FDA-regulated foods, not foods sold in restaurants. However, many of the large national restaurant chains are increasingly providing information about the ingredients in their foods. Your root to the vast volume of this information is restaurant websites.

The FALCPA labeling requirements extend to retail and food-service establishments that package, label, and offer products for consumption, but it does not apply to foods placed in a wrapper or container in response to a customer's order, such as a made-to-order sandwich. If you have a food allergy, the FDA advises you to ask questions about ingredients and preparation and make special requests when eating restaurant foods. Learn more about the FDA allergen regulation at: http://www.fda.gov/food/guidanceregulation/guidancedocumentsregulatoryinformation/allergens/ucm106890.htm#q24

Gluten-Free Labeling in Restaurants

Due to the prevalence of celiac disease in people with type 1 diabetes, as well as the challenges of maintaining a gluten-free eating plan when eating restaurants foods, this book includes information about gluten-free eating in several places. Chapter 6 offers a full rundown on celiac disease and how to eat gluten-free, both at home and in restaurants. Then you'll find *Tips and Tactics for Gluten-Free Eating* in the chapters in Sections 2 and 3.

After a long wait, in 2013 the FDA issued a final rule establishing a federal definition of the term "gluten-free" for food manufacturers that voluntarily label FDA-regulated foods as "gluten-free." This definition, and guidelines for the use of the term "gluten-free," fall within the Food Allergen Labeling and Consumer Protection Act of 2004 discussed above. The definition (outlined in Chapter 6 on page 64) is intended to provide consumers with celiac disease and others who want to avoid gluten with a reliable way to avoid it. Unlike the initial guidelines from FALCPA regarding the other eight allergens, the gluten-free regulation requires food manufacturers who market food as "gluten-free" to meet the FDA's definition of gluten-free, and restaurants who use the term "gluten-free" are expected to meet this definition as well.

Table 8.1 What Nutrition Claims Mean*	
Nutrition Claim	**Meaning**
Cholesterol-Free	Less than 2 mg of cholesterol per serving and 2 g or less of saturated fat per serving
Low-Cholesterol	20 mg or less of cholesterol per serving and 2 g or less of saturated fat per serving
Fat-Free	Less than 0.5 g of fat per serving
Low-Fat	3 g or less of fat per serving
Light or Lite	Cannot be used by restaurants as a nutrient claim, but can be used to describe a menu item, such as "lighter fare" or "light size"
Sodium-Free	Less than 5 mg of sodium per serving
Low-Sodium	140 mg or less of sodium per serving
Sugar-Free	Less than 0.5 g of sugar per serving
Low-Sugar	May not be used as a nutrient claim
Healthy	The food item is low in fat, low in saturated fat, has limited amounts of cholesterol and sodium, and provides significant amounts of one or more key nutrients—vitamins A and C, iron, calcium, protein, or fiber.

*This is not a complete list of FDA allowable nutrition claims. Definitions for nutrition claims are the same as those used for packaged food products. Learn more nutrient claims at: www.fda.gov.

CHAPTER 9

Healthy Drinking Out: Nonalcoholic and Alcoholic Beverages

Your focus when you eat a restaurant meal is typically on the food; however, the type of beverage you choose and the amount you drink is another aspect of restaurant meals you need to deal with, whether you're staring at the menu board in a fast-food restaurant or sitting down for an upscale meal. Yes, meals are typically partnered with a beverage or two. Your beverage choices, both nonalcoholic and alcoholic, deserve as much thought as your food choices. Beverages have the potential to dramatically escalate the calories in a meal ... or not. Learn all about nonalcoholic and alcoholic beverages and how to order them wisely in this chapter. Specific guidance on drinking alcohol safely with diabetes is outlined in Chapter 5 (page 44).

Nonalcoholic Beverages—Challenges and Choices

From fast-food burger-and-fries chains to coffee, bagel, and sandwich shops and walk-up-and-order ethnic restaurants, the thirst quenching options have exploded and sizes have grown. Healthy and less-than-healthy beverages abound. Water, from the tap or bottled, is no longer hard to find. Thank goodness, because it's often the healthiest bet! Many of these restaurants serve both sugar-sweetened and diet sodas (carbonated soft drinks), either from the fountain or in bottles. Drinks from the fountain are typically available in at least three sizes, starting with small (which may well be relatively large at 16 ounces) and going up to large, or even extra-large or larger (in excess of 30 ounces). If restaurants stock bottled or canned beverages, they usually have an array of options, from water to fruit juice, sports drinks, teas, coffees, or sodas. Sometime there's a choice of sugar-sweetened or diet. The sugar-sweetened beverages can pack in a load of carbohydrate grams and calories, yet offer nearly nil nutrition. If you want a hot beverage, most of this ilk of restaurants is at the ready to serve you a variety of coffees or teas, from the basic brew to the specialty types.

In the wide variety of sit-down restaurants, your meal often starts with a complimentary glass of water. But the first question the waitperson asks is typically, "What can I bring you to drink?" The nonalcoholic beverage options usually range from soda (both sugar-sweetened and diet) to milk, fruit juice, coffee, and tea.

Regardless of the type of restaurant foods you eat, the more drinks you pay for, the more the restaurant likes it, because you'll run up your bill on items that require minimal labor to serve. Making health- and calorie-conscious nonalcoholic beverage choices can assist with weight and diabetes control … and keep more money in your pocket. Similar nonalcoholic beverages are served in most restaurants. Table 9.2 on page 104 at the end of this chapter contains key nutrition information for these beverages.

Nutrition and Diabetes Concerns

Before digging further into nonalcoholic beverages, here are a few of the health, nutrition, and diabetes-related concerns surrounding nonalcoholic beverages.

Obesity and Type 2 Diabetes Epidemics—The Beverage Factor

Yes, there's a strong correlation between the increase in availability, over the last few decades, of the types of beverages that contain added sugars (without much nutrition) and the increasing sizes of these beverages, and the expanding waistlines and high incidence rate of prediabetes and type 2 diabetes. According to the *Dietary Guidelines for Americans, 2010,* released by the U.S. Department of Agriculture and the U.S. Department of Health and Human Services, Americans consume about 16% of our calories in the form of all sources of added sugars. That's an average of 300–400 calories or 21 teaspoons of added sugars per day! Over a third of these calories are contributed through sugar-sweetened sodas, energy drinks, and sports drinks. The wider-than-ever variety of beverages like specialty coffee drinks, sweetened iced teas, and those thick smoothies, in large servings, contribute to this problem as well. Americans are sipping and slurping lots of calories without much nutrition bang. That's why a key principle of the *Dietary Guidelines for Americans* is a focus on reducing the intake of added sugars from beverages in order to tighten our calorie-intake belts and hopefully our waistlines.

The easiest way to limit those added sugars (which are all grams of carbohydrate) and calories is to consume fewer and smaller portions of sugar-sweetened beverages—or none at all. People with diabetes who are monitoring grams of carbohydrate generally don't have enough carbohydrate grams to spare on beverages with added sugars.

Chew Calories, Don't Sip Them

Nutrition experts continue to debate whether people consume calories more easily if they're sipped or slurped rather than chewed. When you think about it, it stands to reason that taking the time to chew solid foods, especially sources of carbohydrate, from vegetables, fruits, whole grains, and more, will be more satisfying than quickly and easily sipping them. Typically speaking, a beverage—say a 20-ounce sugar-sweetened soda at 250 calories—can be consumed much more quickly than a small, yet high-volume entrée salad with various ingredients and the same number of calories. And again, you should think about nutrition. High-calorie beverages with added sugars are light on nutrients and much needed fiber. Word to the wise: Chew your calories, don't sip them.

What About High Fructose Corn Syrup and Diabetes?

There are many names for the calorie-containing sweeteners or added sugars used in our foods today. The main sweeteners used in sugar-sweetened beverages are high fructose corn syrup (HFCS) and sucrose from cane or beet sugar. HFCS is a corn-based sweetener that is a blend of glucose and fructose. The blend varies from 42–55% fructose, based on the product. Sucrose, like HFCS, contains equal parts glucose and fructose. Though there have been a number of studies in this area to date, the human studies, though short term and small, consistently show no different impact on measures of health when HFCS or sucrose is consumed compared with other types of sugars. The most recent American Diabetes Association's *Nutrition Therapy Recommendations for the Management of Adults With Diabetes* contains a strong statement suggesting you limit or avoid sugar-sweetened beverages from any calorie-containing sweetener, including HFCS and sucrose, if you want to reduce weight gain and prevent increasing your risk for cardiovascular disease. The recommendations also note that consuming a small amount of fructose naturally occurring in foods like fruit is unlikely to raise triglycerides. High triglycerides can be a risk factor for cardiovascular disease.

What About Sugar Substitutes and Diabetes?

The safety and effectiveness, when it comes to assisting with weight control, of sugar substitutes seems to always be a hot topic because of the potential for an increased use of these products by people looking to limit sugar, carbohydrate grams, and calories. According to the American Diabetes Association's *Nutrition Therapy Recommendations for the Management of Adults With Diabetes,* the U.S. Food and Drug Administration (FDA)—the agency responsible for reviewing the safety of sugar substitutes in the U.S., both initially and over time—has approved seven sugar substitutes for the general public, which includes children and people with diabetes. The major approved sugar substitutes include, in chronological order of approval, saccharin, aspartame, acesulfame-k, sucralose, and stevia-based sweeteners. The most common sugar substitutes found in restaurants contain saccharin, aspartame, sucralose, and stevia. These sweeteners do not, the American Diabetes Association notes, cause a rise in blood glucose unless they are used in foods that contain other nutrients that raise blood glucose—think yogurt, hot cocoa, or fruit cups.

When it comes to their effectiveness in weight control, the American Diabetes Association and other organizations conclude that the jury is still out on whether the use of sugar substitutes assists with long-term weight control. It's not that the research shows that sugar substitutes increase appetite, hunger, or cravings, which has at times been the accusation. The challenge with these products is that when people use beverages or products sweetened with sugar substitutes, they often then eat additional calories to compensate for the calories saved. The American Diabetes Association, other organizations, and nutrition experts conclude that the wise use of sugar substitutes, whether in beverages like diet soda or in other foods, can be part of a comprehensive and successful weight-control plan as long as (this is important!)

you substitute the beverage or food containing a sugar substitute for a sugar-sweetened food.

How Much to Hydrate

For many years, experts preached the guideline of 8 ounces, eight times a day for beverages, but this guideline no longer holds water. In 2004, the Institute of Medicine (IOM), a government health advisory organization, offered an update. The IOM report suggests that fluid needs vary widely from person to person. They vary based on climate and food choices. Most people, the guidelines suggest, can stay hydrated by letting thirst be their guide. When it's warm outside or you are participating in an activity that is causing you to sweat, drink more to stay hydrated. Their general recommendation for fluid is 91 ounces a day for women and 125 for men—about 11 and 16 (8-ounce) cups of liquid for women and men, respectively. The IOM didn't specify how much of the fluid should come from water versus other beverages and foods. (Don't forget that vegetables and fruits contain a good bit of fluid, so the more of these you eat, the more fluid you get.) The panel did note that both caffeinated and noncaffeinated beverages can provide the necessary fluids.

Nonalcoholic Beverage Categories

As you see, with all of these nonalcoholic beverage options, your answer to the question "What do you want to drink?" deserves some healthy contemplation.

Water

Water is likely the healthiest drink in town. It is calorie free, a helpful hydrator, inexpensive (if you drink it from the tap), and plentiful (at least for the moment). When it comes to restaurants, water, either from the tap or bottled, is very accessible. You can purchase a bottle of water in most restaurants that offer a bevy of bottled beverages. In restaurants that rely on fountain drinks, there's usually a spigot you can press for water and they're glad to give you a cup to do so for free. It may be a mini cup, but you'll burn a few calories getting refills. Most sit-down restaurants offer water upon request. In upscale restaurants, they'll pour you a glass, too. Rebuff the offer of bottled flat or sparkling water if you don't want to pad your tab. But, if that's your pleasure, go for it, these options are calorie free too.

Want to add some flavor to your glass of water? In most sit-down restaurants and even some walk-up-and-order spots, you can request a slice of lemon. In many sit-down restaurants, particularly upscale ones serving alcoholic beverages, your options will be a slice of lemon, lime, or orange. Encourage kids to flavor their water with an orange slice or make their own lemonade with lemon wedges and sugar substitute.

Water with gas, fizz, or bubbles has also become plentiful. There are carbonated mineral waters (like seltzer, Perrier, San Pellegrino, or others) or club soda. They're all calorie free and can satisfy that desire for carbonation. Yes, fizz! A slice of lemon or lime or a splash of fruit juice can jazz up these beverages. Note that tonic water, mainly available at bars, contains calories. However diet tonic water, while not generally available in restaurants, contains zero calories.

Milk

Most restaurants, from fast-food to upscale, stock one or more varieties of milk as a beverage choice, with whole milk being more common than fat-free milk. However, with the push to feed kids more healthfully and to increase healthier beverage options, fat-free milk is becoming easier to find. There may be some ethnic restaurants, such as those serving Asian fare, that don't stock milk because it's not a commonly used ingredient in their food.

Nearly everyone in America could benefit from drinking more fat-free milk for the calcium, vitamin D, and other nutrients. Children and adults in this country have a large deficit of calcium and vitamin D. Milk consumption has dramatically decreased over the last few decades, even for children. One key reason? People eat more meals out and, though it is more plentiful in restaurants today, milk is not the beverage of choice. When it comes to children, start young and teach them to select fat-free milk as a beverage option at most restaurant meals (see Chapter 6 for more on this topic).

Most restaurants offer whole or low-fat (2%) milk, with fat-free milk also gaining favor. Choose fat-free if it's available or low-fat if that's your best option. Fat-free milk rings in at 90 calories for 8 ounces, while whole milk has 150 calories for the same amount. The extra calories are nothing but unhealthy fat and cholesterol. Soy milk is also showing up more often today, but it is mainly available in coffee shops as a whitener.

Fruit Juice

Fruit juice—that is, 100% fruit juice—is available at some restaurants. You'll find it at restaurants serving a full breakfast. Sit-down restaurants that have a full bar will have an array of fruit juices as well, such as orange, cranberry, and grapefruit, because they are used as mixers in alcoholic drinks. They'll also be able to pour you a glass of tomato juice or Bloody Mary mix. Fast-food restaurants and coffee and bagel shops typically stock at least orange juice. More recently you see an onslaught of bottled drinks with fruit juice blends, fruit smoothies, mixes of tea and fruit juices, and more. This new wave of drinks provides a range of calories. Both fruit and vegetable juices are healthy vitamin- and mineral-dense beverage choices when served in reasonable serving sizes, such as 4–8 ounces. However, a 12-ounce bottle of fruit juice, the common serving available for purchase in a breakfast or sandwich shop, can load on 160 calories. That's a lot when you want a serving of fruit, which is equivalent to 4 ounces. Bottled juice drinks have a Nutrition Facts label, so to know for sure, read it.

While pure fruit juice or vegetable juice is healthy and nutrient packed, you're better off eating your fruit, rather than gulping it. Other than to treat hypoglycemia, that is. Whole fruit provides volume and fiber and the satisfaction of chewing.

Noncarbonated Sugar-Sweetened Drinks

It's hard to keep up with all the noncarbonated beverages that want to convince you with their healthy looking labels that they're nutritious. However, unless they are made with 100% fruit juice, they're likely not. Many of these beverages—from fruit drinks and punch, to lemonade, energy drinks, and sports drinks—are available in restaurants, mainly coffee, bagel, and sandwich shops, in bottles that range in size from about 16–20 ounces. Sweetened lemonade and fruit punch is also available from fountain spigots in some fast-food and sandwich shops. These drinks are aimed at the taste buds of kids.

The FDA requires that fruit drinks not be called fruit juice if they contain less than 10% fruit juice (and most of them do contain less). Typically, these beverages, like soda, are sweetened with high fructose corn syrup and provide no redeeming nutrition benefits or nutrients. They've got a couple hundred calories of pure refined carbohydrate. You may find the diet counterparts to these fruit drinks and related beverages available at a few types of restaurants. Do make sure you turn the bottle or can around and stare at the nutrition facts, particularly the total carbohydrate count. Make sure that the nutrition facts listed are for the total container rather than for an 8-ounce serving. Look for a drink that contains zero or very few calories per serving. These are most often sweetened with one or more sugar substitutes. If you enjoy a fruit-flavored drink, try to make sure it's a diet variety.

Coffee

Never before has such a big fuss been made over coffee. Nor has it ever been whipped into so many concoctions. Numerous chains from coast to coast make coffee drinks the centerpiece of their menu; baked items and ready-to-eat sandwiches are an afterthought in these restaurants. The national, actually international, leader in this field is Starbucks. The east coast has Dunkin' Donuts and the west coast has Caribou Coffee. Plus, other local and regional coffee chains serve the beverages that people drink all day. Find information about coffee and coffee drinks served in restaurants in Chapter 11 on page 128.

The debates about the health benefits of coffee in general, and caffeine in particular, continue with no absolute conclusions. Some large human studies that have prospectively observed the eating behaviors of adults and their ensuing health, note benefits of drinking coffee (caffeinated or decaf), such as a lower risk of type 2 diabetes. However, there is no conclusion about the health benefits or health risks of caffeine (a component in caffeinated coffee and tea). Some people can handle caffeine until midafternoon and others can drink a cup of java at night before going to sleep with absolutely no effect.

Whether you go for the kick of caffeine or drink it decaf, coffee starts off with essentially zero calories. That's true whether it's a regular brew or deep dark espresso. The calories creep in when scoops of sugar (16 calories per teaspoon) and half-and-half (40 calories per ounce/2 tablespoons) are stirred in. Even more calories tally up when you add in flavored syrups, whipped cream, and (oh, yes) caramel topping. Check out the nutrition totals for a sampling of these drinks in the *Health Busters* section of Chapter 11 (page 135) and an even longer list of *Healthier Bets* (page 138).

It's easy enough to lighten the calorie, carbohydrate, and fat gram load in coffee. And because the drinks are nearly always made to order, you can get your drink as you need it. Start with unadulterated coffee and avoid the sugary

blends that some of the drinks are made from. Next, choose a low-fat whitener, such as low-fat or fat-free milk or soy milk. Do make sure the restaurant
uses calcium-fortified soy milk if it is your regular coffee whitener.

Enjoy some flavorings if they are sugar-free or contain nearly zero calories, which some do. Skip the half-and-half, cream, and/or whipped cream.
Hold off on the caramel topping or high-calorie blended-in ingredients. These
add calories and saturated fat. If you need a touch of sweetness, use a sugar
substitute (whichever suits your taste buds).

Espresso, a rich, dark, thick coffee, is served as a shot or two to finish
off a meal or to sip with a sweet treat. Today, espresso is also the coffee used
to make many of the coffee shop coffee drinks, from cappuccinos, to lattes or
even iced coffee. Espresso has its roots in Italy. Some would define espresso
as "power-packed coffee," which explains why it is typically served in a demitasse (small cup, about 3 ounces) with a twist of lemon to run over the brim
and sugar cubes to cut the biting, bitter taste. Espresso, before anything is
added, contains no calories, fat, or cholesterol. It can be a satisfying tasty treat
to finish off a meal in an upscale or Middle Eastern restaurant.

Tea

The options for tea are wider than ever. Even though tea is one of the most
widely consumed beverages in the world, over the years it has mainly been
consumed as a hot beverage. Yes, that's changed! Today, many types of tea—
from green, black, and oolong to blends of tea like chai, from herbal teas, to
fruit and tea blends (with flavors like lemonade, pomegranate, or raspberry)—
are now available. Plus tea is available hot or iced and by the cup or in a bottle.
Find more about the tea-based beverages served in restaurants in Chapter 11
on page 128.

The debate about the health benefits of tea continues, much like the
debate on coffee but not as robust. Since teas (besides herbal or decaffeinated teas) contain caffeine, tea becomes part of the caffeine discussion noted
above under coffee. However, cup for cup, tea most often contains less caffeine than coffee unless you drink it very concentrated. Generally speaking,
it's a healthy beverage if you just consume the tea and not the extras, like fruit,
milk, and calorie-containing sweeteners that up the calories. Some evidence,
though not conclusive, touts the presence of some disease-preventing anti-
oxidants and phytochemicals in various teas.

In coffee and bagel shops as well as upscale restaurants serving fusion or ethnic fare, you usually have your pick of 6–10 varieties of common tea blends. A few regulars with caffeine are available decaffeinated as well, such as Earl Grey, English Breakfast, and Darjeeling. Then there are usually a couple of decaffeinated herbal teas available, such as chamomile, lemon lift, raspberry zinger, or orange and spice. When going upscale, you often get to choose your tea from a wooden box.

Don't forget chai, which has become popular thanks to the large coffee chains. "Chai" is the word for tea in many areas of the world, including Asia. Chai tea is traditionally made from rich black tea, heavy milk, a combination of various spices, and a calorie-containing sweetener. The current versions of chai tea mimic the traditional and typically contain a hefty hunk of calories.

Then there are many versions of tea mixed with fruit juice or lemonade, like you'll see at Starbucks and other coffee shops served in large plastic cups. You'll find these at bagel and sandwich shops, too. Both types have typically been mixed up with some variety of fruit or fruit juice and calorie-containing sweeteners. Do beware of their healthy-sounding names. When going to purchase one of these drinks, read the label on the bottle or search out the nutrition facts so you know exactly what you'll be sipping.

By all means continue to drink calorie-free hot or iced tea. If you want to keep these drinks calorie free, don't adulterate them with calorie-containing sweeteners, fruit juice, or whiteners. If you do whiten and/or sweeten your tea, follow the same recommendations provided for coffee. Check the nutrition info for a sampling of tea drinks in the *Healthier Bets* section of Chapter 11 on page 138.

Soda/Carbonated Soft Drinks

Soda, soft drink, or pop—the name depends on where in the country you live—is the beverage people drink most frequently with restaurant foods, particularly at walk-up-and-order restaurants. These restaurants like to sell you the largest portion possible because the profit margin is high and gets higher the larger the volume of soda sold. Today, sugar-sweetened soda is typically sweetened with a calorie-containing sweetener called high fructose corn syrup (learn more about HFCS on page 89). Skip sugar-sweetened soda as much as humanly possible, unless it's all you've got to treat hypoglycemia. Aside from its thirst-quenching properties, soda is simply calories with no nutrition. A 20-ounce bottle of soda contains around 250 calories!

Where there's regular soda, there's usually also diet available, whether from the fountain, cans, or bottles. If you've just got to have your fizz, by all means go for the diet option with zip calories. There's nothing nutritionally redeeming about diet soda, but you'll at least be in the zero column for calories. If a sparkling water or club soda with no calories is available, have at it. It's likely an even healthier choice—it's just water.

Smoothies

As more people look for quick-to-guzzle meals and snacks, more restaurants are whipping up smoothies by the blender full. These frothy drinks can be made from a mixture of healthy ingredients, such as low-fat milk or yogurt and pieces of real fruit. However, they're more commonly blends of some healthy ingredients with fruit-flavored syrups or concentrates. They're also generally served in LARGE portions. So, whether they're made with healthy ingredients or not, they usually tip the calorie scale on the high side. Most of the calories in smoothies are from refined carbohydrate with zero fiber. Got to have a smoothie? Find a restaurant that makes them with milk or yogurt and fresh fruit. Then share a small serving with at least one or, better yet, two dining partners. Treat a portion of a smoothie as a sweet treat or snack rather than using it as a meal replacement. Find more on smoothies in Chapter 11 on page 129. And see Table 9.2 (page 104) for nutrition information for nonalcoholic beverages commonly available in restaurants.

Alcoholic Beverages: Challenges and Choices

Restaurant meals are a common time to consume alcoholic beverages. This is particularly true at sit-down restaurants, especially at upscale dining spots. People newly diagnosed with diabetes who enjoy alcohol commonly ask these questions:

▶ Can I continue to enjoy alcoholic beverages?
▶ Which alcoholic beverages are best for people with diabetes?

▶ How can I fit alcoholic beverages into my eating plan?

▶ What are the guidelines for staying safe when drinking alcohol?

You'll find answers to these questions in this book. In this chapter you'll find a discussion about the general and diabetes-specific perks and pitfalls of alcohol intake plus information on how much is safe and healthy to drink. More specific details and tips on how to balance alcoholic beverages, glucose, and restaurant meals are in Chapter 5 on page 49.

For personalized answers about how much and what types of alcoholic beverages are healthy and safe for you to drink, talk directly with your health-care providers.

How Much Alcohol Is Just Enough

The recommendations for alcohol for the general public (from the *Dietary Guidelines for Americans*) and for people with diabetes (from the American Diabetes Association) are the same: no more than a "moderate" amount of alcohol in a single day. "Moderate" is defined as one drink or serving of alcohol (defined below) for women and two drinks/servings for men a day, and this is the maximum amount people should consume in a single day (not an average over a few days at a time). The guidelines encourage refraining from binge drinking, which is defined in the *Dietary Guidelines for Americans* as consuming four or more drinks for women and five or more drinks for men within a 2-hour period. Binge drinking is a particular risk for people with diabetes who take blood glucose–lowering medications that can cause hypoglycemia. To learn more read Chapter 5 (page 44).

Last, but not least, though the recommendation to drink in moderation is a healthy behavior, neither American Diabetes Association nor the *Dietary Guidelines for Americans* recommend you start to drink alcohol if you currently do not drink. There are many other actions you can take to help you get and stay healthy, such as eating healthier, not smoking, and being physically active.

People with a history of alcohol abuse, pregnant woman, people with some medical problems, such as liver disease, pancreatitis, advanced neuropathy (diabetes nerve disease), or severely elevated triglyceride levels, and

Table 9.1 What's in a Serving of Alcohol?				
	Serving Size (fluid ounces)	Alcohol by Volume (%)	Grams of Carbohydrate	Calories
Distilled spirits (vodka, rum, gin, whiskey 80 proof)	1 1/2	30.0	0	97
Beer, regular	12	4.6	13	146
Beer, light	12	4.0	5	99
Wine (dry red or white)	5	13 (average)	2 (average)	123
Liqueur	1 1/2	20–55	20 (varies)	186

Adapted from *American Diabetes Association Guide to Nutrition Therapy for Diabetes.* 2nd ed. Franz MJ, Evert AB, Eds. Alexandria, VA, American Diabetes Association, 2012.

people taking prescription or over the counter medications that can interact with alcohol, should not drink alcohol. Nursing mothers can consume alcohol on occasion, as long as they plan this around feeding times.

Does one type of alcohol provide more health benefits than another? For many years you've heard about the health attributes of red wine; however, research doesn't seem to show that one type of alcohol conveys more health benefits than another. It's simply the effect of drinking alcohol that is beneficial. So, drink the type or types of alcohol you enjoy in moderation.

Benefits and Pitfalls of Alcohol Consumption

Yes, there are health benefits of alcohol! But there are pitfalls, too.

Alcohol's General Health Benefits

Studies show that light to moderate alcohol consumption over time can increase insulin sensitivity and decrease insulin resistance. This effect is at the center of alcohol's beneficial impact on decreasing the risk of metabolic syndrome, prediabetes, and type 2 diabetes and conveying other circulatory benefits. Improved insulin sensitivity can lead to lower fasting glucose and lower risk of heart disease, strokes, death from all causes, and it can improve cognitive function (thinking). Moderate alcohol intake doesn't seem to raise triglycerides (though alcohol is not recommended for people with very elevated triglyceride levels) and may minimally raise HDL ("good") cholesterol. Pretty nice list of health benefits!

However, excess alcohol intake—upwards of three or four drinks a day—does quite the opposite, by increasing the risk of type 2 diabetes and circulatory problems. Once again, the message of moderation prevails.

Diabetes-Specific Benefits of Alcohol

Alcohol's ability to increase insulin sensitivity offers a bit of help to people with prediabetes and those in the first few years of a type 2 diabetes diagnosis, when every little improvement in insulin sensitivity can lower fasting glucose levels. The positive impact of alcohol on heart disease and blood pressure—and the circulatory system in general—is a plus due to the greater risk of people with type 2 diabetes having these conditions. Moderate alcohol consumption, regardless of the type of alcohol, seems to have minimal immediate (acute) or long-term effects on glucose control.

Alcohol's Pitfalls

Yes, there are a few pitfalls to deal with as well. Alcohol contains calories (see Table 9.1) with next to no nutrition to speak of. However, studies show that people who drink in moderation don't gain weight from alcohol. Heavy drinkers may. Calories from alcohol can add up quickly, as you see in Table 9.1. A couple of 12-ounce regular beers contain about 300 calories. If shedding weight is one of your goals, you'll need to employ moderation. You simply can't afford the calories of regular drinking. Plus it's hard to fit nutrient-dense calories into your meal plan if alcohol is replacing them.

Safety is another concern with alcohol. Alcohol is enjoyable to many people due to its fairly rapid cerebral effect on the brain—it creates a loss of some inhibitions and helps some people relax and socialize. This is one reason it's more common to drink alcohol when dining out and lingering over a meal or celebrating an occasion. But this effect on the brain can also impair judgment and physical and mental reactions, which raises concerns about drinking and driving. Bottom line: don't drink and drive. For more specific details about how to manage consuming alcoholic beverages with restaurant meals, read Chapter 5.

Develop Your Alcoholic Beverage Plan

When you'd like to have a serving or two of alcohol, ask yourself these questions:

- ▶ When do you want to fit in an alcoholic beverage?
- ▶ Where do you want to consume it?
- ▶ What do you want to drink?
- ▶ How will you fit it into your eating and diabetes-control plan based on your priorities?

Maybe you decide to drink alcohol only when you dine out on the weekends or with one or two restaurants meals per week. Maybe at other restaurant meals you'll drink nonalcoholic and noncaloric beverages. Or maybe you'll drink alcohol only at home and not when you eat out. Maybe you'll go for wine, beer, or a distilled beverage with no mixer. Or twice a week you'll allot yourself a couple of glasses of wine before and during dinner and you'll take a unit or two less insulin to compensate for the glucose-lowering effect of the alcohol. It's up to you—but do figure out your alcoholic beverage game plan.

Tips to Limit Alcohol Intake

- ▶ Always have a noncaloric beverage by your side. Quench your thirst on this and slowly sip your alcoholic beverage to have it last longer.
- ▶ Need to have an nonalcoholic drink in hand that looks festive at a celebration? Order a club soda or diet tonic water with a splash of cranberry juice and a lime or lemon. Drinking alcohol too? Try alternating an alcoholic drink with a noncaloric, nonalcoholic one.
- ▶ Think about when you enjoy your one or two drinks the most during restaurant meals. Is it as you wait until the food arrives? As you enjoy your meal? To sip on as your meal concludes? As a sweet end to a meal (think a liqueur or dessert wine)? Order your alcoholic beverage when you enjoy it most. Don't sip it down beforehand.
- ▶ Order alcohol in small quantities: wine by the glass rather than the bottle (unless you have enough people to share), beer by the can or 12-ounce glass rather than by the pint or pitcher.

Alcoholic Beverage Categories

If a restaurant serves alcohol, the types they serve usually don't differ much, other than variations in the types of wine, beer, and liqueurs they serve. Table 9.3 on page 106 contains the calories and key nutrition information for common alcoholic beverages.

Beer

It might be labeled Singha in Thai restaurants, Dos Equis in Mexican dining spots, or Bud or Mick in a local American bar and grill. Beer is a brewed and fermented drink. Most beers are created by blending malted barley and other starches and flavoring them with hops. However, with microbreweries multiplying, new methods of brewing beer as well as new beer ingredients are being found. Though beer might be light, dark, or caramel in color and gutsy or mellow in taste, from a calorie stance, beer is beer. The calories can add up fast: 12 ounces of regular beer contain about 150 calories. Light beer (that is light in calories, not color) can cut calories down to about 100 calories for 12 ounces.

Wine

Whether it's red, white, or rosé, domestic, French, or Italian, wine contains about 100 calories for 5 ounces. If you typically split a bottle of wine, you might want to reduce the quantity by ordering wine by the glass. Remember to order it at the time during the meal you most want it. One calorie-conscious strategy, if you enjoy it, is to order a wine spritzer with white, red, or rosé. But make sure the spritzer is made with noncaloric club soda rather than a clear sugar-sweetened soda. Ask the bartender to mix it half and half rather than the usual three-fourths wine and one-fourth soda.

Champagne

This beverage is classified as a wine and is named after its origins in Champagne, France. Champagne is slightly higher in calories than most wines, and the calories depend on its dryness. Drier champagne is slightly higher in calories. Champagne shows up at brunches in mimosas, where it is teamed with orange juice, or on its own as a celebratory drink to welcome a new couple into married life or to toast other life celebrations and accomplishments.

Distilled Beverages

Rum, gin, vodka, and whiskey are all classified as distilled spirits. Interestingly, like wine, they all contain about the same number of calories—about 100 calories per jigger (or 1 1/2 ounces) for 80-proof liquor. Many people have the misconception that rum, scotch, and other slightly sweeter distilled spirits are higher in calories. That's not true. If hard liquor is what you prefer, enjoy it in moderation. Don't get caught up in the misconception that wine and beer have many fewer calories than distilled liquor. You simply get more volume for your calories with wine and beer.

The problem with distilled spirits is that they are often mixed with other high-calorie nonalcoholic liquids, such as fruit juices, tonic water (regularly sweetened), milk or cream, syrups, or other high-calorie liqueurs. For example, a piña colada (5 ounces) has 250 calories and a Kahlua and cream (3 ounces) has 200 calories. It's best to limit drinks that are combinations of distilled spirits, liqueurs, fruit juice, regular soda, tonic water, or cream unless you've got calories and grams of carbohydrate to spare. Order distilled spirits on the rocks with a splash of water, club soda, or diet soda.

Liqueur and Brandy

Another category of alcoholic beverages is liqueurs, cordials, and brandies. Liqueurs and cordials synonymously describe beverages such as the familiar Kahlua, Amaretto, Grand Marnier, Chambord, or one of the many brandies available. You sip these straight up or on the rocks as after-dinner drinks or in combination with other distilled spirits in a mixed drink. Brandy is created from distilled wine or the mash of fruit. The most familiar brandy is Cognac.

Liqueurs, cordials, and brandies ring in at about 185 calories per jigger (1 1/2 ounces). That's a substantial number of calories for a small amount of liquid. A good way to enjoy liqueurs and get more ounces for your calories is to make liqueur part of a coffee drink, such as Irish coffee or Kahlua and coffee. By adding a shot of liqueur to black coffee, you increase the volume substantially. Ask the server to hold the whipped cream and sugar. One of these coffee drinks at the end of a meal may quench your sweet tooth. As others are downing their mega-calorie confections, you can sip your relatively low-calorie, no-fat dessert. Cheers! (See Table 9.3 for nutrition information for alcoholic beverages commonly available in restaurants.)

Table 9.2 Nutrition Information for Nonalcoholic Beverages*

Beverage	Amount	Cal.	Fat (g)	Sat. Fat (g)	Chol. (mg)	Sod. (mg)	Carb. (g)	Pro. (g)	Exchanges/Choices˟
Coffee, black (regular and decaffeinated)	12 oz	4	0	0	0	7	0	0	Free Food
Tea, (hot, nothing added)	12 oz	4	0	0	0	11	1	0	Free Food
Cola (regular)	20 oz	239	0	0	0	81	67	0	4 1/2 Other Carbohydrate
Cola (diet)	20 oz	2	0	0	0	69	1	0	Free Food
Soda, non cola (regular)	20 oz	246	0	0	0	116	64	0	4 Other Carbohydrate
Soda, non cola (diet)	20 oz	0	0	0	0	83	0	0	Free Food
Iced tea (unsweetened)	12 oz	0	0	0	0	6	0	0	Free Food
Lemonade (regular)	12 oz	181	0	0	0	8	48	0	3 Other Carbohydrate
Lemonade (sugar-free)	12 oz	9	0	0	0	15	2	0	Free Food
Milk (whole)	8 oz	146	8	5	24	98	13	8	1 Whole Milk
Milk (reduced-fat/2%)	8 oz	122	5	3	20	100	12	8	1 Reduced-Fat Milk

(table continues on next page)

Table 9.2 Nutrition Information for Nonalcoholic Beverages* *(continued)*

Beverage	Amount	Cal.	Fat (g)	Sat. Fat (g)	Chol. (mg)	Sod. (mg)	Carb. (g)	Pro. (g)	Exchanges/Choices^
Milk (low-fat/1%)	8 oz	105	2	2	10	127	12	8	1 Fat-Free Milk, 1/2 Fat
Milk (fat-free)	8 oz	90	0	0	5	120	12	8	1 Fat-Free Milk
Milk, chocolate (low-fat)	8 oz	160	3	2	8	152	26	8	1 Fat-Free Milk, 1 Starch
Almond milk (unflavored, unsweetened)	8 oz	60	3	0	0	150	0	1	1 Fat
Soy milk (regular, plain)	8 oz	90	4	1	0	100	8	6	1/2 Carbohydrate, 1 Fat
Apple juice	8 oz	110	0	0	0	20	28	0	2 Fruit
Orange juice	8 oz	112	0	0	0	4	26	2	2 Fruit
Cranberry juice	8 oz	140	0	0	0	35	36	0	2 1/2 Fruit
V8 vegetable juice	8 oz	50	0	0	0	420	10	2	2 Vegetable

*Consider the nutrition information for these beverages as an estimate and not specific for the actual restaurant beverage you drink. Use specific information from the restaurant serving the beverage when it is available.
^Calculated based on the information provided in American Diabetes Association and Academy of Nutrition and Dietetics: *Choose Your Foods: Food Lists for Diabetes*, 2014.

Table 9.3 Nutrition Information for Alcoholic Beverages*

Beverage	Amount	Cal.	Fat (g)	Sat. Fat (g)	Chol. (mg)	Sod. (mg)	Carb. (g)	Pro. (g)	Exchanges/Choices⁺
Beer (regular)	12 oz	150	0	0	0	14	13	2	1 Alcohol Equivalent + 1 Carbohydrate
Beer (light)	12 oz	103	0	0	0	14	6	1	1 Alcohol Equivalent + 1/2 Carbohydrate
Wine, Pinot Grigio	5 oz	112	0	0	0	0	4	0	1 Alcohol Equivalent
Wine, Chardonnay	5 oz	118	0	0	0	0	4	0	1 Alcohol Equivalent
Wine, Pinot Noir	5 oz	115	0	0	0	0	3	0	1 Alcohol Equivalent
Wine, Merlot	5 oz	117	0	0	0	0	4	0	1 Alcohol Equivalent
Champagne	5 oz	96	0	0	0	0	2	0	1 Alcohol Equivalent
Vodka	1.5 oz	96	0	0	0	0	0	0	1 Alcohol Equivalent
Tequila	1.5 oz	96	0	0	0	0	0	0	1 Alcohol Equivalent
Gin	1.5 oz	96	0	0	0	0	0	0	1 Alcohol Equivalent
Rum	1.5 oz	96	0	0	0	0	0	0	1 Alcohol Equivalent

(table continues on next page)

Table 9.3 Nutrition Information for Alcoholic Beverages* *(continued)*

Beverage	Amount	Cal.	Fat (g)	Sat. Fat (g)	Chol. (mg)	Sod. (mg)	Carb. (g)	Pro. (g)	Exchanges/Choices^
Whiskey	1.5 oz	96	0	0	0	0	0	0	1 Alcohol Equivalent
Gin and tonic	6 oz	143	0	0	0	17	12	0	1 Alcohol Equivalent
Martini	2.2 oz	135	0	0	0	1	0	0	1 Alcohol Equivalent
Old Fashioned	4 oz	177	0	0	0	30	38	0	1 Alcohol Equivalent + 2 1/2 Carbohydrate
Rum and coke	6 oz	144	0	0	0	18	15	0	1 Alcohol Equivalent + 1 Carbohydrate
Margarita	4 oz	185	0	0	0	700	9	0	1 1/2 Alcohol Equivalent + 1/2 Carbohydrate
Manhattan	3.5 oz	130	0	0	0	0	3	0	2 Alcohol Equivalent
Mojito	3.5 oz	149	0	0	0	0	6	0	1 Alcohol Equivalent

*Consider the nutrition information for these beverages as an estimate and not specific for the actual restaurant beverage you drink. Use specific information for the beverage served when it is available.

^Calculated based on the information provided in American Diabetes Association and Academy of Nutrition and Dietetics: *Choose Your Foods: Food Lists for Diabetes*, 2014.

CHAPTER 10

How to Make This Book Work for YOU

S o far, you've learned about the health and nutrition pitfalls of restaurant foods and meals and gathered skills and strategies to combat these pitfalls. In this last chapter of Section 1, you'll learn how to make the rest of the book, the chapters in Sections 2 and 3, work for you. Section 2 covers restaurants under the umbrella of American fare. Section 3 covers restaurants that serve ethnic fare.

On the Menu

Eat Out, Eat Well aims to include the broad landscape of restaurants that line America's highways and byways, main streets, and city streets and to help you make healthier choices in these restaurants, whether you eat in the restaurants or take out.

Think of this *On the Menu* section as an introduction. It paints a picture of the types of restaurants included in that chapter. In some chapters the types of restaurants will be quite obvious. For example, in Chapter 14: Sandwiches, Subs, Soups, and Snacks (page 222), you know what you'll find. But you may wonder whether you'll find breakfast sandwiches in this chapter or in Chapter 11: Breakfast, Brunch, Bagels, and Bakeries (page 124). Or you may go to Chapter 19: Italian (page 361), figuring you'll find pizza, but because pizza has become such a ubiquitous restaurant food in America, it's got its own in-depth chapter—Chapter 20: Pizza (page 390).

The Menu Profile

The *Menu Profile* in each chapter offers a detailed description of the menu items served in each type of restaurant covered in Sections 2 and 3. You'll find details on the nutrition strengths and pitfalls of the specific category of restaurant covered in each chapter and whether it's easy or a downright challenge to eat a healthy meal at that type of restaurant.

Nutrition Snapshot

The nutrition numbers are telling, perhaps convincing. In most of the chapters in Sections 2 and 3 you'll find two tables with snapshots of nutrition information—*Health Busters* and *Healthier Bets.* There is no *Nutrition Snapshot* section for Chapter 16: Going Upscale—Fine Dining or Chapter 24: Indian, because there's too little nutrition information available from these generally independent, single-location restaurants.

A note about serving size in these tables: For many of the items listed in *Health Busters* and *Healthier Bets,* the serving size is specific (for example, "1 bagel" or "2 pieces"), but when the serving size is listed as "1 portion" that means that the nutrition information given is based on one portion of the item *as served* by the restaurant.

Health Busters

In the *Nutrition Snapshot* section you'll find a chart with about 15–25 *Health Busters.* These are foods or menu items that break the proverbial calorie, carbohydrate, fat, and/or sodium bank, and you'll see why when you look at the nutrition counts. Use the *Health Busters* for shock value and to help you realize just how easy it is to exceed your nutrition limits with restaurant foods.

Healthier Bets

The second list under the *Nutrition Snapshot* section is *Healthier Bets,* which will help you identify a sampling of healthier restaurant options for the restaurant type covered in each chapter. This is a list of about 25–35 foods or menu items selected based on the specified nutrition criteria developed for this book (see Table 10.1 on page 111). These *Healthier Bets* are just a sampling of healthier choices from these restaurants. For much more complete restaurant nutrition information get the *Eat Out, Eat Well* companion app.

When possible, the nutrition information in the *Nutrition Snapshot* section is specific, meaning you'll see the name of the chain restaurant that serves that food listed next to the menu item. For some menu items, particularly those in the ethnic restaurant chapters, the nutrition information will be more generic and not restaurant specific (think pad thai in Thai restaurants or hummus in a Middle Eastern restaurant). The nutrition information for *Health Busters* and *Healthier Bets* has been made available through Food-Care Inc. (http://www.foodcare.com), a "community nutrition transformation company" that brands nutrition apps.

More About Healthier Bets

As you'll learn throughout this book, you can make many restaurant foods healthier just by practicing the skills and strategies detailed in Chapter 4 (page 29). Also check out the *Menu Samplers* in each chapter in Sections 2 and 3 for ideas about putting healthier meals together (read description on page 115). The following nutrition information is provided for *Healthier Bets*: calories, carbohydrate, fiber, protein, fat, saturated fat, cholesterol, sodium. See Table 10.1 for the full nutrition criteria for *Healthier Bets*.

The diabetes exchanges/choices for the *Healthier Bets* and *Menu Samplers* have been calculated and are provided based on *Choose Your Foods: Food Lists for Diabetes*, 2014. There is no one right way to fit restaurant foods into your eating plan. Figuring out what food group the grams of carbohydrate come from to calculate your total grams of carbohydrate or exchanges/choices, depending on the approach you use, for each item in *Healthier Bets* and *Menu Samplers* is the biggest challenge. The following approach was used in this book: When it appears that the grams of carbohydrate come from a starch—be it potato, bread, or starchy vegetable—choices are listed as Starch. If the carbohydrate comes from a vegetable, fruit, or milk, the exchanges/choices are designated as such. One food group in *Choose Your Foods: Food Lists for Diabetes* is called "Sweets, Desserts and Other Carbohydrates." This group contains foods such as sweets, frozen desserts, spaghetti sauce, jam, and maple syrup. The calories and carbohydrate grams in many of these foods come from added sugars. Therefore, in calculating the exchanges/choices for this book, we've designated foods that fit into the Other Carbohydrate group as such. Exchanges/choices for fast-food shakes and frozen and regular desserts, for example, are listed as Other Carbohydrate.

Table 10.1   Healthier Bets Nutrition Criteria

Category	Calories	Carbohydrate (g)	Fiber (g)	Protein (g)	Fat (g)	Saturated Fat (g)	Cholesterol (mg)	Sodium (mg)
Appetizers*	<400	<45	>3	<20	<20	<6	<75	<750
Lunch or Dinner Entrées—with side items (per serving)	<600	<60	>3	<30	<20	<8	<75	<1,000
Lunch or Dinner Entrées—individual items, no sides (per serving)	<300	<30	>1	<20	<15	<4	<50	<500
Salads—Entrée/Main Dish (per serving, including dressing)	<600	<45	>4	<25	<20	<8	<75	<750
Pizza (serving 2 slices medium pizza), Sandwiches (including breakfast sandwiches), Subs (per 6-inch sub), and Hamburgers (per sandwich)	<450	<50	>4	<25	<20	<8	<100	<800
Side Items—fruit, vegetables (raw, including salads without dressing, and cooked), grains, legumes, starches, and meats (pork or turkey sausage or bacon) (per serving)	<200	<20	>2	<10	<5	<3	<50	<500

(table continues on next page)

Table 10.1 Healthier Bets Nutrition Criteria *(continued)*

Category	Calories	Carbohydrate (g)	Fiber (g)	Protein (g)	Fat (g)	Saturated Fat (g)	Cholesterol (mg)	Sodium (mg)
Side Items (Fried)—such as french fries, hash browns, chicken pieces, fried chicken, onion rings, and potato chips (per serving)	<200	<20	>2	<10	<10	<4	<50	<500
Soups (per serving)	<250	<30	>2	<10	<10	<4	<50	<800
Salad Dressings, Cream Cheeses, Spreads, and Condiments (per tablespoon)	<50	<10	>0	<5	<5	<2	<50	<250
Breads—such as rolls, biscuits, bagels, croissants, scones, donuts, muffins, pretzels, and scones (per serving)	<300	<45	>2	<8	<10	<4	<50	<500
Kids' Meals (complete meals with sides)	<300	<45	>3	<20	<15	<6	<50	<500
Fruit Smoothies and Fruit and Yogurt Parfaits (per serving)	<300	<30	>2	<8	<10	<8	<50	<500
Desserts (per serving)^	<300	<30	>2	<8	<10	<8	<50	<500

*Appetizers are often larger portions which are intended for splitting among several diners. A whole order/serving of a healthy appetizer can be a good option instead of ordering an entrée. These nutrition criteria are for a whole order.

^To lessen the calorie and carbohydrate load of desserts, consider splitting and sharing them, eating them only on occasion, and balancing extra carbohydrate with insulin adjustments (if you take insulin and can afford the calories).

For protein dishes, the exchanges/choices were calculated based on the group that the protein itself fits into, regardless of how it's prepared. For example, fish fillet sandwiches and chicken fingers both fall under the Lean Protein choice category even though they have a lot of fat by the time they are served. On the other hand, sausage, in any form, is classified as a High-Fat Protein because that's the food group sausage fits into. If the dish has several types of protein, then Medium-Fat Protein is used.

Beverages

Chapter 9 (page 87) offers a full discussion of beverages served at restaurants. At the end of that chapter you'll find nutrition information for common non-alcoholic and alcoholic beverages.

Condiments

You'll find a chart at the end of this chapter (Table 10.3 on page 119) with the nutrition information for the condiments you commonly find in restaurants, such as ketchup, mustard, mayonnaise, cream cheese, honey, and basic salad dressings. Chapter 15, dedicated to salads, offers details about choosing and using salad dressings (page 250).

Accuracy of Restaurant Nutrition Information

Do be aware that the nutrition information from chain restaurants is close but not exact. The same is true for nutrition information on packaged foods. Many restaurant chains state that their nutrition information (if it's made available) is based on the specific ingredients and preparation they use. But, think about it: the same restaurant chain, especially if it is a larger chain, has locations all over the country and perhaps the world. Different ingredients and foods are purchased from different food vendors and wholesalers. For example, a Wendy's in California might purchase lettuce, tomatoes, and hamburger buns from food suppliers in California, whereas a Wendy's in Connecticut buys foods from another company. The same is true internationally. Granted, the differences between the products is probably not significant because these large restaurant chains have very detailed specifications on the ingredients and food items they use or have made for them. The nutrition information used in this book is for the foods served by these restaurants in the U.S., not in their international locations.

Adding to the inaccuracy of nutrition information is the fact that restaurant foods are prepared by different people on different days. Even in the same restaurant and even in chain restaurants that pride themselves on quality control, on different days you might get a bit more or less cheese on your pizza, more pickles or ketchup on your hamburger, or a slightly smaller or larger steak even though you ordered the 6-ounce filet. Wherever and whenever humans are involved, portions aren't exact. Use your eyes to always assess the foods and portions you eat alongside looking at the nutrition information provided by a restaurant. Using all the information you have at your fingertips will help you make the best decision about your carbohydrate and calorie counts and/or the blood glucose–lowering medication you take.

Green-Flag and Red-Flag Words

Most of the chapters in Sections 2 and 3 contain the lists *Green-Flag Words* and *Red-Flag Words*. As you'll see, these words are ingredients, cooking methods, menu descriptors, and menu items that you'll commonly see on the menus of the particular type of restaurants covered in the chapter. Review these carefully. Knowledge of these words will help you navigate restaurant menus to decide what you want and don't want to eat.

Healthy Eating Tips and Tactics

Throughout *Eat Out, Eat Well* you'll find tips and tactics to help you eat healthier restaurant meals and snacks. The *Healthy Eating Tips and Tactics* sections in most of the chapters in Sections 2 and 3 assemble a convenient go-to list of healthy eating strategies for the particular type of restaurants covered in that chapter.

Get It Your Way

In each of the chapters in Sections 2 and 3, you'll find a list of special requests pertinent to the type of restaurant being discussed. You'll be able to use this list to make special requests and get your food as you want and need it. For helpful tips and strategies for making special requests, see page 35 in Chapter 4.

Tips and Tactics for Gluten-Free Eating

In most chapters in Section 2 and 3, you'll find tips and tactics for going gluten-free in that type of restaurant. To learn more about celiac disease and following a gluten-free eating plan, read Chapter 6 (page 56).

Tips and Tactics to Help Kids Eat Healthy

In most chapters in Section 2 and 3, you'll also find tips and tactics to help the kids in your life eat restaurant meals heathfully, whether or not they have diabetes. The earlier children and teens master these skills, the better it will be for their weight and health. To learn more about healthy restaurant eating with kids, read Chapter 7 (page 72).

What's Your Solution?

Eating healthier restaurant meals entails a variety of skills and strategies. It's not just about gazing at a menu or menu board and picking out the healthier choice. To be successful takes willpower (or "won't power") and application of the 10 skills and strategies detailed in Chapter 4 (page 29). To help you test your knowledge and skills, each of the chapters in Sections 2 and 3 present you with a common situation pertinent to the particular type of restaurant, followed by a few possible solutions. The answers (yes, there may be more than one right answer!) are found at the end of each chapter. Use the tips, skills, and strategies integrated into the pages of this book to help you find the best solutions to these situations.

Menu Samplers

One of the most challenging aspects of eating healthy restaurant meals is figuring out how to put them together. To illustrate how to assemble healthier meals in the types of restaurants covered in the book, under *Menu Samplers* you'll find six sample meals based on the nutrition criteria in Table 10.2 on page 117. The *Menu Samplers* in each chapter show how to mix and match foods to achieve your nutrition goals and how to apply the 10 skills and strategies for healthier restaurant eating that are outlined in Chapter 4 (page 29).

Note that the nutrition criteria may be less strict than what you would consider healthy for a meal you prepare at home. The reality is that most restaurant meals tend to be higher in calories, fat, and sodium. Plus, fruit, vegetables, and milk may be nowhere on the menu. Keep in mind that you can make special requests to have high-fat or high-sodium ingredients left in the kitchen, or you can axe restaurants that make it particularly hard to eat healthy from your list of options. Zero in on restaurants that make it easy for you to eat healthy—that's a self-defense strategy.

Why include six meals in each chapter? Because there's no longer one "diabetic diet" or any one-size-fits-all approach to diabetes meal planning and achieving good health. Plus, typically speaking, women require fewer calories than men. For this reason you'll find three meal samplers for women and three for men, One of each for each of the three types of menus—Light 'N' Healthy, Hearty 'N' Healthy, and Lower Carb 'N' Healthy. See Table 10.2 for the *Menu Samplers* nutrition criteria. Read more about today's healthy eating goals to manage diabetes in Chapter 2 (page 9).

Light 'N' Healthy

The Light 'N' Healthy *Menu Samplers* are designed for women and men who have weight loss as one of their diabetes and nutrition goals. The Light 'N' Healthy meals are based on the following calorie percentages: about 45–55% of the calories come from carbohydrate, 15–25% from protein, and 25–35% from fat, with more total calories allotted for men than women. This calorie split among carbohydrate, protein, and fat—our main sources of calories— is what's common and comfortable for many Americans. This is a moderate amount of carbohydrate from healthy sources. These meals are not high in carbohydrate.

Hearty 'N' Healthy

The Hearty 'N' Healthy *Menu Samplers* are designed for women and men who want to *maintain* a healthy weight. Like the Light 'N' Healthy samplers, these *Menu Samplers* are based on calorie percentages of about 45–55% of the calories from carbohydrate, 15–25% from protein, and 25–35% from fat, with more calories allotted for men than women. This calorie split among carbohydrate, protein, and fat—our main sources of calories—is what's common and

Table 10.2 Menu Sampler Nutrition Criteria

	Based On	Calories^	Carbohydrate (g)	Protein (g)	Fat (g)*	Cholesterol (mg)#	Sodium (mg)#
Light 'N' Healthy	For Women	1,500 calories per day	400–600	45–83	15–38	11–23	No more than 100 (total per day; no more than 200)	No more than 1,500 (total per day; no more than 2,300)
	For Men	2,000 calories per day	600–800	68–110	23–50	17–31	No more than 100 (total per day; no more than 200)	No more than 1,500 (total per day; no more than 2,300)
Hearty 'N' Healthy	For Women	2,000 calories per day	600–800	68–110	23–50	17–31	No more than 100 (total per day; no more than 200)	No more than 1,500 (total per day; no more than 2,300)
	For Men	2,500 calories per day	700–900	79–128	38–56	20–35	No more than 100 (total per day; no more than 200)	No more than 1,500 (total per day; no more than 2,300)
Lower Carb 'N' Healthy§	For Women	1,500 calories per day	400–600	No more than 45–68	20–45	11–23	No more than 100 (total per day; no more than 200)	No more than 1,500 (total per day; no more than 2,300)
	For Men	2,000 calories per day	600–800	No more than 68–90	30–60	17–31	No more than 100 (total per day; no more than 200)	No more than 1,500 (total per day; no more than 2,300)

^Total calories per meal are based on the estimated calorie needs in U.S. Department of Agriculture and U.S. Department of Health and Human Services: *Dietary Guidelines for Americans, 2010.* Available at http://www.health.gov/dietaryguidelines/dga2010/DietaryGuidelines2010.pdf..

*An effort was consistently made to minimize the amount of saturated and trans fat in all meals. This can be a challenge in restaurant meals. If you eat a restaurant meal that is high in fat, balance this out with healthier meals other times of the day.

#According to American Diabetes Association: Nutrition Therapy Recommendations for the Management of Adults with Diabetes, *Diabetes Care* 37 (Suppl. 1): S120–S143, 2014.

§Research shows that eating a lower percentage of calories as carbohydrate may help some people lose more weight initially, but research also shows that this pattern of eating doesn't result in better long-term weight loss, weight maintenance, or glycemic control.

comfortable for many Americans. This is a moderate amount of carbohydrate from healthy sources. Hearty 'N' Healthy meals are not high in carbohydrate.

Lower Carb 'N' Healthy

The Lower Carb 'N' Healthy *Menu Samplers* are designed for women and men who have weight loss as one of their diabetes and nutrition goals. These *Menu Samplers* are based on calorie percentages of no more than 45% of calories from carbohydrate, 20–30% from protein, and 25–35% from fat, with more calories allotted for men than women. This calorie split among carbohydrate, protein, and fat—our main sources of calories—is a bit lower in carbohydrate than what is common and recommended for many Americans.

Menu Lingo

Most of the chapters in section 3 contain *Menu Lingo,* a cuisine glossary. Here you'll find explanations for unfamiliar terms, such as for ingredients, preparation methods, or menu offerings, that are commonly used in the particular type of restaurants covered.

Table 10.3 Nutrition Information for Common Restaurant Condiments*^

Condiment	Amount	Cal.	Fat (g)	Sat. Fat (g)	Chol. (mg)	Sod. (mg)	Carb. (g)	Pro. (g)	Exchanges/ Choices
Bacon (thinly sliced, cooked)	1 slice	43	3	1	9	185	0	3	1 Fat
BBQ Sauce (tomato based)	1 Tbsp	53	0	0	0	390	13	0	1 Carbohydrate
Butter, stick (salted)	1 tsp	34	4	2	10	27	0	0	1 Fat
Cheese, American	1-oz slice	106	9	6	27	422	1	6	1 High-Fat Protein
Cheese, Swiss	1-oz slice	108	8	5	26	54	2	8	1 High-Fat Protein
Cheese, Mozzarella	1 oz, shredded	81	5	3	15	172	1	8	1 Medium-Fat Protein
Cream Cheese (regular)	1 Tbsp	51	5	3	16	43	0	1	1 Fat
Cream Cheese (light)	1 Tbsp	30	2	1.5	8	75	1	2	1/2 Fat
Guacamole	1 oz	44	4	2	0	200	3	0	1 Fat
Half & Half (regular)	2 Tbsp/1 oz	39	3	2	11	12	1	1	1 Fat

(table continues on next page)

Table 10.3 Nutrition Information for Common Restaurant Condiments*^ *(continued)*

Condiment	Amount	Cal.	Fat (g)	Sat. Fat (g)	Chol. (mg)	Sod. (mg)	Carb. (g)	Pro. (g)	Exchanges/ Choices
Half & Half (fat-free)	2 Tbsp/1 oz	17	0	0	1	29	3	1	Free Food
Honey	1 tsp	21	0	0	0	0	6	0	Free Food
Jam/jelly (regular)	1 Tbsp	56	0	0	0	6	14	0	1 Carbohydrate
Jam (fruit spread)	1 Tbsp	40	0	0	0	0	10	0	1 Carbohydrate
Ketchup	1 Tbsp	15	0	0	0	167	4	0	Free Food
Maple Syrup (pure)	1 Tbsp	52	0	0	0	2	13	0	1 Carbohydrate
Margarine (regular stick)	1 tsp	33	4	1	0	31	0	0	1 Fat
Margarine (regular tub)	1 tsp	33	4	1	0	41	0	0	1 Fat
Mayonnaise (regular)	1 Tbsp	90	10	2	5	90	0	0	1 Fat
Mayonnaise (light)	1 Tbsp	49	5	1	5	101	1	0	1 Fat
Mustard (regular)	1 tsp	3	0	0	0	57	0	0	Free Food
Mustard (honey)	1 tsp	7	0	0	0	16	1	0	Free Food

(table continues on next page)

Table 10.3	Nutrition Information for Common Restaurant Condiments*^ (continued)								
Condiment	Amount	Cal.	Fat (g)	Sat. Fat (g)	Chol. (mg)	Sod. (mg)	Carb. (g)	Pro. (g)	Exchanges/ Choices
Non-Dairy Creamer	1/2 oz/ 1 Tbsp	13	1	0	0	0	0	0	Free Food
Oil, Olive	1 tsp	39	5	1	0	0	0	0	1 Fat
Oil, Vegetable (any type)	1 tsp	40	5	1	0	0	0	0	1 Fat
Pancake Syrup (regular)	1 Tbsp	52	0	0	0	2	14	0	1 Carbohydrate
Pancake Syrup (light)	1 Tbsp	25	0	0	0	27	7	0	1/2 Carbohydrate
Pickles	1 spear, dill (1.2 oz)	4	0	0	0	300	1	0	Free Food
Relish (sweet pickle-type)	1 Tbsp	20	0	0	0	122	5	0	Free Food
Salsa (tomato based)	1 Tbsp	4	0	0	0	99	1	0	Free Food
Sour Cream (regular)	1 Tbsp	26	3	2	5	5	1	0	1/2 Fat
Sour Cream (light)	1 Tbsp	16	2	1	4	9	1	0	Free Food

(table continues on next page)

Table 10.3 Nutrition Information for Common Restaurant Condiments*^ (continued)

Condiment	Amount	Cal.	Fat (g)	Sat. Fat (g)	Chol. (mg)	Sod. (mg)	Carb. (g)	Pro. (g)	Exchanges/Choices
Sour Cream (light)	1 Tbsp	16	2	1	4	9	1	0	Free Food
Soy Sauce (regular)	1 tsp	4	0	0	0	333	1	0	Free Food
Soy Sauce (low-sodium)	1 tsp	4	0	0	0	142	1	0	Free Food
Sriracha	1 Tbsp	20	0	0	0	580	5	0	Free Food
Steak Sauce	1 Tbsp	15	0	0	0	280	3	0	Free Food
Sugar	1 tsp	16	0	0	0	0	4	0	Free Food
Sweet and Sour Sauce	1 oz	39	0	0	0	65	12	0	1 Carbohydrate
Tartar Sauce	1 Tbsp	60	6	1	3	110	2	0	1/2 Fat
Teriyaki sauce	1 tsp	5	0	0	0	200	1	0	Free Food
Tzatziki Sauce (Middle Eastern yogurt-based sauce)	1 oz	50	4	4	0	80	2	0	1 Fat
Vinegar (all types)	1 Tbsp	1	0	0	0	1	0	0	Free Food

*The nutrition information provided in this table for these condiments is an estimate and not specific for the actual brand or restaurant condiment you consume. Use the specific information for the condiments you use when it is available and particularly if you use these in a restaurant you frequent.

^Most nutrition information for this table was obtained from U.S. Department of Agriculture, National Nutrient Database for Standard Reference, Release 26: http://www.ars.usda.gov/nutrientdata.

SECTION 2

American Fare

CHAPTER 11

Breakfast, Brunch, Bagels, and Bakeries

Restaurants where you can eat breakfast—from grabbing a bowl of oatmeal to-go on a weekday to enjoying a relaxed weekend brunch—also generally serve lunch and dinner. These restaurants and their menus fall into several categories, within which you'll find national and large regional chains and independently owned locations ready to feed you the most important meal of the day.

There are the increasingly popular chain coffee shops, like Starbucks, Dunkin' Donuts, Tim Hortons, Caribou Coffee, Au Bon Pain, Le Pain Quotidien, Panera Bread, and more. They'd be pleased to welcome you for breakfast as well as lunch or dinner. Then there are bagel shops. The large chains include Einstein Bros. Bagels, Bruegger's, and Manhattan Bagels. They've also widened their menus to invite you in for breakfast and other meals or a quick pick-me-up. Don't forget the fast-food restaurants that fought for and won over the many breakfast eaters who are in a hurry and in need of an easy-to-eat breakfast sandwich. With so many Americans on a quest to get food fast and to be able to eat it while walking, driving, or texting, the breakfast menus of these types of restaurants now seem to overlap.

There are also chain and independent restaurants that encourage you to sit down and take the time to savor breakfast. You more commonly frequent these on weekends or on vacations. Large chains known for serving sit-down breakfast are IHOP, Waffle House, and Denny's. These chains would gladly serve you lunch and dinner too.

Hotels, from upscale to moderately priced establishments, offer breakfast to help you kick off your day. In upscale hotel restaurants you'll either find a typical breakfast menu or you'll be encouraged to enjoy their cold and/or hot buffet, which may include made-to-order omelets or eggs, fruit, breakfast breads and pastries, hot and cold cereals, breakfast meats, and more. There's usually a breakfast buffet included with the price of your low- to moderately priced hotel room.

You can find the foods these types of restaurants serve for lunch and dinner in the three chapters that follow: Chapter 12: Family Fare, Chapter 13: Fast Food—Burgers, Chicken, and More, and Chapter 14: Sandwiches, Subs, Soups, and Snacks.

While you can easily get your fill of refined grains, carbohydrate, fat, cholesterol, and saturated fat in breakfast/brunch restaurants, bagel shops, and bakeries, it's easier than ever, albeit with some effort, to exit these restaurants having enjoyed a healthy breakfast or with grab-and-go healthy option in hand.

Ⓨ On the Menu

Over the last few decades, breakfast has moved from one's kitchen table to one of the number of restaurants. Breakfast has also transitioned, especially during the hustle-bustle of work or school days, from a sit-down affair to an eat-on-the-run meal. What's on the menu for breakfast has changed dramatically, too. During the week, you may order an easy-to-handle breakfast sandwich or wrap with a steaming cup of hot coffee or a cappuccino to down while you get to your destination. On weekends or when you're away for vacation or business travel, you may take a few more minutes to eat at a sit-down restaurant or hotel buffet.

Breakfast is the meal that breaks the night fast. You may think of breakfast, especially during the work week, as your lightest meal of the day. But, by the time you down an oversized muffin, an ever expanding bagel with a thick layer of cream cheese slathered on by the person behind the counter, or a breakfast sandwich, you may have unknowingly consumed upwards of 600 calories. Yes, breakfast can be more calories than you think.

As you try to eat a healthy breakfast, the challenge is to find quick and easy choices that are moderate in carbohydrate, are relatively light in fat and calories, and help you fit in foods from the often lacking food groups—whole grains, fruits, and dairy foods. (Vegetables are often lacking, too, because they're not usually part of breakfast unless they are tucked into an omelet, topped on a bagel, or enjoyed in a breakfast smoothie.) Either intuitively or because your mother always said so, you realize that breakfast is one of the most important meals of the day. Unfortunately, it's the meal that people most frequently skip. You've heard that you need fuel (meaning food) to activate your brain for the day. When you have diabetes, it's important to balance out the nutrients you eat through the day, and if you take a blood glucose–lowering medication that can cause hypoglycemia, skipping or delaying a meal can put you at risk of hypoglycemia.

There's research to suggest that eating breakfast regularly is a plus for weight control. Data collected from the National Weight Control Registry, a registry of nearly 10,000 people who've lost weight and kept it off (at least 30 pounds for at least 1 year), report that eating breakfast regularly has been an important strategy for keeping lost pounds off. Interestingly, regular breakfast eaters are also regular exercisers. Yes, healthy behaviors tend to flock together. In the long-term Look AHEAD study of overweight or obese people with type 2 diabetes, eating breakfast regularly was a behavior that people who began the study at a lower body mass index regularly practiced.

In addition to eating breakfast regularly, take a realistic approach to the foods you order and calories you eat. Shoot for consuming at least 20–30% of your daily calories. If eating breakfast helps you achieve your diabetes, nutrition, and weight goals, that's great! If you think you'd be more successful getting a larger percent of your calories at breakfast, however, then try that.

Nutritionally speaking, starting your day off with a healthy breakfast that contains whole grains, fruit, and dairy foods—common breakfast foods—can make it easier for you to eat the number of daily servings of these foods you need. And yes, if you get a sufficient supply of these foods, you'll more easily meet your nutritional needs for vitamins, minerals, and dietary fiber.

If you find that your energy and satiety last longer if you include a small amount of protein in your breakfast, then do so. But according to the *Nutrition Therapy Recommendations for the Management of Adults With Diabetes,* there's no longer a dictate about eating some protein at every meal. You'll likely want to reserve the minimal amount of protein you should consume each day for lunch and dinner. If you load up on protein in the morning by eating a two- or three-egg omelet with cheese or have an egg sandwich with breakfast meat, you'll have a rough time holding to your protein allotment for the day.

According to the *Dietary Guidelines for Americans,* the recommendation for protein is 10–35% of your calories. You don't need more than 0.4 grams of protein per pound of body weight. Most Americans eat more protein than needed.

While you can be more creative at home with lean sources of protein, finding a healthy breakfast protein is more challenging at restaurants, where your choices are pretty much eggs, cheese, bacon, or sausage. Do consider that more restaurants, from coffee shops to bagel places and sit-down restaurants, now make egg whites or egg substitutes available. And keep in mind that a cup of milk provides as much protein as an ounce of meat. Greek yogurt has a little bit more protein than regular yogurt, but it's tough to find plain Greek yogurt beyond the supermarket aisle.

If you're grabbing breakfast on the run several mornings a week at a local fast-food restaurant, coffee shop, or bagel joint, you may want to assess the whens, whys, wheres, and whats of your restaurant excursions (see page 30). After putting this healthy restaurant eating strategy of into action, give some thought to a few quick-to-fix breakfasts you can prepare at home and eat at home or take to go. This will make eating healthier breakfasts easier.

When it comes to those breakfast spreads in moderately priced hotels, try to put yourself in auto pilot mode, especially if you have to frequent hotels for business travel. You know the food lineup all too well. Have your mind made up about what you'll eat before you enter. Don't survey the offerings, just go straight to the foods that fit your needs, prepare them, and sit and eat.

As for more elaborate "all-you-can-eat" breakfast or brunch buffets, the best advice is to avoid them if at all possible. If the restaurant offers a menu to order from, then go along willingly—order healthfully while your partners indulge at the buffet. If not, request a change of venue. Then steer them in the direction of a restaurant that also has a menu from which you can eat healthfully. If your arm is twisted or there's just not another choice, there are some healthier ways to tackle the breakfast buffet. First, survey the situation; peruse the buffet and check out the foods lining the buffet. See if you can limit your choices by simply partaking in the cold buffet. If you've got to choose from the whole buffet, plan what and how much you'll eat carefully. Try a bowl of fresh fruit or a salad as a first course to take the edge off your appetite. Return just once to fill your plate. Take larger portions of the healthier items and tastes (tablespoons) of the appealing items you've just got to taste. Lastly, drink plenty of no-calorie fluids and enjoy the relaxing environment and company.

The Menu Profile

Coffee

Coffee—it's not just a plain cup of joe any longer. Your choices are wide and deep, whether it's the coffee blends or the variety of specialty drinks available, your choice of whiteners and sweeteners, or whether you like it hot or cold. Plus, coffee has become a drink for any time of the day. And it is served in more locations today than ever before, from large chain coffee, bagel, and sandwich shops to McDonald's—which serves a variety of coffees that resembles a Starbucks or Dunkin' Donuts lineup, from lattes, to mochas, to caramels, and more. Oh yes, their calorie counts resemble Starbucks' too, at up to 400–500 calories, without a whole heck of a lot of nutrition.

When it comes to hot coffee, consumers can choose among regular or espresso, café au lait, cappuccino, café latte, café mocha, and caramel latte (a favorite of many). You've got a choice of sizes, too—from small (which is still relatively large at 12 ounces), to large at about 20 ounces. Dunkin' Donuts has an extra-large size (24 ounces)! The coffee drinks contain varying mixtures and strengths of coffee and different kinds of whitener, from whole milk to low-fat (2%), fat-free, or soy milk. As a policy, Starbucks whitens with 2% milk unless you request otherwise. To sweeten your coffee, should you want to, most restaurants offer a variety of low-calorie sweeteners or sugar substitutes. For more on sugar substitutes see page 90 in Chapter 9.

There are also plenty of iced coffee drinks, such as mocha, caramel, and dolce lattes, available from this same genre of restaurants. Dunkin' Donuts has their trademarked Coolattas. In the larger sizes, which in some cases are even bigger portions than large hot coffees, with the works added in, their calories top out at 400–500.

Word to the wise on coffee drinks: the plainer, the better; the lower fat the milk, the better; and the lower the carbohydrate count of the sweeteners and syrups you use, the better. Unadulterated coffee contains almost zero calories. Save your calories for nutrition-dense foods and meals. Find further discussion about coffee and coffee drinks in Chapter 9 on page 94.

Tea

The large chain coffee shops, from Starbucks to Caribou Coffee, have widened their variety of tea-based beverages, both hot and iced, caffeinated and herbal (non-caffeinated). Many of these drinks have syrup, juice, flavorings, and sometimes whipped cream added to them. There's green tea, chai tea, shaken tea, tea mixed with lemonade, and even chai tea mixed with cocoa. You'll see these drinks served by the cup or pre-mixed and sold in bottles, particularly in coffee, bagel, and sandwich shops. The vast majority are loaded with calories. They are not as high in calories as some of the coffee drinks noted above, but they can top 200–300 calories for the large size. The fast-food restaurants and coffee shops will gladly serve you "sweet" tea—a combo of no-calorie tea and calorie-containing sweetener. But, no need to give up tea! Bottles of unsweetened iced tea or tea sweetened with one or a combination of sugar substitutes are available (see Chapter 9 to learn more). Plus a cup of hot tea sweetened with a sugar substitute is always an option.

Similar words to the wise apply to both tea and coffee. Drink it plain. Use fat-free milk to lighten, when possible, and a sugar substitute if you want a sweet taste. Try not to sip and slurp all of your precious calories. To learn more about how to fit coffee and tea into your healthy eating plan and check out the health benefits of these beverages, see Chapter 9.

Smoothies

Another healthy (sounding) slurpable beverage that has made its way onto the menus of coffee shops, bagel shops, and a smattering of fast-food restaurants (and many of the restaurants covered in Chapter 14) is the so-called "fruit" smoothie. Smoothies are often large and calorie-dense. Generally speaking, they're a combination of real fruit (sometimes) and juice concentrates mixed with other calorie-containing sweeteners and ingredients. In their various sizes, from medium to large, they can run 200–300-plus calories. Worse yet, they contain essentially refined non–nutrient-dense carbohydrate. You're better off with a good old piece of fresh fruit—many fewer calories, more fiber, and more to chew. For more information on smoothies, check out Chapter 9 on page 97.

Fruit and Juice

When you sit down to breakfast at an upscale restaurant or hotel, you're usually greeted with the offering of fresh-squeezed orange juice. Fruit juice—typically orange, as it is the ubiquitous breakfast fruit beverage—is present at breakfast buffets, both moderately priced and upscale. But you can bet it's not always fresh squeezed. You'll also find 12-ounce containers of fruit juice in coffee shops, bagel shops, and fast-food restaurants. McDonald's sizes of juice range from 12–22 ounces, which is more than anyone, particularly a person with diabetes, needs in one sitting. Even 12 ounces is three servings of fruit!

Yes, it's better to eat fruit than drink it. For one, you'll get more fiber from eating fruit. Fruit is finally becoming available at a wider array of restaurants that serve breakfast. In a sit-down breakfast restaurant you may find a half grapefruit, berries, or a bowl or platter of fresh fruit in the menu. They love to serve huge portions, so be sure to split it up among diners.

At coffee and bagel shops, you'll typically find whole pieces of fruit, which are your best nutritional bargain due to both portion and price. You can order a side of sliced apples at McDonald's and Burger King. They also often serve fresh fruit cups in a plastic container. The portions served are often just about right or they are equal to about one and a half fruit servings.

Fruit, due to its perishability and the labor needed to cut and process it, can be very expensive to purchase in restaurants. If you're trying to eat more fruit and still have change left in your pocket, eat your fruit at home before you leave the house. Or grab a piece of fruit and eat it while you walk to the bus or drive to work. If your glucose level can't handle fruit early in the day, then enjoy the fresh fruit with lunch or as a snack. If you're traveling, consider stopping in to a supermarket and buying a few pieces of fruit that don't need refrigeration—apples, oranges, or bananas.

Fruit and Yogurt Parfaits

Another entry in the relatively healthy, easy-to-eat category of restaurant foods is fruit and yogurt parfaits. You'll find them in the popular coffee and sandwich shops as well as in some fast-food restaurants, such as McDonald's. Generally in a plastic container, parfaits consist of layers of low-fat or fat-free yogurt (regular or Greek), some fresh berries, and a couple tablespoons of granola. The calories for parfaits run from about 150–300 per serving, with larger portions having more calories and grams of carbohydrate. Larger parfaits could suffice as a complete breakfast. The smaller ones or half of a large serving make for a reasonably healthy side item.

Cereal—Cold/Dry and Hot

Cold/dry cereals used to be a regular on breakfast menus, but today those little boxes have disappeared. Cold/dry cereal tends to be found on the breakfast buffets of moderately priced hotels. There you'll find several types of cereal in pour-yourself dispensers or in large containers. Typically they offer Raisin Bran, Fruit Loops, Rice Krispies, and Corn Flakes. None are stellar nutritionally, but Raisin Bran tops the list with its whole grains and reasonable fiber content. Cold/dry cereal is an easy food to tote along on your travels. If you've got a healthy one that you enjoy, pack it.

Conversely, hot cereal, particularly oatmeal, has now become very available in popular coffee and sandwich shops and some fast-food restaurants. That's good news because it's a healthy breakfast option. And there's more good news: the portions are relatively small. But you typically get more than just oatmeal when you order it in a restaurant, and you may need to make some special requests, if possible, to get your oatmeal your way. Restaurants start with a reasonable serving of oatmeal, somewhere between 1/2–1 cup. Then they typically add fresh or dried fruit, nuts and/or seeds, and a sweetener, such as brown sugar or agave syrup. You'll need to resort to making special requests to get what you want on your oatmeal. Oatmeal is also typically the hot cereal of choice at other breakfast locales, including hotel breakfast buffets. You may find it made from scratch or in those ready-to-eat packages. Go for made from scratch. Skip the packages.

Breakfast Entrées

Pancakes, French toast, and waffles are all basically made from the same ingredients: flour (and, in most restaurants, generally not whole-wheat flour or flour made from other healthy whole grains), water, egg, a bit of sugar, and a leavening agent. Before the whipped butter and syrup are loaded on, these breakfast entrées really aren't nutritional disasters, but they typically contain a lot of refined carbohydrate. A big problem is the portions. These foods are often stacked high. To solve that problem, share an order or order a "short stack" of pancakes made with whole-grain flour or whole grains. You may be more likely to find these options at an independent health-oriented breakfast restaurant. Ask the server to hold the butter and syrup. Make a special request to get them topped with fresh fruit or get an order of fruit served on the side. If sugar-free syrup is available and it meets the mark with your taste buds, then pour a small amount.

Eggs

The biggest problem with eggs is their cholesterol content, just over 200 milligrams per egg, which all comes from the yolk. But they're low in saturated fat (depending on the size of the egg, about 1–2 milligrams per egg). The current

American Diabetes Association guideline for cholesterol is 300 milligrams per day, which is consistent with the federal government's *Dietary Guidelines for Americans*. Most people's lipid levels can tolerate a few eggs each week. But do check with your health-care providers for individual advice.

Eggs can be a challenge in sit-down restaurants that cook them to order because they're usually served in duplicate or triplicate and with sides of break-fast potatoes, toast, and often breakfast meat. Omelets are often made with three eggs and contain high-fat ingredients. You are best off sharing an omelet filled with veggies and lean protein, such as ham. That way, you end up eating about one and a half eggs. In restaurants that present you with a menu, you can usu-ally order one or two eggs à la carte. Poached eggs will be the lowest in fat. The availability of egg substitutes or egg whites in both sit-down and walk-up-and-order restaurants has increased. Using these substitutes will greatly decrease cholesterol and, in the case of egg whites, calories. Today it's becoming more common to find hard-boiled eggs served at hotel buffets or for sale at coffee and bagel shops. Hard-boiled eggs are easy to make and portable. Consider making a supply at home and carrying them along with you if you can.

Bagels, Breads, Donuts, Danishes, Muffins, Pastries, Pretzels, and More

The range of bread and baked-good options available for breakfast has wid-ened over the years and varies based on restaurant type. Coffee shops serve a range from simple to savory and sweet, which may include bagels, crois-sants, muffins, pound cake, fruit breads, scones, pretzels (see these covered in Chapter 14), fritters, and more. Bagel shops? Well yes, their specialty is bagels with all sorts of ingredients mixed in. Fast-food restaurants like to stuff eggs, cheese, and breakfast meat between a biscuit, bagel, or English muffin (breakfast sandwiches, which are covered on page 133). In sit-down restau-rants specializing in breakfast you'll usually find white and whole-grain bread and bagels, and wider menus usually serve biscuits, croissants, and Danish pastries. Unfortunately, the list is long on breads made with refined grains, which are low in fiber. These are better left on the baker's shelf. That's all the more reason to opt for a breakfast prepared at the home front when possible.

Another issue with breakfast breads and pastries is portion size. For example, muffins today are about double the size of the muffins your grand-mother used to make. On average, these "mega muffins" contain somewhere in the range of 350–500 calories and a load of carbohydrate. If the muffin is huge, split it into two servings. Share it or save half for another meal.

Bagels are also bigger than ever in both size and prevalence. An average bagel in a bagel or coffee shop is equivalent to at least four or five slices of bread or 350–450 calories and is a carbohydrate load. Most people are under the impression that a bagel is equivalent to two slices of bread or about 160 calories. If you let the server spread the cream cheese of your choice on your bagel, they'll use several tablespoons. Before you know it, you've eaten 500–600 calories. Try these bagel noshing tips: find a bagel shop that serves relatively small bagels and offers whole-grain options. You may want to scoop out some excess dough to save on carbohydrate grams. Then take advantage of the light spreads and order spreads on the side. Try to spread only a thin layer. Finally, consider splitting a bagel in half and complementing one half of the bagel with fruit, a hard-boiled egg, and/or yogurt, if available.

Croissants, biscuits, donuts, pastries, coffee cakes, cinnamon and sticky buns, and other options combine fat grams and carbohydrate grams and rack up excess calories. Put these on your once-in-a-while list. Scones are another once-in-a-while treat. They are a quick bread believed to have originated in Scotland and are traditionally served with tea. Today, scones have become a staple at coffee shops and are much larger than their traditional Scottish counterparts. They contain in the range of 300–400 calories and are nearly all carbohydrate and fat. They're definitely not whole grain. They're best skipped.

For healthier options choose items that are not made with a lot of fats, sugar, or refined grains. Healthier breakfast breads, which contain ostensibly no fat, are bread, bagels, and English muffins. If you can choose whole-grain varieties, all the better. With the pressure to provide healthier offerings, a few whole-grain rolls and bagels are creeping onto menus, but they remain few and far between. Be careful about what you load on top. Request that any bread be served dry. Keep margarine, butter, cream cheese, and other fats to a minimum. At home, all-fruit jam works well, but they're hard to find in restaurants. And, when you eat out, try to choose breakfast breads or pastries that are served in reasonable portions, versus mega sizes.

Breakfast Sandwiches

A food item will catch on if you can hold it while multitasking. That's sure true for breakfast sandwiches. Introduced in fast-food restaurants, today they line the menu boards of bagel and sandwich shops. Each of these restaurants is trying to capture the breakfast business. With this quest comes creativity. Today, breakfast sandwiches tend to offer the same range of fillers—eggs, cheese, and breakfast meats (either sausage, bacon, ham, or Canadian bacon), but the choice of outer layers or wrappers has expanded. Beyond the usual biscuit, croissant, English muffin, or bagel, you'll now find breakfast paninis, sandwiches served on focaccia, flatbread, or sourdough bread, and breakfast wrapped in a tortilla. Breakfast sandwiches range in calories from about 300–400 in fast-food outlets to closer to 400–500 in bagel shops. The more cheese and meat added on, the more fat and calories.

The pressure to offer healthier options has given rise to healthier breakfast sandwiches. Typically these feature sandwiches on a bagel thin or flatbread (a few are whole grain) or wrapped in a tortilla. To stuff in between, you'll choose from egg whites, egg whites mixed with vegetables, and turkey bacon or sausage. All in all, it's great to see these options when you're in a pinch and a breakfast sandwich on the run is your healthiest option.

Breakfast Sides

Breakfast sides vary based on the type of restaurant you visit. Fast-food restaurants push their fried potatoes. Bagel and coffee shops promote fruit, juice, yogurt, and fruit and yogurt parfaits. These restaurants like to stuff breakfast meats into one of their many varieties of breakfast sandwiches. Sit-down restaurants often offer you a choice of a breakfast meat and hash browns as sides with egg dishes or a side of meat with breakfast entrées such as waffles, pancakes, etc.

The usual breakfast meats are bacon, sausage, ham, and Canadian bacon. Ham and Canadian bacon are leaner but contain a fair amount of sodium. Slightly healthier breakfast meats made from turkey are creeping onto a few menus and being used in healthier breakfast sandwiches. Today, health experts recommend keeping these types of processed meats to a minimum due to sodium and other ingredients introduced in processing.

Next, breakfast potatoes. Whether they're called hash browns or home fries, breakfast potatoes are another example of taking a nutritious food and dosing it with unnecessary fat and sodium in the cooking process. The fast-food varieties of breakfast potatoes are usually deep-fried as opposed to pan-fried and derive more of their calories from fat.

Nutrition Snapshot

Health Busters

Category	Restaurant Name	Dish Name	Serving Size	Cal.	Total Fat (g)	Carb. (g)	Sod. (mg)
Bagels	Noah's Bagels	Three Cheese Gourmet	1 bagel	490	18	58	1040
Bagels	Honey Dew Donuts	Everything	1 bagel	380	4.5	73	700
Bagels	Panera Bread	Cinnamon Crunch	1 bagel	420	6	81	430
Breads and Pastries	Einstein Bros Bagels	Chocolate Chip Coffee Cake	1 piece	800	36	114	270
Breads and Pastries	Panera Bread	Pecan Roll	1 piece	740	39	89	320
Breads and Pastries	Cinnabon	Cinnabon Classic	1 piece	880	36	127	830
Breads and Pastries	Starbucks	Banana Walnut Bread	1 piece	490	19	75	210
Muffins	Manhattan Bagel	Banana Nut	1 muffin	630	34	74	530
Muffins	Bob Evans	Carrot Raisin	1 muffin	642	35	77	788

(table continues on next page)

Health Busters

Category	Restaurant Name	Dish Name	Serving Size	Cal.	Total Fat (g)	Carb. (g)	Sod. (mg)
Sandwiches	Chick-Fil-A	Sausage, Egg & Cheese Biscuit	1 portion	670	45	45	1420
Sandwiches	Hardee's	Loaded Breakfast Burrito	1 portion	770	49	39	1790
Sandwiches	Jack in the Box	Steak & Egg Burrito w/Salsa	1 portion	820	50	57	1620
Pancakes, Waffles, etc.	IHOP	Create Your Own Viva La French Toast Combo, Cinn-A-Stack	1 portion	1300	73	121	1580
Pancakes, Waffles, etc.	Denny's	Lumberjack Slam	1 portion	1350	50	80	2820
Pancakes, Waffles, etc.	Burger King	BK Ultimate Breakfast Platter	1 portion	1450	84	134	2920
Eggs	IHOP	Big Steak Omelette	1 omelet	1220	82	54	2270
Eggs	Ruby Tuesday	Western Omelet	1 omelet	1381	65	18	2172
Fruit and Yogurt Parfaits	Starbucks	Strawberry & Blueberry Fat-Free Yogurt w/Real Fruit (topped w/crunchy granola)	1 portion	300	3.5	60	130

(table continues on next page)

Health Busters

Category	Restaurant Name	Dish Name	Serving Size	Cal.	Total Fat (g)	Carb. (g)	Sod. (mg)
Fruit and Yogurt Parfaits	IHOP	Simple & Fit Fresh Fruit & Yogurt Bowl	1 portion	320	3	73	45
Fruit and Yogurt Parfaits	Bob Evans	Fresh Fruit Plate with Low Fat Strawberry Yogurt	1 portion	353	2	84	73
Coffee Drinks (Hot)	Caribou Coffee	Medium Mint Condition w/ Milk Chocolate 2% Milk and Whipped Cream	16 oz	580	31	68	145
Coffee Drinks	Starbucks	Salted Caramel Mocha	16 oz	420	16	66	290
Coffee Drinks	Panera Bread	Caramel Latte	16 oz	475	21	73	238
Coffee Drinks (Cold)	Panera Bread	Frozen Mocha	16.25 oz	540	17	94	130
Coffee Drinks (Cold)	Caribou Coffee	Medium Mocha Cooler w/Dark Chocolate Skim Milk and Whip	16 oz	570	18	103	130
Coffee Drinks (Cold)	Dunkin' Donuts	Frozen Caramel Coolatta with Cream	Medium	800	40	107	200

Healthier Bets

Category	Restaurant Name	Dish Name	Serving Size	Cal.	Total Fat (g)	Sat. Fat (g)	Carb. (g)	Pro. (g)	Fiber (g)	Chol. (mg)	Sodium (mg)	Exchanges/ Choices
Donuts	Krispy Kreme	Yeast-Glazed Cinnamon	1 donut	210	12	3	24	2	1	5	100	1 1/2 Other Carbohydrate, 2 Fat
Donuts	Dunkin' Donuts	Sugar Raised Donut	1 donut	230	14	6	22	3	1	0	330	1 1/2 Other Carbohydrate, 2 1/2 Fat
Bagels	Noah's Bagels	Cranberry Orange Bagel	1 bagel	250	1	0	54	9	3	0	520	3 1/2 Starch
Bagels	Noah's Bagels	Everything Bagel Thin Singles	1 bagel	150	2	0	25	4	1	0	390	2 Starch
Bagels	Panera Bread	Sesame Bagel	1 bagel	310	3	0	59	10	2	0	460	4 Starch

(table continues on next page)

Healthier Bets

Category	Restaurant Name	Dish Name	Serving Size	Cal.	Total Fat (g)	Sat. Fat (g)	Carb. (g)	Pro. (g)	Fiber (g)	Chol. (mg)	Sodium (mg)	Exchanges/ Choices
Pastries	Panera Bread	Pastry Ring— Apple Cherry Cheese	1 piece	230	10	6	30	3	1	35	160	2 Other Carbohydrate, 2 Fat
Pastries	Au Bon Pain	Chocolate and Creme Torsade	1 piece	250	12	7	30	4	1	30	220	2 Other Carbohydrate, 2 1/2 Fat
Breads	Coco's Bakery	English Muffin incl. Butter And Jam	1 whole	280	12	7	37	5	2	30	320	2 1/2 Starch, 2 Fat
Breads	Coco's Bakery	Wheat Toast	1 whole	320	13	7	45	8	6	30	480	3 Starch, 2 Fat
Breads	Panera Bread	Orange Mini Scone	1 piece	180	7	4.5	27	3	1	25	270	2 Starch, 1 1/2 Fat
Breads	Panera Bread	Cornbread Muffie	1 piece	220	9	1.5	32	3	1	30	240	2 Starch, 1 1/2 Fat

(table continues on next page)

Healthier Bets

Category	Restaurant Name	Dish Name	Serving Size	Cal.	Total Fat (g)	Sat. Fat (g)	Carb. (g)	Pro. (g)	Fiber (g)	Chol. (mg)	Sodium (mg)	Exchanges/ Choices
Breads	Hardee's	Made from Scratch Biscuit	1 piece	260	13	3	37	5	1	0	750	2 1/2 Starch, 2 Fat
Sandwiches	Starbucks	Turkey Bacon & White Cheddar Classic	1 sand- wich	320	7	2	43	18	3	20	700	3 Starch, 2 Lean Protein
Sandwiches	Burger King	Croissan'- wich Egg & Cheese	1 sand- wich	280	15	7	25	12	1	160	620	1 1/2 Starch, 2 Medium-Fat Protein
Sandwiches	McDonald's	Egg McMuffin	1 sand- wich	300	12	5	30	18	2	260	820	2 Starch, 2 Medium-Fat Protein
Pancakes, Waffles, etc.	IHOP	Baby Cakes	1 portion	210	6	1.5	25	13	2	35	760	2 Starch, 1 Fat

(table continues on next page)

Healthier Bets

Category	Restaurant Name	Dish Name	Serving Size	Cal.	Total Fat (g)	Sat. Fat (g)	Carb. (g)	Pro. (g)	Fiber (g)	Chol. (mg)	Sodium (mg)	Exchanges/ Choices
Pancakes, Waffles, etc.	Denny's	Pancakes, Hearty Wheat	1 portion	310	1.5	0	64	10	8	15	950	4 Starch
Pancakes, Waffles, etc.	Bob Evans	Plain Crepe (no topping)	1 crepe	255	14	6	27	5	1	67	285	2 Starch, 2 Fat
Meats	Coco's Bakery	Turkey Sausage	1 patty	70	4	1.5	0	8	0	15	260	1 Medium-Fat Protein
Meats	IHOP	Ham	2 slices	60	1.5	0.5	1	10	0	35	630	1 1/2 Lean Protein
Hot Cereals	Starbucks	Starbucks Perfect Oatmeal	1 portion	140	2.5	0.5	25	5	4	0	105	1 1/2 Starch, 1/2 Fat
Hot Cereals	Burger King	Quaker Oatmeal Original	1 portion	140	3.5	1	23	5	3	5	100	1 1/2 Starch, 1/2 Fat

(table continues on next page)

Healthier Bets

Category	Restaurant Name	Dish Name	Serving Size	Cal.	Total Fat (g)	Sat. Fat (g)	Carb. (g)	Pro. (g)	Fiber (g)	Chol. (mg)	Sodium (mg)	Exchanges/ Choices
Hot Cereals	Au Bon Pain	Apple Cinnamon Oatmeal (small)	1 portion	190	3	0	37	6	4	0	5	2 Starch, 1/2 Fat
Eggs	Bob Evans	Veggie Omelet with Fresh Fruit Dish & Wheat Toast w/ Jelly	1 omelet	311	6	2	43	22	4	1	581	1 Starch, 2 Fruit, 3 Lean Protein
Eggs	IHOP	Simple & Fit Spinach, Mushroom & Tomato Omelette w/ Fresh Fruit	1 omelet	330	12	4.5	31	29	5	30	690	2 Starch, 4 Lean Protein

(table continues on next page)

Healthier Bets

Category	Restaurant Name	Dish Name	Serving Size	Cal.	Total Fat (g)	Sat. Fat (g)	Carb. (g)	Pro. (g)	Fiber (g)	Chol. (mg)	Sodium (mg)	Exchanges/ Choices
Coffee Drinks	Starbucks	Cool Lime Refresher	16 oz	50	0	0	13	0	0	0	0	1 Other Carbohydrate
Coffee Drinks	Panera Bread	Hot Coffee	16.75 oz	5	0	0	0	1	0	0	10	Free Food
Tea Drinks	Panera Bread	Tropical Hibiscus Herbal Iced Tea	20.75 oz	0	0	0	0	0	0	0	0	Free Food
Tea Drinks	Panera Bread	Green Tea with Passion Fruit and Papaya	20.75 oz	130	0	0	31	0	0	0	10	2 Other Carbohydrate
Tea Drinks	Starbucks	Full Leaf Chai Tea	16 oz	0	0	0	0	0	0	0	0	Free Food

(table continues on next page)

Healthier Bets

Category	Restaurant Name	Dish Name	Serving Size	Cal.	Total Fat (g)	Sat. Fat (g)	Carb. (g)	Pro. (g)	Fiber (g)	Chol. (mg)	Sodium (mg)	Exchanges/ Choices
Fruit and Yogurt Parfaits	McDonald's	Fruit 'n Yogurt	1 portion	160	2	1	31	4	1	5	85	1 Fruit, 1/2 Low-Fat Milk, 1/2 Other Carbohydrate
Fruit and Yogurt Parfaits	Bob Evans	Blueberry Banana Mini Fruit & Yogurt	1 portion	177	1	0	39	4	3	3	61	1 1/2 Fruit, 1/2 Nonfat Milk, 1/2 Other Carbohydrate,
Fruit Cup/ Fresh Fruit	IHOP	Jr. Fresh Fruit Dish	1 portion	80	0	0	21	1	2	0	0	1 1/2 Fruit
Fruit Cup/ Fresh Fruit	Starbucks	Seasonal Harvest Fruit Blend	1 portion	90	0	0	24	1	4	0	0	1 1/2 Fruit
Fruit Cup/ Fresh Fruit	Panera Bread	Seasonal Fruit Cup	1 portion	60	0	0	17	1	n/a	0	15	1 Fruit

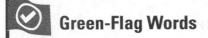 **Green-Flag Words**

Ingredients:

- All-fruit jam or spread
- Coffee and tea (without added syrups, flavorings, whipped cream, etc.)
- Dry cereals (whole-grain, high-fiber)
- Egg—served as one
- Fruit (fresh piece of fruit, cut fruit, 100% juice, dried for oatmeal)
- Oatmeal
- Turkey bacon, turkey sausage, Canadian bacon, ham
- Vegetables—in an omelet, egg white sandwich, or even in veggie cream cheese
- Whole-grain bagels
- Whole-grain or low-fat breads, flatbread, tortilla
- Yogurt (nonfat plain or Greek)

Cooking Methods/Menu Descriptions:

- Omelet—loaded with vegetables, light on cheese; split or share

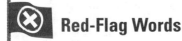 **Red-Flag Words**

Ingredients:

- Bacon
- Hash browns
- Sausage
- Scones, donuts, cinnamon buns, biscuits, Danish pastries, croissants
- Specialty coffee and tea drinks (with added syrups, flavorings, whipped cream, etc.)

Cooking Methods/Menu Description:

- Fried
- Omelet (loaded with cheese and breakfast meats)
- Smothered with cheese

🍎 Healthy Eating Tips and Tactics

▶ Stick to coffee without a lot of added cream, whole milk, or sugar. These extras add fat and empty calories. Use a sugar substitute.

▶ Choose a bagel shop serving smaller bagels (~45 grams of carbohydrate) versus larger bagels (60 grams of carbohydrate or more).

▶ Opt for one of the light bagel spreads, but keep in mind that they are hardly calorie or fat free. Still spread them thinly.

▶ Request an omelet made with two eggs (instead of three).

▶ Eat breakfast. Skipping breakfast just keeps your engine in low gear and may help you rationalize overeating the rest of the day. Plus, if you take glucose-lowering medications that can cause low blood glucose, skipping breakfast may put you at risk for hypoglycemia (see Chapter 8, page 78).

▶ In a breakfast sandwich, choose ham, egg, and/or cheese. Pass on bacon or sausage.

▶ If jam or jelly is an option, use a thin layer of that instead of margarine, butter, or cream cheese. Jams and jellies contain no fat and just a small amount of carbohydrate.

▶ Minimize portions by splitting servings. Share with your dining partner or save half for another meal rather than overeating. (Think pancakes, omelet, bagel, etc.)

👍 Get It Your Way

▶ Order bagel spreads on the side so that you can control how much is spread.

▶ Request that your bagel be scooped out (the excess dough removed).

▶ Order butter or margarine on the side.

▶ Opt for fat-free milk in hot or dry cereal, coffees, and teas.

▶ Order a breakfast sandwich on a bagel thin, tortilla, or flatbread.

▶ Hold the cheese in an omelet or on a breakfast sandwich.

Tips and Tactics for Gluten-Free Eating

▶ Fresh eggs are naturally gluten-free. Try soft or hard cooked eggs, or fresh eggs prepared in a clean pan with olive oil rather than butter or margarine. Other egg dishes, such as omelets, may contain flour or may be cross-contaminated with gluten-containing ingredients. Ask your server.

▶ Ask to check the labels of prepared foods that you may order or that will be used in your meal for gluten-containing additives (especially in all processed breakfast meats).

▶ Fresh fruit and dairy foods (milk, yogurt) are good choices. You may want to bring your own gluten-free breakfast cereal to add to yogurt or have with milk.

▶ If breakfast potatoes are on the menu, make sure they do not have a seasoning mix with flour added to help them brown.

▶ Unless the bakery or bagel shop has a designated separate area to bake gluten-free products, then their products will most likely be contaminated with gluten. Residual flour can remain airborne for several hours. Question the bakery's methods carefully.

▶ Discuss gluten-free choices with your waitperson or the manager at an all-you-can-eat buffet or brunch. Ask what seasonings are added to foods that they identify as gluten-free. Watch for cross-contamination with serving utensils that may have been used for gluten-containing dishes.

▶ Because of all the gluten-containing foods commonly served for breakfast, it can be tough to eat gluten-free. You may want to carry a homemade gluten-free nutrition bar or a commercial one that you know is gluten-free.

Tips and Tactics to Help Kids Eat Healthy

▶ Order family style in a sit-down breakfast restaurant and split servings to get a balanced meal with reasonably sized portions. Consider a three-egg vegetable omelet with cheese, a short stack of whole-grain pancakes, and a bowl of fruit.

► Opt for berries for your fruit and split them. Kids like berries in part because they're finger foods.
► Start them early on the healthier and smaller breakfast sandwiches—on English muffin, bagel thins, or flatbread.
► Split a bagel, an order of whole-grain toast, or a muffin.
► Limit their exposure to high-fat and high-calorie breakfast sweets.
► At a hotel breakfast buffet: With older kids, decide on what they'll eat before they load their plate. With younger kids, accompany and guide them. Teach them to serve themselves just the food they want and need. Encourage them not to waste food (it's a teachable moment!).

⑦ What's Your Solution?

You're on a family vacation and you're traveling by car. You are staying at a moderately priced hotel that offers a breakfast buffet. (You know it's not ideal, but it's included in the price of the room.) You accompany your family to breakfast. You survey the situation. It's the usual spread—make-your-own Belgian waffles with syrup, apples, bananas, a few dry cereal options, oatmeal packets, hard-boiled eggs, containers of fruit yogurt, breads to toast (including whole-grain bread), bagels, and a range of milk options.

What is a breakfast option from this spread that will meet your nutrition needs and satisfy your taste buds?

a) Raisin bran dry cereal, fat-free milk, a hard-boiled egg, and half a banana
b) Half of a Belgian waffle with a sliced half a banana on top and a fruit yogurt on the side
c) Bagel with cream cheese, a sliced apple, 1 cup of fat-free milk
d) Two hard-boiled eggs, one slice of whole-grain bread with butter, and half an apple sliced

See page 155 for answers.

Menu Samplers

Light 'N' Healthy

Menu Samplers Section	Menu Item	Amount	Calories	Fat (g)	% Calories from Fat	Saturated Fat (g)	Chol. (mg)	Sodium (mg)	Carb. (g)	Fiber (g)	Protein (g)	Exchanges/Choices
Light 'N' Healthy (Women)	Oatmeal with dried fruit and nut topping	1 order	254	3		0.8	0	256	52	5	7	2 Starch, 1 Fruit, 1 Fat
	Side of bacon	2 strips	110	6		2.3	60	1010	2	0	13	2 Lean Protein
	Cafe latte with reduced-fat milk	1 medium (16 oz)	190	7		4.5	30	150	18	0	12	1 1/2 Reduced-Fat Milk
Totals			554	16	26	8	90	1416	72	5	32	2 Starch, 1 Fruit, 1 1/2 Reduced-Fat Milk, 2 Lean Protein, 1 Fat

(table continues on next page)

Light 'N' Healthy

Menu Samplers Section	Menu Item	Amount	Calories	Fat (g)	% Calories from Fat	Saturated Fat (g)	Chol. (mg)	Sodium (mg)	Carb. (g)	Fiber (g)	Protein (g)	Exchanges/ Choices
Light 'N' Healthy (Men)*	Ham, egg, and cheese breakfast sandwich on English muffin	1 order	350	17		6.8	180	1244	31	1	20	2 Starch, 3 Medium-Fat Protein
	Cafe latte with reduced-fat milk	1 small (9 oz)	150	6		3.5	25	115	14	0	10	1 1/2 Reduced-Fat Milk
	Fruit and yogurt parfait (made with 1% or fat-free yogurt)	1 cup	150	1.9		0.6	7	101	37	2	7	1 Fruit, 1 Fat-Free Milk
Totals			**650**	**25**	**35**	**11**	**212**	**1460**	**82**	**3**	**37**	**2 Starch, 1 Fruit, 1 1/2 Reduced-Fat Milk, 1 Fat-Free Milk, 3 Medium-Fat Protein**

(table continues on next page)

Hearty 'N' Healthy

Menu Samplers Section	Menu Item	Amount	Calories	Fat (g)	% Calories from Fat	Saturated Fat (g)	Chol. (mg)	Sodium (mg)	Carb. (g)	Fiber (g)	Protein (g)	Exchanges/ Choices
Hearty 'N' Healthy (Women)	Whole-grain pancakes	2 pancakes	340	17		3	38	1160	35	3	9	2 1/2 Starch, 3 Fat
	Table syrup (regular)	2 table-spoons	106	0		0	0	24	28	0	0	2 Other Carbohydrate
	Turkey sausage	2 links	144	8		2	62	315	2	0	18	2 1/2 Lean Protein
Totals			**590**	**25**	**38**	**5**	**100**	**1499**	**65**	**3**	**27**	**2 1/2 Starch, 2 Other Carbohydrate, 2 1/2 Lean Protein, 3 Fat**

(table continues on next page)

Hearty 'N' Healthy

Menu Samplers Section	Menu Item	Amount	Calories	Fat (g)	% Calories from Fat	Saturated Fat (g)	Chol. (mg)	Sodium (mg)	Carb. (g)	Fiber (g)	Protein (g)	Exchanges/ Choices
Hearty 'N' Healthy (Men)*	French toast	2 slices	326	6		6	154	560	38	2	8	2 1/2 Starch, 1 Fat
	Table syrup (regular)	2 table- spoons	106	0		0	0	24	28	0	0	2 Other Carbohydrate
	Turkey sausage	2 links	141	8		2	62	315	2	0	18	2 1/2 Lean Protein
	Fruit cup	8 oz	78	0		0	0	15	20	3	1	1 1/2 Fruit
	Fat-free milk	8 oz	90	0		0	5	130	13	0	8	1 Fat-Free Milk
	Margarine	1 teaspoon	34	3.8		0.6	0	0	0	0	0	1 Fat
Totals			**775**	**18**	**21**	**9**	**221**	**1044**	**101**	**5**	**35**	**2 1/2 Starch, 1 1/2 Fruit, 1 Fat-Free Milk, 2 Other Carbohydrate, 2 1/2 Lean Protein, 2 Fat**

(table continues on next page)

Lower Carb 'N' Healthy

Menu Samplers Section	Menu Item	Amount	Calories	Fat (g)	% Calories from Fat	Saturated Fat (g)	Chol. (mg)	Sodium (mg)	Carb. (g)	Fiber (g)	Protein (g)	Exchanges/ Choices
Lower Carb 'N' Healthy (Women)*	Hashbrown	1 patty	150	9		1.5	0	310	15	2	1	1 Starch, 2 Fats
	Whole-wheat toast	2 slices	170	2		0.2	0	320	32	3	7	2 Starch
	Canadian bacon	2 slices	120	10		2	50	310	0	0	6	1 Medium-Fat Protein, 1 Fat
	Poached egg	1 egg	80	5		1.5	210	80	0	0	7	1 Medium-Fat Protein
	Jam (regular)	1 table-spoon	50	0		0	0	10	13	0	0	1 Other Carbohydrate
Totals			**570**	**26**	**41**	**5.2**	**260**	**1030**	**60**	**5**	**21**	**3 Starch, 1 Other Carbohydrate, 2 Medium-Fat Protein, 3 Fat**

(table continues on next page)

Lower Carb 'N' Healthy

Menu Samplers Section	Menu Item	Amount	Calories	Fat (g)	% Calories from Fat	Saturated Fat (g)	Chol. (mg)	Sodium (mg)	Carb. (g)	Fiber (g)	Protein (g)	Exchanges/Choices
Lower Carb 'N' Healthy (Men)*	Garden veggie omelet	1/2 order (split the whole order with your dining partner)	354	24		9	330	590	13	2	18	2 Vegetable, 3 Medium-Fat Protein, 2 Fat
	Whole-wheat toast	2 slices	170	2		0	0	320	32	3	7	2 Starch
	Fat-free milk	8 oz	90	0		0	5	130	13	0	8	1 Fat-Free Milk
	Butter	1 pat (square)	36	4		2.6	11	29	0	0	0	1 Fat
Totals			650	30	41	12	346	1069	58	5	33	2 Starch, 1 Fat-Free Milk, 2 Vegetable, 3 Medium-Fat Protein, 1 Fat

*This meal is above the cholesterol goal for the day due to the amount of cholesterol in eggs.

ⓘ What's Your Solution? Answers

a) Of the choices available, this is a reasonably healthy breakfast that is balanced in carbohydrate, protein, and fat.

b) This will provide several hundred calories more than you've likely allotted for breakfast. Plus, it tips the scale on carbohydrate.

c) This is a reasonable choice given the limited options, but it is a carbohydrate load. Consider eating just half the bagel.

d) This is a reasonably healthy breakfast if you want to keep your carbohydrate grams low and don't have cholesterol concerns.

CHAPTER 12

Family Fare

amily-fare restaurants offer moderately priced food in a casual atmosphere. Many national chains specialize in family fare, including Applebee's, Bob Evans, Denny's, and Cracker Barrel. Typically, you sit down and order off a menu in these restaurants. But there are walk-up-and-order types that serve family fare too, such as Boston Market. Independently owned and operated restaurants are also plentiful. Even in our nation of restaurant franchises, local diners and mom-and-pop corner restaurants are alive and well.

In this chapter, the food focus is traditional American fare, which offers something for everyone: from meat-and-potatoes meals to Americanized versions of popular ethnic dishes (Italian, Mexican, Chinese, and others). Of course, many traditional ethnic fare restaurants are great for family meals, too. Explore those in the chapters of Section 3.

On the Menu

Family restaurants aim to offer a virtual potpourri of foods and flavors. Several chains and independents are just as happy to serve you breakfast as they are lunch, dinner, or late night snacks. These restaurants hardly limit their menu to American specialties. They globe trot to bring you Mexican fajitas or salads, Italian pastas or pizzas, and Chinese pot stickers or stir-fry dishes. This can help to widen the variety of healthier choices available in family-fare restaurants.

The menus, which are sometimes multiple pages, will tantalize you with descriptive wording for everything from appetizers and entrées to desserts and beverages. If you're at a restaurant like Bob Evans, Denny's, or Perkins, you can expect to find everything from country-fried steak and club sandwiches to entrée-size salads on the menu. (The breakfast options at these restaurants are covered in Chapter 11.) At restaurants like Applebee's, Cracker Barrel, Red Robin, Ruby Tuesday, TGI Fridays, and the plethora of others that specialize in American fare, you'll find the standard rundown of burgers, sandwiches, and salads. The entrée section of the menus expands to include options like pasta, grilled meats, and some dishes influenced by south-of-the-border flavors. Steakhouses, like LongHorn Steakhouse and Ponderosa, feature narrower menus that focus on large cuts of red meat, potatoes, and salads or a trip to the salad bar. Then there are the more upscale steakhouses like Outback Steakhouse, Morton's, and Ruth's Chris, which offer the aforementioned options but serve you tableside.

Eating at one of these family-fare restaurants can be challenging for health-oriented diners. The food, from appetizers through desserts, is typically loaded with fat—think about fried mozzarella sticks, french fries, supersized nachos with lots of cheese, mayonnaise-based sauces, and gravy-topped entrées. And then there's the large portions (often large enough for two). These restaurants often focus on protein (meat) over vegetables—think half-pound hamburgers, a half chicken, a rack of ribs, and large servings of seafood. Specials, such as half-priced appetizers and 50-cent wings, may tempt you to splurge. Plus, the wait staff is skilled at further testing your willpower by pushing beverages, appetizers, extra sides, and desserts.

That being said, one benefit of family-fare restaurants is that the menus are generally vast enough that there are a scattering of healthier choices, especially if you put healthy eating strategies into high gear. Another benefit: slowly but surely, some of these restaurants are attempting to cater to health-conscious diners by identifying "lighter fare" and "smaller portion" options on their menus. These options usually have 600 calories or less. Though you'll need to skip around the menu and be creative, family-fare restaurant meals can fit into your healthy eating plan.

Your winning strategy in theses restaurants will be to implement a portion-control plan. Take a preventive approach by using portion-control strategies from the start—when you order. Opt for a soup or salad and half-sandwich combination. Or entertain splitting orders with a dining partner. If you can't convince anyone to split or share, go it alone. Split a large dinner salad or entrée with yourself by requesting a take-home container when you place your order. As soon as you're served, pack up half of your food for tomorrow's lunch or dinner. This will reduce the amount of food in front of you from the start, so you aren't tempted to overeat by nibbling your way to a clean plate.

The Menu Profile

Appetizers

Silverware and napkins are generally all that greet you at the table in lower-priced family restaurants. When you go more upscale, bread and butter are served. Then you're asked: "Can I bring you an appetizer?" The crunchy fried variety of appetizers are easy to find and lethal in terms of fat and calories. Even healthy onions and mushrooms are battered, dipped, and fried; they're not-so-healthy by the time they arrive at your table. Super-sized nachos are a frequent offering. They're fried tortilla chips with high-fat goodies topped on—cheese, sour cream, and guacamole—which often exceed 1500 calories. Other appetizers that add insult to injury are fried mozzarella sticks, buffalo chicken wings (fried and traditionally served with blue cheese dressing), and that battered deep-fried whole onion served up with creamy dressing in a well-known steakhouse.

A few redeeming appetizers that can work well as a portion-controlled main dish are shrimp cocktail (peel-and-eat shrimp with cocktail sauce), oysters on the half shell, a cup of chili, and Mexican pizza. You might even find a platter featuring raw vegetables with creamy dip. Unfortunately, the dip is 100% fat, but here's menu creativity at work: ask for a side of low-calorie salad dressing instead. If your dining partners order high-fat appetizers, order a lighter appetizer or garden or spinach salad as your healthier appetizer. That's easier than just keeping your hands to yourself when the greasy little tidbits arrive.

Soups

Soups are divided down the middle between healthy and fat-dense. Here's a rule of thumb: if you can see through it or it's loaded with beans and vegetables, it's likely a healthier soup. If it's white and/or creamy, it's likely loaded with fat. Common soup options are the high-fat French onion, which is healthy before the cheese is loaded on top (there's no reason you can't get it minus the bread and cheese to keep it healthy, but it will still be high in sodium), New England clam chowder, potato, and broccoli and cheese soup. Healthier choices are chicken vegetable, black bean, chili (hold the cheese), and Manhattan clam chowder. Take, for example, two of the soup options at O'Charley's (a chain restaurant): a bowl of chicken noodle soup has just 170 calories, while the cream of tomato option has 570 calories, thanks to all that cream (even though the tomato base makes you think it's healthy). If sodium is a concern, it's best to avoid any soup. It's generally loaded with sodium, even in small servings.

Sandwiches

Sandwiches are regular listings at restaurants serving family fare. Unfortunately, they're usually stacked with an excess of protein and/or fat. Watch out for the healthy-sounding tuna or chicken salad. These options are often packed with mayonnaise and, therefore, tip the fat scale. Stick with unadulterated meats— turkey, roast beef, ham, and chicken. Ask to have the mayonnaise held and request a side of mustard, low-calorie salad dressing, honey-mustard, barbecue sauce, or ketchup. Mexican salsa, hot sauce, or horseradish work as well. Half a sandwich with soup or a salad might be plenty. Or you could substitute a baked potato for the half sandwich and pair that with soup and/or salad.

When you're trying to zero in on a sandwich choice, observe the sandwich toppers. Take, for example, the Jack Daniel's Chicken Sandwich at TGI Fridays. It may look healthy at first glance. After all, it's a grilled chicken sandwich. But thanks to its toppings—bacon, mixed cheeses, fried onion strings, and mayo—it tallies up to more than 1100 calories! A healthier choice at TGI Fridays is the Grilled Chicken Sandwich with a side of steamed broccoli, which you can enjoy for a tally of 480 calories. Keep to the healthy preparation (charbroiled, teriyaki, or barbecued) and stick to the healthy toppers, such as sautéed onions, mushrooms and/or peppers, and jalapeños. Other sandwiches to avoid are Reubens, Philadelphia cheese steaks, clubs, and melts. They ooze with fat and a big culprit in that is cheese.

Another problem with sandwiches is their typical side dishes: potato chips, pasta salad, French fries, and/or creamy coleslaw. These are all loaded with fat and calories, even before the restaurant adds extra toppings. The

Loaded Waffle Fries at Friendly's, for example, have more than 1700 calories, 62% of which are from fat! If you must have fries, choose the smallest size without any toppings or split them with a dining partner. Better yet, opt for a baked potato, rice pilaf, a green salad, steamed or sautéed vegetables, or a side of fruit instead.

Burgers

On to one of America's favorite foods: burgers. A family menu without hamburgers would be sacrilegious. Portions of protein (meat) start off at over 6 ounces or, more often, 8 ounces prior to cooking. That delivers around 5–6 ounces cooked to your table. And if you choose a classic bacon cheese-burger, which is offered at pretty much every family restaurant in the country, you'll eat anywhere from 900–1400 calories, not counting any sides! Order a smaller-size burger (typically about 3 ounces of cooked meat) and forgo the bacon and cheese in favor of lettuce, tomato, and sautéed onion, peppers, and mushrooms.

Steaks and Ribs

You can find various cuts of steak at many family restaurants. Control your calorie and fat intake by staying smart with your portion sizes and choosing healthier cuts. Sirloin is a much leaner cut than the fattier T-bone or porter-house. The 6-ounce sirloin at Ponderosa has a very respectable 310 calories, about half of which are from fat. On the other hand, order the 1-pound T-bone and you'll be getting nearly 1,000 calories with about 70% of the calories from fat.

Ribs are a similar story. Take Famous Dave's, for example, famous for its rib dishes. An order of The Big Slab, which is 12 ribs, has 1810 calories, more than half of which are from fat. Ouch! Satisfy your protein craving with a smaller portion. The 4-bone serving has a much more reasonable 600 calories.

Entrées

Entrées, beyond the burgers, steaks, and ribs, vary tremendously in family restaurants. You'll spot entrée salads, chicken and fish prepared a number of ways, and a number of mixed dishes (think pastas, stir-fries and other rice dishes) on the menu. Fortunately, healthy items abound—seek and you shall find.

You might be inclined to skirt around hot entrées because you think salads and sandwiches are lighter and lower in calories. Interestingly, you might do better with chicken or beef fajitas, chicken or vegetable stir-fry, or a barbequed chicken breast, especially if you split them or take half home. No doubt, some nutritional disasters lurk in the hot entrée section, but if you can enjoy a healthy meal if you choose wisely. When in doubt, do your homework and check out the nutrition information before you order. Today you can do this from your seat with an app on your smart phone. You'll find some nutrition sneak peeks in *Nutrition Snapshot* (page 164).

Salads

The salad choices on family-fare menus have grown. This is great for the health-conscious diner, but you've still got to be careful and creative to control the extras loaded on top of the healthy bed of greens. Some restaurants serve salads in fried tortilla shells. Request that yours arrives sans (without) shell. The shell is just too crunchy and tempting to have within arm's reach. Many restaurants also top their salads with fried chicken, bacon, and other fried toppings. Try to avoid these toppings.

If you choose a salad, let the lists of *Green-Flag Words* and *Red-Flag Words* (page 178) guide you. A salad with all the fixings can run upwards of 1,000 calories. Consider a Cobb salad: on top of greens you find chicken or turkey breast, crisp bacon, avocado, blue cheese, hard-boiled egg, black olives, and tomatoes. You see a few red-flag words and a few green-flag words in this description. If you like the basic ingredients of a salad, request that the chef leave a few of the higher-fat items in the kitchen. Ask to replace them with ingredients of the healthy variety, such as tomatoes, onions, or peppers. Read the salad ingredients carefully. Tell your waitperson what you want kept in and left out of your salad.

Also be mindful of the dressings you find in restaurants. Dressing easily can transform a salad from healthy to a nutritional disaster. America's favorites—ranch, thousand island, and blue cheese—ring in at 70 calories for each level, not heaping, tablespoon. Here are a few ways to dress successfully:

- ▶ Take advantage of reduced-calorie or fat-free dressings.
- ▶ Order any dressing on the side so that you control the quantity you eat.
- ▶ Request a side of vinegar or lemon wedges to dilute the dressing.

For more details and nutrition information on salad dressings and suggestions for a healthy approach, read all about salads in Chapter 15, beginning on page 250.

Desserts

Desserts in family-fare restaurants are best passed by because, simply stated, they're usually not worth the calories. Cheesecake, decadent chocolate cake, apple pie à la mode, and ice cream sundaes are the usual options. Once in a while, you'll see fruit sorbet or sherbet or frozen yogurt. Some decent choices are fruit pie (hold the ice cream or whipped cream), sorbet, sherbet, and frozen yogurt, but they still contain a good many carbohydrate grams and calories without much nutrition. If you eat dessert, remember that portions are huge, so order dessert knowing that at least two people should dig in.

Kids' Menus

Family restaurants are known for providing a kids' menu, which caters to what we perceive are kids' favorite foods—chicken fingers (fried), hamburgers, and hot dogs, of course, all served with fries. Then there may be macaroni and cheese, pizza, or pasta with tomato sauce. Many restaurants now offer healthier children's options, while simultaneously offering higher-fat and higher-calorie options. Take Applebee's, for example. The Applebee's kids' menu features healthy options like grilled chicken, steamed broccoli, and vanilla yogurt with strawberries. On the other end of the spectrum, the menu also includes two mini cheeseburgers, fried mozzarella sticks, and ice cream sundaes. Read Chapter 6 (page 56) to learn more about the downfalls of kids' menus and how to raise kids with healthier restaurant eating habits.

Senior Menus

Some restaurants also have meal options geared toward matured audiences. In general, these cost slightly less than their equivalents on the regular menu, and they may have healthier sides or be slightly smaller in portion size (and, therefore, lower in calories). Denny's, for example, has a menu for adults aged 55 years and older. On it, you'll find items such as the Senior Grilled Tilapia and the Senior Country Fried Steak, which is 3 ounces smaller than the version on the regular menu.

Lighter Menus

Fortunately, many restaurants now feature lighter items on the menu, but you never know if these will be short or long lived. If they don't sell well, they'll be off the menu in no time. Typically, these items are lower in calories but not necessarily lower in sodium. Still, they are a strong ally in sticking to your healthy eating plan. At Applebee's, you'll find options under 550 calories, such as Roma Pepper Steak, Savory Cedar Salmon, and Lemon Parmesan Shrimp. Cracker Barrel's "Wholesome Fixin's" menu features meals under 600 calories, such as Buttermilk Oven Fried Chicken Breast and Spice Rubbed Pork Chop, complete with healthy side dishes. Even the more casual family-fare restaurants have jumped on the bandwagon. Take the Friendly's menu, for example, which features items under 565 calories, such as Turkey Tips and Asian Chicken Salad. Then there's the Denny's "Fit Fare" menu—which includes options such as Tilapia Ranchero and Loaded Veggie Omelet— and Cheesecake Factory's SkinnyLicious menu with a host of calorie-conscious small plates and snacks. Most of these are healthy choices.

Nutrition Snapshot

Health Busters

Category	Restaurant Name	Dish Name	Serving Size	Cal.	Total Fat (g)	Carb. (g)	Sod. (mg)
Appetizers	Applebee's	Spicy Chili Cheese Nachos	1 whole	1610	103	125	3240
Appetizers	Chili's	Texas Cheese Fries w/Chili & Ranch	1 whole	2120	144	117	5920
Appetizers	Outback Steakhouse	Bloomin' Onion	1 whole	1949	161	115	4099
Appetizers	T.G.I. Friday's	Loaded Potato Skins	1 whole	2030	131	161	1010
Soups	Ninety Nine Restaurant	Seafood Chowder, Crock	1 bowl	490	34	30	880
Soups	LongHorn Steakhouse	Loaded Baked Potato Soup (bowl)	1 bowl	470	33	23	1260
Salad (Entrée)	Applebee's	Oriental Chicken Salad, Regular	1 salad with dressing	1380	99	91	1430
Salad (Entrée)	Chili's	Quesadilla Explosion Salad	1 salad with dressing	1300	86	75	2070

(table continues on next page)

Health Busters

Category	Restaurant Name	Dish Name	Serving Size	Cal.	Total Fat (g)	Carb. (g)	Sod. (mg)
Salad (Entrée)	Outback Steakhouse	Aussie Chicken Cobb Salad Crispy w/Honey Mustard Dressing	1 salad with dressing	1302	99	64	2119
Entrées	Applebee's	Hand-Battered Fish & Chips	1 portion	1570	106	108	2000
Entrées	Chili's	Shiner Bock BBQ Ribs	Full rack	2310	123	168	6340
Entrées	Outback Steakhouse	No Rules Parmesan Pasta with Grilled Scallops	1 portion	1306	71	86	2005
Entrées	Buffalo Wild Wings	Ribs & More Ribs	1 portion	2380	158	88	2980
Steaks	Sizzler	Rib Eye (14 oz)	1 portion	1055	66	1	942
Steaks	LongHorn Steakhouse	LongHorn Porterhouse 20 oz	1 portion	1200	85	1	2180
Burgers	Applebee's	Bourbon Black and Bleu	1 portion	1670	103	111	3170
Burgers	Chili's	Southern Smokehouse w/ Ancho Chile BBQ w/Fries	1 portion	2290	139	163	6500
Burgers	T.G.I. Friday's	Kansas City BBQ	1 portion	1510	85	137	4330

(table continues on next page)

Health Busters

Category	Restaurant Name	Dish Name	Serving Size	Cal.	Total Fat (g)	Carb. (g)	Sod. (mg)
Sandwiches	Applebee's	Fried Green Tomato & Turkey Club	1 whole	1210	68	94	3980
Sandwiches	Chili's	Philly Cheesesteak w/Fries	1 whole	1810	121	133	4410
Sandwiches	Friendly's	Country Club Chicken	1 whole	1300	73	121	1840
Desserts	Applebee's	Chocolate Chip Cookie Sundae	1 portion	1540	74	210	910
Desserts	Outback Steakhouse	Chocolate Thunder from Down Under	1 portion	1554	105.5	133.4	561.6
Desserts	Friendly's	Hunka Chunka PB Fudge Sundae	1 portion	1770	107	164	1050

Healthier Bets

Category	Restaurant Name	Dish Name	Serving Size	Cal.	Total Fat (g)	Sat. Fat (g)	Carb. (g)	Pro. (g)	Fiber (g)	Chol. (mg)	Sodium (mg)	Exchanges/ Choices
Appetizers	Bob Evans	Grilled Chicken Breast w/ Baked Potato & Broccoli Florets	1 whole	413	8	2	57	40	9	77	632	2 Starch, 3 Vegetable, 4 Lean Protein
Appetizers	Outback Steakhouse	Grilled Shrimp on the Barbie	1 whole	295	16	3	23	17	4	9	867	1 1/2 Other Carbohydrate, 2 1/2 Lean Protein, 1 1/2 Fat
Appetizers	Ruby Tuesday	Fire Wings	1 whole	178	11	n/a	4	16	1	n/a	603	2 1/2 Medium-Fat Protein
Soups	Bob Evans	Bean Soup (bowl)	1 bowl	198	3	1	28	14	8	8	1118	2 Starch, 1 Lean Protein
Soups	Boston Market	Chicken Tortilla Soup without Toppings	1 bowl	160	8	1.5	13	10	2	35	1640	1/2 Starch, 1 Vegetable, 1 1/2 Medium-Fat Protein

(table continues on next page)

Healthier Bets

Category	Restaurant Name	Dish Name	Serving Size	Cal.	Total Fat (g)	Sat. Fat (g)	Carb. (g)	Pro. (g)	Fiber (g)	Chol. (mg)	Sodium (mg)	Exchanges/ Choices
Soups	Denny's	Vegetable Beef Soup	1 bowl	140	5	0	17	7	3	10	1290	3 Vegetable, 1 Medium-Fat Protein
Soups	Applebee's	Chicken Noodle Soup (bowl)	1 bowl	150	4	1	16	14	1	n/a	1160	1 Starch, 2 Lean Protein
Salads (Entrée)	Denny's	Chicken Deluxe Grilled	1 salad (no dressing)	340	13	6	13	44	4	110	530	3 Vegetable, 5 1/2 Lean Protein
Salads (Entrée)	Chili's	Grilled Chicken	1 salad (no dressing)	420	22	6	21	38	5	n/a	660	1 Starch, 1 Vegetable, 4 1/2 Medium-Fat Protein
Salads (Entrée)	T.G.I. Friday's	Strawberry Fields	1 salad (no dressing)	600	46	10	39	11	6	n/a	610	1 Starch, 1 Fruit, 1 Vegetable, 1 1/2 High-Fat Protein, 6 1/2 Fat

(table continues on next page)

Healthier Bets

Category	Restaurant Name	Dish Name	Serving Size	Cal.	Total Fat (g)	Sat. Fat (g)	Carb. (g)	Pro. (g)	Fiber (g)	Chol. (mg)	Sodium (mg)	Exchanges/ Choices
Salads (Entrée)	LongHorn Steakhouse	Grilled Salmon Salad— Mixed Greens	1 salad (no dressing)	560	27	9	29	50	n/a	n/a	690	1 Starch, 2 Vegetable, 7 1/2 Lean Protein, 1 Fat
Salads (Side)	Bob Evans	Specialty Garden	1 salad (no dressing)	123	7	3	10	6	2	16	337	2 Vegetable, 1 1/2 Fat
Salads (Side)	Applebee's	Applebee's House	1 salad (no dressing)	230	15	7	12	13	3	n/a	400	1/2 Starch, 1 Vegetable, 2 High-Fat Protein
Salads (Side)	Elephant Bar	Organic Field Greens	1 salad (no dressing)	310	28	7	8	10	2	25	370	1 1/2 Vegetable, 1 1/2 High-Fat Protein, 3 Fat

(table continues on next page)

Healthier Bets

Category	Restaurant Name	Dish Name	Serving Size	Cal.	Total Fat (g)	Sat. Fat (g)	Carb. (g)	Pro. (g)	Fiber (g)	Chol. (mg)	Sodium (mg)	Exchanges/ Choices
Salad Dressing	T.G.I. Friday's	Caesar Vinaigrette	2 Tbsp	120	12	1.5	3	0	0	n/a	580	2 1/2 Fat
Salad Dressing	T.G.I. Friday's	Low Fat Balsamic Vinaigrette	2 Tbsp	80	3	0	15	0	0	n/a	290	1 Starch
Salad Dressing	Ponderosa Steakhouse	Buttermilk Ranch Dressing	2 Tbsp	151	15	2	2	0	0	14	284	3 Fat
Salad Dressing	Ponderosa Steakhouse	Creamy Italian Dressing	2 Tbsp	105	10	1	3	0	0	0	374	2 Fat
Salad Dressing	Ponderosa Steakhouse	Honey Mustard Dressing	2 Tbsp	107	9	1	7	0	0	0	197	1/2 Starch, 1 Fat
Burgers	Applebee's	Kids' Mini	1 burger	390	27	7	23	15	1	n/a	500	1 1/2 Starch, 2 High-Fat Protein, 1 Fat

(table continues on next page)

Healthier Bets

Category	Restaurant Name	Dish Name	Serving Size	Cal.	Total Fat (g)	Sat. Fat (g)	Carb. (g)	Pro. (g)	Fiber (g)	Chol. (mg)	Sodium (mg)	Exchanges/ Choices
Burgers	Chili's	Pepper Pals Little Mouth	1 burger	330	18	7	23	19	1	n/a	630	1 1/2 Starch, 3 Medium-Fat Protein
Burgers	Buffalo Wild Wings	Bean Burger	1 burger	310	7	1.5	50	17	n/a	n/a	700	3 Starch, 2 Lean Protein
Sandwiches	Boston Market	Rotisserie Chicken Carver (half)	1/2 whole	380	18	4.5	33	22	2	50	880	2 Starch, 3 Medium-Fat Protein
Sandwiches	Chili's	Pepper Pals Grilled Chicken	1 whole	230	5	0.5	21	22	1	n/a	230	1 1/2 Starch, 2 1/2 Lean Protein
Sandwiches	Buffalo Wild Wings	Grilled Chicken	1 whole	470	7	3	50	51	3	120	750	3 Starch, 5 1/2 Lean Protein
Sandwiches	T.G.I. Friday's	Chicken (Kids)	1 whole	290	13	3.5	24	19	1	n/a	700	1 1/2 Starch, 2 1/2 Medium-Fat Protein

(table continues on next page)

Healthier Bets

Category	Restaurant Name	Dish Name	Serving Size	Cal.	Total Fat (g)	Sat. Fat (g)	Carb. (g)	Pro. (g)	Fiber (g)	Chol. (mg)	Sodium (mg)	Exchanges/ Choices
Sandwiches	Lone Star Steakhouse	Grilled Cheese	1 whole	252	12	8	27	9	1	37	618	2 Starch, 1 High-Fat Protein
Entrées (Complete Meals)— Seafood	Bob Evans	Potato Crusted Flounder with Baked Potato & Broccoli Florets	1 portion	442	11	4	66	29	9	27	551	3 Starch, 3 Vegetable, 3 Lean Protein
Entrées (Complete Meals)— Seafood	Outback Steakhouse	2 Lobster Tails with Tangy Tomato Salad (no croutons) and Broccoli (no butter)	1 portion	416	9	3	31	52	7	342	912	1 Starch, 2 Vegetable, 6 1/2 Lean Protein

(table continues on next page)

Healthier Bets

Category	Restaurant Name	Dish Name	Serving Size	Cal.	Total Fat(g)	Sat. Fat (g)	Carb. (g)	Pro. (g)	Fiber (g)	Chol. (mg)	Sodium (mg)	Exchanges/ Choices
Entrées (Complete Meals)— Seafood	Outback Steakhouse	Simply Grilled 8 oz Mahi with Rice Garnish and Steamed Veggies	1 portion	472	12	6	37	53	8	79	1042	2 Starch, 2 Vegetable, 7 1/2 Lean Protein
Entrées (Complete Meals)— Poultry	Boston Market	1/4 White Rotisserie Chicken (No Skin) w/Garlic Dill New Potatoes and Fresh Steamed Vegetable	1 portion	420	8	2	33	54	6	145	860	1 Starch, 2 Vegetable, 7 Lean Protein

(table continues on next page)

Healthier Bets

Category	Restaurant Name	Dish Name	Serving Size	Cal.	Total Fat (g)	Sat. Fat (g)	Carb. (g)	Pro. (g)	Fiber (g)	Chol. (mg)	Sodium (mg)	Exchanges/ Choices
Entrées (Complete Meals)— Poultry	Outback Steakhouse	Grilled Chicken on the Barbie & Fresh Seasonal Mixed Veggies	1 portion	401	7	2	21	60	7	142	1045	3 Vegetable, 7 1/2 Lean Protein
Entrées (Complete Meals)— Steak/ Beef	Boston Market	Beef Brisket (4 oz) w/Fresh Steamed Vegetables and Cornbread	1 portion	470	20	6	38	33	4	105	880	2 Starch, 2 Vegetable, 3 1/2 Medium-Fat Protein

(table continues on next page)

Healthier Bets

Category	Restaurant Name	Dish Name	Serving Size	Cal.	Total Fat (g)	Sat. Fat (g)	Carb. (g)	Pro. (g)	Fiber (g)	Chol. (mg)	Sodium (mg)	Exchanges/ Choices
Entrées (Complete Meals)— Steak/ Beef	Outback Steakhouse	6 oz Sirloin with Broccoli (no butter) and Tangy Tomato Salad (no croutons)	1 portion	404	12	6	30	46	6	109	500	1 Starch, 2 Vegetable, 6 Lean Protein
Entrées (Complete Meals)— Pork	Outback Steakhouse	Wood-Fire Grilled Pork Chop	1 portion	381	12	4	17	48	0	143	1655	1 Starch, 6 1/2 Lean Protein
Entrées (Complete Meals)— Pork	Outback Steakhouse	Sweet Glazed Pork Tenderloin	1 portion	303	9	3	14	42	0	102	788	1 Starch, 5 1/2 Lean Protein

(table continues on next page)

Healthier Bets

Category	Restaurant Name	Dish Name	Serving Size	Cal.	Total Fat (g)	Sat. Fat (g)	Carb. (g)	Pro. (g)	Fiber (g)	Chol. (mg)	Sodium (mg)	Exchanges/ Choices
Entrées (Complete Meals)— Pasta	Bob Evans	Spaghetti with Meat Sauce, Savor Size	1 portion	468	22	7	47	20	3	29	1067	3 Starch, 2 Medium-Fat Protein, 2 Fat
Entrées (Complete Meals)— Pasta	Boston Market	Mac & Cheese Entrée	1 portion	230	9	6	27	9	1	25	850	2 Starch, 1 Medium-Fat Protein
Entrées (Complete Meals)— Vegetarian	Ruby Tuesday	Petite Spaghetti Squash Marinara-Fit & Trim	1 portion	177	9	n/a	17	5	5	n/a	667	2 Starch, 3 Vegetable, 2 Lean Protein
Entrées (Complete Meals)— Vegetarian	Denny's	Fit Fare Veggie Skillet	1 portion	330	9	1.5	44	20	9	0	1450	2 Starch, 2 Vegetable, 2 Lean Protein

(table continues on next page)

Healthier Bets

Category	Restaurant Name	Dish Name	Serving Size	Cal.	Total Fat (g)	Sat. Fat (g)	Carb. (g)	Pro. (g)	Fiber (g)	Chol. (mg)	Sodium (mg)	Exchanges/Choices
Kids' Meals	Applebee's	Kids' Kraft Macaroni and Cheese	1 portion	300	9	2.5	45	11	2	n/a	570	3 Starch, 1 Medium-Fat Protein
Kids' Meals	Buffalo Wild Wings	Kids' Boneless Wings (4)	4 pieces	288	20	5	0	24	0	104	264	3 1/2 Medium-Fat Protein, 1/2 Fat
Kids' Meals	T.G.I. Friday's	Spaghetti	1 kids portion	310	7	0.5	52	10	4	n/a	710	3 1/2 Starch, 1 Fat
Desserts	Bob Evans	Vanilla Ice Cream	1 portion	111	6	4	13	2	0	24	36	1 Other Carbohydrate, 1 Fat
Desserts	Ruby Tuesday	Chocolate Chip Cookie	1 cookie	180	9	n/a	24	2	1	n/a	190	1 1/2 Other Carbohydrate, 1 1/2 Fat
Desserts	Famous Dave's	Ice Cream Sundae	1 portion	270	14	9	33	3	1	55	65	2 Other Carbohydrate, 2 1/2 Fat
Desserts	Ponderosa Steakhouse	Macaroons	1 portion	112	5	5	15	2	1	5	44	1 Other Carbohydrate, 1 Fat

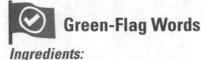

Green-Flag Words

Ingredients:

- ► BBQ sauce
- ► Cocktail sauce
- ► Horseradish
- ► Jalapeños
- ► Lettuce, sliced tomatoes, raw onions
- ► Low-calorie or fat-free salad dressing
- ► Mustard, honey mustard
- ► Sautéed onions, peppers, mushrooms
- ► Spicy Mexican beef or chicken

Cooking Methods/Menu Descriptions:

- ► Barbecued
- ► Cajun or blackened
- ► Charbroiled or grilled
- ► Marinated
- ► Marinated in teriyaki sauce
- ► Mesquite-grilled
- ► Steamed
- ► Stir-fried

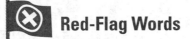

Red-Flag Words

Ingredients:

- ► Bacon (strips, crumbled, crisp)
- ► Blue cheese (crumbled, topped with, salad dressing)
- ► Butter or cream
- ► Cheese (grated, melted, topped with, smothered in, sauce)
- ► Guacamole
- ► Mayonnaise, garlic mayonnaise, aioli, "special or house" sauce
- ► Sausage
- ► Sour cream

Cooking Methods/Menu Descriptions/Names:

- ▶ Alfredo
- ▶ Battered and fried
- ▶ Deep-fried
- ▶ Golden fried, crispy fried
- ▶ Large, jumbo, piled high, stacked
- ▶ Lightly fried
- ▶ Loaded or topped with cheese, bacon, or sour cream
- ▶ Rolled in bread crumbs and fried or sautéed
- ▶ Served in or on crisp tortilla shell

At the Table:

- ▶ Butter, margarine
- ▶ Mayonnaise
- ▶ Sour cream

Healthy Eating Tips and Tactics

- ▶ Decline the bread basket if one is offered. Or, if others want it, keep it beyond your arm's reach.
- ▶ Combine a soup, salad, and side dish or combine an appetizer and a salad for a healthy portion-controlled meal. Hold the entrée and large portions.
- ▶ Split everything with your dining partner, from appetizer to dessert.
- ▶ Order off the "lighter" menu if there is one. Or create your own lighter fare by limiting high-fat toppings and choosing healthier sides.
- ▶ Request a take-home container when you order your meal. Pack up a portion of your meal to take home as soon as your food arrives.

Get It Your Way

- ▶ Ask for your salad dressing on the side—all of the time.
- ▶ Ask that high-fat salad toppers be used lightly or left in the kitchen.

▶ Request to substitute for high-fat, high-calorie sides with lower-fat, lower-calorie items: substitute a baked potato for french fries or onion rings, request a sandwich on whole-wheat bread rather than on a croissant, or opt for mustard rather than mayonnaise. Each and every change improves the healthiness of your meals.

▶ Request some lemon or lime slices, vinegar, or soy or teriyaki sauce on the side to flavor menu items without adding tons of calories.

Tips and Tactics for Gluten-Free Eating

▶ Fresh unprocessed meat, poultry, fish, and seafood are naturally gluten-free; however, preparation methods and some processed meats may contaminate these food with gluten.

▶ Prime rib with au jus may contain gluten, and self-basting turkeys and imitation bacon bits may contain hydrolyzed vegetable protein (HVP) or textured vegetable protein (TVP) and therefore the ingredient label should be checked.

▶ Avoid all breading, flour dusting, gravies, or stuffing for meats.

▶ Sauces typically contain gluten. It is safest to avoid sauces.

▶ Order proteins that have been roasted, grilled, or baked on cleaned surfaces. If necessary, ask that a clean pan be used for preparation.

▶ Mashed potatoes, hash browns, or other potato dishes may contain gluten if they are made from mixes or are prepackaged. A baked potato or sweet potato is a good choice.

▶ French fries may be fried in oil that is also used for gluten-containing foods, so they may be contaminated.

▶ Rice may be prepared in a gluten-containing broth; ask if it is made with only water or if it can be. Brown or wild rice is a good choice if available.

▶ Plain steamed vegetables with fresh herbs and lemon or a salad without croutons, bacon bits, or gluten-containing salad dressings are good bets.

▶ If you want or need dessert, opt for fresh fruit, sorbet, ice cream, or frozen yogurt. On the prepared items, ask to check the food and ingredient label to assure that the food is gluten-free. Mention that all you want is the ice cream with nothing else on the side; no cookies or brownies.

Tips and Tactics to Help Kids Eat Healthy

▶ Employ the same healthy eating strategies for kids that you use elsewhere (see Chapter 7 for ideas). Have a plan and talk about this plan with your child before you set foot in the restaurant.

▶ Order wisely. Choose entrées that are grilled, opt for healthier sides like steamed veggies, and avoid high-fat toppings.

▶ Decline the kids' menu. Order off the regular menu to expose your child to healthier flavors and ingredients.

▶ Split portions with your child (or among your children).

▶ Avoid desserts, which are often offered at a steep discount as part of kids' menus. If your child tries to negotiate something special, promise a trip to the dollar store. (Go for non-food rewards.)

What's Your Solution?

Nearly every Saturday evening, you go out to eat with your family. It's one of your favorite times of the week because it always feels like a celebration. Your family typically starts with a big appetizer platter and then everyone orders their favorite dish. For years, you've been ordering the 9-ounce sirloin with butter sauce and two sides: French fries and cole slaw. It's only once a week, so this has never seemed like a big deal. But you have recently been diagnosed with type 2 diabetes and you've been encouraged to trim off some pounds, so you know that your routine needs some tweaking.

Which of the following healthy eating strategies could you implement?

a) You stay quiet about your strategy. After all, you don't want to ruin the fun. Just do the best you can.

b) Announce to your family that there will be no longer be any appetizers ordered because you just can't be tempted by them. Mandate that everyone order off the new "light" menu.

c) Eat just one or two healthier items off the appetizer platter. Order the sirloin, but request that the cream sauce be left in the kitchen (hold the butter sauce). Ask for a baked potato, instead of fries.

d) Share your needs and plan with your family in advance. Get their input. Order a smaller appetizer for everyone to share. Request the sirloin with no sauce, fries, and steamed veggies. Ask the waitperson to bring a take-home container with your meal and put half your meal in it to enjoy tomorrow.

See page 189 for answers.

Menu Samplers

Light 'N' Healthy

Menu Samplers Section	Menu Item	Amount	Calories	Fat (g)	% Calories from Fat	Saturated Fat (g)	Chol. (mg)	Sodium (mg)	Carb. (g)	Fiber (g)	Protein (g)	Exchanges/ Choices
Light 'N' Healthy (Women)	Sirloin steak	1/2 6 oz (cooked) full sirloin	156	5		1.9	49	54	0	0	26	3 1/2 Lean Protein
	Grilled zucchini	1 cup	51	3		2.3	11	143	6	2	2	1 Vegetable, 1 Fat
	Glazed carrots	1 cup	90	3		2	10	190	15	2	0.5	2 Vegetable, 1 Fat
	Whole-wheat roll	1 roll, 1 oz	74	1		0	0	147	14	2	3	1 Starch
	Baked potato	1/2 potato	128	0		0	0	14	29	3	4	2 Starch
	Sour cream	1 Tbsp	26			1.6	5	6	0	0	1	1/2 Fat
Totals			525	12	21	8	75	554	64	9	36	3 Starch, 3 Vegetable, 3 1/2 Lean Protein, 2.5 Fat

(table continues on next page)

Light 'N' Healthy

Menu Samplers Section	Menu Item	Amount	Calories	Fat (g)	% Calories from Fat	Saturated Fat (g)	Chol. (mg)	Sodium (mg)	Carb. (g)	Fiber (g)	Protein (g)	Exchanges/ Choices
Light 'N' Healthy (Men)	Meat chili	1 bowl (about 10 oz)	408	20		10.5	58	1090	35	7	23	2 Starch, 2 1/2 Medium-Fat Protein, 1 Fat
	House salad (greens and 1–3 additional vegetables) without croutons and cheese	2 cups	16	0		0	0	0	3	1	1	1 Vegetable
	Whole-wheat roll	2 rolls (1 oz each)	148	2		0	0	280	27	5	6	2 Starch
	Oil and vinegar dressing	1 Tbsp olive oil	120	14		2	0	0	0	0	0	3 Fat
Totals			**692**	**36**	**47**	**12.5**	**58**	**1370**	**65**	**13**	**30**	**4 Starch, 1 Vegetable, 2 1/2 Medium-Fat Protein, 4 Fat**

(table continues on next page)

Hearty 'N' Healthy

Menu Samplers Section	Menu Item	Amount	Calories	Fat (g)	% Calories from Fat	Saturated Fat (g)	Chol. (mg)	Sodium (mg)	Carb. (g)	Fiber (g)	Protein (g)	Exchanges/ Choices
Hearty 'N' Healthy (Women)	Spaghetti and meatballs	1/2 order (about 1.5 cups)	500	17		7	49	880	59	4	25	4 Starch, 3 Medium-Fat Protein
	House salad (greens and 1–3 additional vegetables) without croutons and cheese	2 cups	16	0		0	0	0	3	1	1	1 Vegetable
	Oil and vinegar dressing	1 Tbsp olive oil	120	14		2	0	0	0	0	0	3 Fat
	Breadstick	1 breadstick (4 inches long)	140	5		1	0	260	19	1	5	1 Starch, 1 Fat
Totals			**776**	**36**	**42**	**10**	**49**	**1140**	**81**	**6**	**31**	**5 Starch, 1 Vegetable, 3 Medium-Fat Protein, 4 Fat**

(table continues on next page)

Hearty 'N' Healthy

Menu Samplers Section	Menu Item	Amount	Calories	Fat (g)	% Calories from Fat	Saturated Fat (g)	Chol. (mg)	Sodium (mg)	Carb. (g)	Fiber (g)	Protein (g)	Exchanges/ Choices
Hearty 'N' Healthy (Men)	Classic hamburger (with toppings including ketchup, mustard, tomato, lettuce, onion)	1/2 burger (split whole 1/2 lb burger)	410	26		10	70	700	25	3	23	1 1/2 Starch, 3 Medium-Fat Protein
	Baked potato	1 medium	242	1		0.3	0	190	53	7	8	3 Starch
	Shredded cheese	1 oz	109	8		6	30	185	1	0	7	1 High-Fat Protein
Totals			**761**	**35**	**41**	**16**	**100**	**1075**	**79**	**10**	**38**	**4 1/2 Starch, 4 Medium-Fat Protein, 1 Fat**

(table continues on next page)

Lower Carb 'N' Healthy

Menu Samplers Section	Menu Item	Amount	Calories	Fat (g)	% Calories from Fat	Saturated Fat (g)	Chol. (mg)	Sodium (mg)	Carb. (g)	Fiber (g)	Protein (g)	Exchanges/ Choices
Lower Carb 'N' Healthy (Women)	Glazed salmon	1/2 order (3 oz cooked)	307	10		1.5	70	740	29	1.5	24	2 Starch, 3 Lean Protein
	Steamed broccoli florets	1 cup	34	1		0	0	98	5	2	2	1 Vegetable
	Seasoned rice	1/2 order (1/2 cup)	130	0		0	0	500	26	1	3	2 Starch
Totals			**471**	**11**	**21**	**1.5**	**70**	**1338**	**60**	**4.5**	**29**	**4 Starch, 1 Vegetable, 3 Lean Protein**

(table continues on next page)

Lower Carb 'N' Healthy

Menu Samplers Section	Menu Item	Amount	Calories	Fat (g)	% Calories from Fat	Saturated Fat (g)	Chol. (mg)	Sodium (mg)	Carb. (g)	Fiber (g)	Protein (g)	Exchanges/ Choices
Lower Carb 'N' Healthy (Men)	Roasted chicken/half chicken dinner	quarter chicken breast without skin (5 oz)	270	2.5		1	134	100	1	0	47	6 Lean Protein
	Green bean casserole	1/2 cup	85	4.5		2	5	450	9	2	1	2 Vegetable, 1 Fat
	Corn bread	2 oz	145	5		1.4	16	295	22	3	2	1 1/2 Starch, 1 Fat
	Steamed seasoned spinach (non-cream sauce)	1/2 cup	140	10		6	25	440	9	5	6	1 Vegetable, 2 Fat
	Cinnamon apples	1/2 6-oz serving	120	1.5		0	0	135	27	2	0	2 Fruit
Totals			**760**	**24**	**28**	**10**	**180**	**1420**	**68**	**12**	**60**	**1 1/2 Starch, 2 Fruit, 3 Vegetable, 6 Lean Protein, 4 Fat**

(i) What's Your Solution? Answers

a) Every family communicates differently. In general, having a clear plan, sharing your goals with your family, and sticking to them is an effective way to succeed. Also asking for their buy-in and assistance can help. Do keep in mind that you may have an unwilling family member in your midst.

b) You will likely meet a lot of resistance and won't be able to sustain this drastic change for long. Try less extreme changes that you and your family can maintain without feeling deprived.

c) This is a healthier option. You are showing portion control with the appetizer, and you're cutting down fat (and calories) by changing your potato choice and skipping the butter sauce.

d) You've got the hang of this! Your whole family is eating healthier by cutting back on calories with a smaller, lighter appetizer. And you saved calories and fat grams by only eating half of your entrée. Allowing yourself fries will help keep you from feeling deprived. Added bonus: you get to enjoy the rest of the sirloin tomorrow in the comfort of your own home and prepared any way you like it … perhaps as a steak sandwich or topped on a salad.

CHAPTER 13

Fast Food—Burgers, Chicken, and More

F ast-food restaurants can churn out your meal in minutes (sometimes less) and offer you a relatively low-cost meal. These restaurants dot the highways, byways, and streets of cities and towns across America—actually, most of the world. They're generally easy to find, no matter where you live. On the plus side, you likely know these restaurants and their menus well.

The restaurants in this chapter include the large chain restaurants best known for serving their mainstays—burgers, chicken sandwiches, fried chicken, french fries, and soda. Today, lots of restaurants in America serve food fast and it's all covered in this book. You'll find information about other foods served fast (e.g., pizza, Mexican, Chinese, and other ethnic cuisines) in the related fare-specific chapters in Sections 2 and 3. Most of these fast-food chains also serve breakfast. You'll find breakfast foods covered in Chapter 11, beginning on page 124.

(♨) On the Menu

Fast-food restaurants began lining America's highways in the 1950s and 1960s. Their menus of burgers, fries, and soda were augmented over the years with items like chicken pieces (nuggets, tenders, and the like), chicken sandwiches (grilled, broiled, or deep-fried), breakfast items, and desserts. But it was the invention of the super-sized burger, fries, and soda combos, also known as meal deals, in the 1990s that greatly expanded fast-food restaurants' profits and our waistlines. These double or triple mammoth burgers and fried chicken sandwiches, loaded with cheese and bacon, continue to be present on these restaurants' menus.

Today, however, it is easier than ever to use the words "fast food" and "healthy" in the same breath. Yes, believe it, then try it! Fast-food restaurants have been trying to introduce healthier options for years. They've tried and failed a number of times. Not all the fault is on their side—people weren't buying. Of late, they've received increasing pressure, legislatively, from health authorities and consumers to make healthy changes to their menus and come clean with nutrition information. Here are some of the health-conscious changes that are, or are in the process of, being implemented by fast-food restaurants:

▶ Tucked within the Affordable Care Act (also known as Obamacare) is a regulation that requires chain restaurants with 20 or more outlets serving the same menu to post the calories on their menu or menu board. (Learn more about restaurant nutrition labeling in Chapter 7, which begins on page 72.) The availability of calories on the menu board can (but doesn't always) make it easier for you to choose lower-calorie options. Making restaurants disclose their calories counts has motivated some restaurants to lower the calories of some popular menu options and offer a few healthier sandwiches and sides.

▶ Trans fat, in the form of partially hydrogenated oil, has been reduced or eliminated in many restaurants and will likely (eventually) be completely phased out due to an FDA regulation proposed in late 2013. But as with all government regulations, putting this regulation into action will take time.

▶ Lower-fat items, such as leaner burgers (Burger King has a veggies burger, Carl's Jr. has a turkey burger), grilled chicken sandwiches, baked potatoes, lower-fat salad dressings, and low-fat milk, are more commonly available today.

▶ More fruits, vegetables, and whole grains are now on fast-food menus. For example, several chains offer an assortment of entrée-size and side salads, and Wendy's even sells half-size salads, which often are just enough for a healthy meal. Plus, several restaurants offer a fresh fruit option, such as apple slices or a fruit cup, as a side option or with kids' meals. McDonald's has publicly committed to test more fruit and vegetable side options, so we may soon see more healthful options added to the menu there and at other leading fast-food chains.

Let's commend these steps! And, more importantly, let's buy these items to keep them on the menu.

Despite this handful of positive changes and the fact that you can eat healthier fast-food meals if you try, the bitter truth is that fast-food meals are generally high in total fat, saturated fat, and sodium. They're also lower in healthy sources of carbohydrate than desirable. Even the nutritious potato, when placed on the fast-food menu, becomes drenched in oil from the deep-fryer, and/or surrounded by lots of unhealthy cheese, bacon, and sour cream. There's not much green and crunchy in an order that consists of a burger, fries, and a shake, though the pictures they promote can fool you. At least a side or garden salad can help complement a burger with something crunchy other than fries. Fruit—other than apple slices, the occasional fruit cup, fruit juice, or fruit mixed in a high-sugar dessert—simply doesn't make a showing on most fast-food menus.

Minimize Fried Foods

Fried foods are plentiful, but it's important to minimize the amount you eat to cut down on total fat and decrease calories. Try to offset one fried food with a grilled or non-fried item. For example, opt for a small order of french fries (or share a medium order) with a no-frills hamburger or a grilled chicken sandwich. Or complement a piece or two of fried chicken with a plain baked potato (preferably shared because they are large), a garden salad, and baked beans or an ear of corn. Obviously, you're better off avoiding all fried foods, but that's easier said than done.

Watch Out for "Sneaky" Fat

Be mindful of all the ways fat grams can sneak into your meal. Think about these popular additions to hamburgers and chicken sandwiches: cheese, bacon, "special sauce"—which most often is mayonnaise-based—or just plain mayonnaise. All of these are just about 100% fat and contain some unhealthy saturated fat. Even with the healthier options of salads and baked potatoes, fat is in toppings like salad dressing and cheese.

Consider the fast-food packets of salad dressing; many contain 4 table-spoons of dressing and upward of 200 calories! So, if you pour on the whole packet, you can quickly destroy the health benefits of a salad with more calories from the dressing than the salad itself. The same logic holds true for the no-fat baked potato to which fat-dense cheese sauce, sour cream, and/or bacon bits are added. But one positive aspect of the healthier food choices—grilled chicken sandwiches, salad, and potatoes—is that you're in the driver's seat and can control the toppings by using special requests or just not overdoing it with add-ons.

Limit Sodium

The high sodium content of fast-food meals is another pitfall. The sodium gauge rises as foods are coated in salty batters or as pickles, special sauces, bacon, cheese, and salad dressing are added. Not to mention the salt shaker used on french fries. Consider Burger King's Original Whopper with cheese, which contains more than 1,200 milligrams of sodium—a bit over half of what's recommended for an entire day! It's not unusual to see a fast-food meal quickly rise above the desirable daily sodium count of 2,300 milligrams. Some of the sodium in fast-food meals is difficult to cut down because of the high-sodium ingredients used in some foods before they even enter the restaurant's back door. The chicken fillet used in grilled or fried sandwiches, for example, contains anywhere from 400 to a whopping 1,300 milligrams of sodium, depending on the restaurant, prior to being placed on the grill or in the deep fryer. Cut your sodium intake where you can by cutting down on high-sodium ingredients (salad dressing, cheese, special sauces, and bacon). Order french fries unsalted and make it a small order. Keep in mind that you can decrease your sodium count by just eating less food.

Have a Plan

Surprisingly, the art of preplanning is actually easier in fast-food restaurants for several reasons. You aren't greeted with a menu to peruse that tempts your taste buds. You know only too well what's on the menu board at each restaurant from California to New York and well beyond.

One important healthy restaurant eating strategy is to decide what you'll order before you cross the threshold or hit the drive-thru speaker; have an action plan in mind. The smells, meal deals, and visual cues might tempt you to vacillate, but hold firm. If you have a willing partner, give him or her your order prior to walking in and then offer to snag a table to avoid the cues that may lead you astray.

Control Your Portions

Another advantage of fast-food restaurants when it comes to controlling portions is that you don't have to wait to eat. It's order and chow down. No bread and butter or chips and salsa greet you at the table, and there are no high-fat appetizers to tempt you. Also, dessert receives almost no attention. You can keep portions small by ordering items with the words "small," "regular," "junior," or "single." Skirt around the words that mean large portions: "giant," "super," "jumbo," "double," "triple," "big," and "extra-large." A single hamburger has between 2 and 3 ounces of cooked meat, just about the right portion for lunch or dinner.

Eat Mindfully

Lastly, try to eat mindfully in order to really enjoy each and every bite. To do this, monitor your pace of eating. Granted, getting the job of eating done quickly is the main goal of your fast-food stop. And the environment of a fast-food restaurant fosters a quickened pace. But take at least 15–20 minutes for a meal. Chew your food and put down your utensils every few bites. Savor the tastes of different foods. Train yourself over time to eat more mindfully. Mindful eating has the potential to help with weight management because you may eat less. Avoid drive-thrus—there's nothing positive about them. They cause you to eat quickly, and, when you go through a drive-thru, you are likely multitasking and can't focus solely on eating mindfully. You hardly taste the food as you shovel it in.

The Menu Profile

Hamburgers

A trend in hamburgers is giant loaded burgers. Most fast-food burger chains offer double, triple, quad (4 patties), biggie, or monster burgers. And high-fat toppings, such as cheese, bacon, and special sauces, are commonplace. The vegetable toppings remain minimal—a bit of lettuce and tomato and, oh yes, sometime a pickle or two. The good news is that small- and regular-size burgers remain on all menus and kids' meals are getting healthier. (Don't be shy about ordering one, there's no age cutoff at fast-food restaurants like there is in sit-down restaurants.)

The frequent additions of cheese, special sauces (usually mayonnaise-based), and bacon add fat and calories, whereas pickles, onions, lettuce, tomatoes, mustard, and ketchup increase flavor without the fat. Compare the nutrition info of a plain hamburger at Burger King, with about 230 calories and 9 grams of fat (35% of calories from fat), to the

Double Whooper with Cheese, with about 1070 calories and 70 grams of fat (almost 60% of calories from fat). Keeping your burgers plain and simple will help you with your healthy eating goals. See *Little Changes Make a Big Difference* (page 198) for examples of how small adjustments can make your fast-food meal healthier.

Chicken Sandwiches

Restaurant chains that got their start with burgers and fries now also serve both a grilled and fried chicken sandwich. Make these sandwiches healthier (lower in fat) by skipping the special sauce. Generally, if you can manage to get them to hold the "special sauce" (translated, this means more fat grams), then the grilled chicken sandwich is healthier than a loaded hamburger, fried chicken sandwich, or fried chicken pieces (nuggets or tenders). You might also find grilled chicken in a wrap at several chains. Do look for the word "grilled" in the description. If you see the descriptor "crispy," the chicken is fried. And if you don't see a descriptor at all, chances are the chicken is fried. Most restaurants that serve a grilled chicken sandwich also serve fried chicken pieces with your choice of sauces. Take advantage of this. Try one of the low-fat dipping sauces, such as barbecue or honey mustard, on your grilled chicken sandwich. Yes, they contain a few grams of carbohydrate. For that matter, do the same with a burger. Keep in mind, however, that mustard is your best bet for condiments when it comes to calories and carbohydrate.

Chicken Nuggets or Tenders

Fried chicken pieces were first introduced by McDonald's and are now stocked by many other chains. They're a hit with kids because they're a finger food and easy to eat. No matter what restaurant serves them, they are essentially chicken that is coated and deep-fried. (An occasional restaurant may offer these grilled.) Loaded with around 50% of calories from fat, there are just too many healthier options available today to even think of eating these.

Fried Chicken

A few chains specialize in serving fried chicken to the masses. Several of them tried serving roasted chicken, but it didn't last. Kentucky Fried Chicken, or KFC (as they want to be called to avoid the "F" word), is the leader in this field. Then there are some other hamburger chains that also serve fried chicken, such as Hardee's and Roy Rogers. There's little nutritionally redeeming about fried chicken. If you eat fried chicken once in a blue moon, set a limit of one or two pieces. From a fat count standpoint, you're best off with the breast minus the wing, but if you only eat it once in a while, eat the parts you enjoy the most. Complement the chicken with healthier sides, such as mashed potatoes, corn on the cob, green beans, or baked beans, rather than more fried offerings.

Fried Fish Sandwiches

Fish is healthy, of course, but not when it's lost among batter, oil, tartar sauce, and (to add insult to injury) a slice of cheese. Fried fish sandwiches are among the least healthy item on a fast-food menu. Without counting the French fries, these sandwiches run between 400–550 calories and about 45% of the calories are from fat. It's too bad that grilled fish just doesn't seem to be an option when it comes to fast food. Hold off on fish until you can prepare it at home or order it grilled or broiled in a sit-down restaurant so you really get to eat some healthy fish.

French Fries

It seems that crispy golden french fries accompany nearly every fast-food sandwich. Yes, they are hard to pass up, especially once you enter the restaurant and take a whiff. As a vegetable, potatoes do offer nutritional value, and a small or regular order of french fries isn't overly loaded with calories at about 200–300 per order. However, about 40 to 45% of those calories are from fat, thanks to the cooking method. If you've just got to have some, order a small serving (think kids' size) or split a larger order.

Baked Potatoes

Baked potatoes have been a healthier alternative on several fast-food menus for a while now. Wendy's is the national burger chain that most promotes the availability of baked potatoes. But, once again, you start off with a strong nutritional bet, a potato, and restaurants find a multitude of ways to drive up the fat with added butter, margarine, cheese, bacon, sour cream, chili, or a combination of these. The best of the toppings, though none of them are wonderful, are broccoli or chili, without the cheese. If the cheese sauce adds a lot of flavor for you, then request a small amount. At Wendy's, it's easy to order a plain baked potato and a small chili. With these items you're set for a filling and healthy meal. Or, instead of french fries with a sandwich, you can split a baked potato with a dining partner—they are large.

Salads

A variety of salad options are available at most national chains, including McDonald's, Burger King, Wendy's, Carl's Jr., Steak 'n' Shake, Culver's, and Chick-fil-A. Clearly a side or garden salad, when matched with a sandwich instead of French fries, improves the healthfulness of a fast-food meal. Wendy's even offers half-size salads, making them a perfect choice for a side, a lighter meal for those in need of more calories, and a sufficient meal for those on a tighter calorie budget. And speaking of lighter meals, opt for a meal-size salad as your entrée whenever you can. Do watch out, however, for high-fat add-ons, such as sour cream, fried chicken, Chinese noodles, nuts, and the like. Next, use the ridiculously large serving of salad dressing (generally provided in packets on the side) sparingly. Choose a low-fat or fat-free salad dressing if you like the taste. But drizzle these judiciously. They might not have the calories and fat of regular dressing, but their sodium count can be sky high. If you like a particular regular dressing best, leave more in the packet than you put on your relatively small salad. Learn more about salads and salad dressings in Chapter 15 (page 250).

Sides

Other than french fries, side salads, and baked potatoes, fast-food restaurants are expanding side items on the menu. At fried chicken–focused restaurants, you will often find sides like biscuits and mayonnaise-based cole slaw, both of which are high in fat. Healthier options, such as steamed veggies, baked beans, ready-to-eat carrots, apple slices, and fresh fruit cups, are appearing at more restaurants, making it easier for you to improve the nutritional content of your meal. Use your buying power to support these options. Hopefully, restaurants will respond to the demand by introducing ever more healthy options.

Shakes

The shakes at fast-food restaurants pack a lot of calories from carbohydrate (mainly from sugars), which can certainly raise glucose levels. But they are reasonably low in fat. The servings are large. Treat them as you would ice cream or any other dessert: order a small size on occasion as a dessert to satisfy a sweet tooth. Request an extra cup and split it with another diner.

Desserts

Desserts are easy to avoid in fast-food restaurants. They don't receive or deserve much play because their tastes are marginal at best. On occasion, if you just feel the urge, order a small ice cream or frozen yogurt cone or an order of cookies. Do split or share when you are able. Skip the pies, sundaes, and cheesecakes. Save your calories and precious carbohydrate grams for something more splurge-worthy.

Beverages

By far, one of the best beverage picks at a fast-food restaurant is low-fat or fat-free milk. Sometimes, 100% fruit juice, most commonly apple or orange, is available. Juice can be a decent choice if you pay attention to serving size. Avoid the sugar-loaded lemonade, fruit punch, and sugar-sweetened beverages in favor of no-calorie diet beverages, unsweetened iced or hot coffee or tea, or just good old water. Check out Chapter 9 (page 87) for a complete rundown on nonalcoholic beverages.

Little Changes Make a Big Difference

Small changes in the foods you order at a fast-food restaurant can add up to a big nutritional difference. Changes in the size of a food item, its preparation method, its toppings, or even its accompanying side dish or beverage can easily help you create a healthier fast-food meal. Here are two examples of how a few changes can make your meal both healthy and satisfying:

Food Choice	Calories	Fat (g) (total)	Fat (g) (unsaturated)	Carbohydrate (g)	Sodium (mg)
CHANGE THIS ORDER:					
Quarter-Pound Hamburger with Cheese	520	26	14	41	1100
French Fries (medium)	380	19	16.5	48	270
Regular Soda (21 oz)	200	0	0	55	5
Totals	1620	45	30.5	144	1375

(table continues on next page)

Food Choice	Calories	Fat (g) (total)	Fat (g) (unsaturated)	Carbohydrate (g)	Sodium (mg)
TO THIS ORDER:					
Hamburger (Single without Cheese)	250	9	5.5	31	480
French Fries (small)	230	11	9.5	29	160
Diet Soda (21 oz)	0	0	0	0	20
Totals	480	20	15	60	660
CHANGE THIS ORDER:					
Fried Chicken Sandwich with Bacon and Sauce	590	27	21	57	1380
French Fries (medium)	380	19	16.5	48	270
Vanilla Shake (12 oz)	530	15	5	86	160
Totals	1500	61	42.5	191	1810
TO THIS ORDER:					
Grilled Chicken Sandwich with No Mayo and 1 Tbsp Barbecue Sauce	350	3.5	2.5	53	990
Side salad with Low-Fat Vinaigrette (half-packet)	38	1.5	1.5	5.5	220
Nonfat Vanilla Latte (12 oz)	190	0	0	39	115
Totals	578	5	4	97.5	1325

📷 Nutrition Snapshot

Health Busters

Category	Restaurant Name	Dish Name	Serving Size	Cal.	Total Fat (g)	Carb. (g)	Sod. (mg)
Hamburgers	Dairy Queen	1/2 lb Flame Thrower Grill Burger	1 burger	1000	74	40	1610
Hamburgers	Five Guys Burgers and Fries	Hamburger	1 burger	700	43	39	430
Hamburgers	Burger King	Triple Whopper Sandwich	1 burger	1140	75	51	1110
Cheeseburgers	Five Guys Burgers and Fries	Bacon Cheeseburger	1 burger	920	62	40	1310
Cheeseburgers	Burger King	Triple Whopper Sandwich with Cheese	1 burger	1230	82	53	1550
Cheeseburgers	Hardee's	2/3 lb Monster Thick-burger	1 burger	1290	92	47	2840
Chicken Sandwiches	Wendy's	Asiago Ranch Chicken Club	1 sandwich	690	36	56	1630
Chicken Sandwiches	Burger King	Tendercrisp Chicken Sandwich	1 sandwich	750	45	58	1560

(table continues on next page)

Health Busters

Category	Restaurant Name	Dish Name	Serving Size	Cal.	Total Fat (g)	Carb. (g)	Sod. (mg)
Chicken Sandwiches	Wendy's	Spicy Guacamole Chicken Club	1 sandwich	770	42	58	1790
Fried Chicken (Pieces)	Burger King	Homestyle Chicken Strips (5 pc)	5 pieces	610	32	57	2340
Fried Chicken (Pieces)	McDonald's	Chicken Selects Premium Breast Strips (5 pc)	5 strips	640	38	36	1240
Fried Chicken (Pieces)	Kentucky Fried Chicken	Popcorn Chicken Value Box	1 box	680	41	53	1850
Fried Fish Sandwiches	Carl's Jr.	Carl's Catch Fish Sandwich	1 sandwich	700	37	73	1300
Fried Fish Sandwiches	Popeye's Chicken & Biscuits	Catfish Po'Boy	1 sandwich	800	50	65	2015
Wrap Sandwiches	Carl's Jr.	The Green Burrito—Steak	1 burrito	830	30	104	2890
French Fries	Burger King	French Fries	Large order	500	22	72	710
French Fries	McDonald's	French Fries	Large order	500	25	63	350
French Fries	Five Guys Burgers and Fries	French Fries	Large order	1314	57	181	1327

(table continues on next page)

Health Busters

Category	Restaurant Name	Dish Name	Serving Size	Cal.	Total Fat (g)	Carb. (g)	Sod. (mg)
French Fries	Arby's	Curly Fries	Large order	630	35	74	1420
Sides	Arby's	Mozzarella Sticks	6 pieces	650	33	56	2670
Sides	Burger King	Onion Rings	1 large	500	25	64	1310
Sides	Wendy's	Bacon Cheese Potato	1 potato	520	20	65	870
Milkshakes, Ice Cream Drinks	McDonald's	McFlurry with M&M's Candies (16 fl oz cup)	1 portion	860	31	127	260
Milkshakes, Ice Cream Drinks	Chick-fil-A	Banana Pudding Milkshake	1 large	1010	31	173	580
Milkshakes, Ice Cream Drinks	Dairy Queen	Malt, Peanut Butter	1 large	1350	72	143	910
Milkshakes, Ice Cream Drinks	Sonic, America's Drive-In	Reese's Peanut Butter Cups Sonic Blast	1 large	1730	83	219	1020
Milkshakes, Ice Cream Drinks	Wendy's	Caramel Frosty Shake	1 large	1000	19	195	500
Desserts	Burger King	Oreo Sundae	1 portion	440	12	77	390
Desserts	Dairy Queen	Peanut Buster Parfait	1 portion	710	31	96	350

Healthier Bets

Category	Restaurant Name	Dish Name	Serving Size	Cal.	Total Fat (g)	Sat. Fat (g)	Carb. (g)	Pro. (g)	Fiber (g)	Chol. (mg)	Sodium (mg)	Exchanges/ Choices
Hamburgers	Dairy Queen	Deluxe Hamburger	1 burger	350	14	7	34	17	1	50	680	2 Starch, 2 1/2 Medium-Fat Protein
Hamburgers	Sonic, America's Drive-In	Jr. Burger	1 burger	340	17	6	34	15	1	35	640	2 Starch, 2 Medium-Fat Protein, 1 Fat
Hamburgers	Wendy's	Jr. Hamburger	1 burger	250	10	4	25	15	1	35	620	1 1/2 Starch, 2 Medium-Fat Protein
Hamburgers	Whataburger	Justaburger	1 burger	290	15	4.5	26	15	1	33	727	1 1/2 Starch, 2 Medium-Fat Protein, 1 Fat
Hamburgers	White Castle	Original Slider	1 burger	140	6	2.5	13	7	1	10	360	1 Starch, 1 Medium-Fat Protein

(table continues on next page)

Healthier Bets

Category	Restaurant Name	Dish Name	Serving Size	Cal.	Total Fat (g)	Sat. Fat (g)	Carb. (g)	Pro. (g)	Fiber (g)	Chol. (mg)	Sodium (mg)	Exchanges/ Choices
Hamburgers	McDonald's	Hamburger	1 burger	250	9	3.5	31	12	2	25	520	2 Starch, 1 Medium-Fat Protein, 1 Fat
Hamburgers	Burger King	Hamburger	1 burger	260	10	4	28	13	1	35	490	2 Starch, 1 Medium-Fat Protein, 1 Fat
Hamburgers	Jack in the Box	Hamburger	1 burger	290	12	4.5	32	14	1	30	570	2 Starch, 2 Medium-Fat Protein
Cheese-burgers	Wendy's	Jr. Cheese-burger	1 burger	290	13	6	26	17	1	45	820	1 1/2 Starch, 2 1/2 Medium-Fat Protein
Cheese-burgers	McDonald's	Cheese-burger	1 burger	300	12	6	33	15	2	40	750	2 Starch, 2 Medium-Fat Protein

(table continues on next page)

Healthier Bets

Category	Restaurant Name	Dish Name	Serving Size	Cal.	Total Fat (g)	Sat. Fat (g)	Carb. (g)	Pro. (g)	Fiber (g)	Chol. (mg)	Sodium (mg)	Exchanges/ Choices
Cheese-burgers	Burger King	Cheese-burger	1 burger	300	14	6	28	16	1	45	710	1 1/2 Starch, 2 1/2 Medium-Fat Protein
Chicken Sandwiches	Wendy's	Ultimate Chicken Grill	1 sand-wich	390	10	3.5	43	34	3	100	880	3 Starch, 3 1/2 Lean Protein
Chicken Sandwiches	McDonald's	McChicken	1 sand-wich	360	16	3	40	14	2	35	830	2 1/2 Starch, 2 Medium-Fat Protein, 1 Fat
Chicken Sandwiches	Carl's Jr.	Charbroiled BBQ Chicken Sandwich	1 sand-wich	390	7	1.5	50	30	3	60	990	3 Starch, 3 1/2 Lean Protein
Chicken Pieces (Fried or Grilled)	Chick-fil-A	Nuggets (8 Count)	8 pieces	260	12	2.5	11	28	1	70	990	1 Starch, 3 1/2 Lean Protein, 1/2 Fat

(table continues on next page)

Healthier Bets

Category	Restaurant Name	Dish Name	Serving Size	Cal.	Total Fat (g)	Sat. Fat (g)	Carb. (g)	Pro. (g)	Fiber (g)	Chol. (mg)	Sodium (mg)	Exchanges/ Choices
Chicken Pieces (Fried or Grilled)	Church's Chicken	Nuggets (6 count)	6 pieces	280	18	3	18	13	1	40	540	1 Starch, 2 Lean Protein, 2 1/2 Fat
Chicken Pieces (Fried or Grilled)	Arby's	Prime-Cut Chicken Tenders	2 tenders	230	11	1.5	17	17	1	30	650	1 Starch, 2 1/2 Lean Protein, 1 Fat
Wrap Sand-wiches	McDonald's	Chipotle BBQ Snack Wrap (grilled)	1 sand-wich	250	8	3.5	27	16	1	40	670	2 Starch, 2 Lean Protein
Wrap Sand-wiches	Jack in the Box	Chicken Fajita Pita Made w/ Whole Grain (w/salsa)	1 sand-wich	330	11	5	35	24	4	65	990	2 Starch, 3 1/2 Lean Protein

(table continues on next page)

Healthier Bets

Category	Restaurant Name	Dish Name	Serving Size	Cal.	Total Fat (g)	Sat. Fat (g)	Carb. (g)	Pro. (g)	Fiber (g)	Chol. (mg)	Sodium (mg)	Exchanges/ Choices
Wrap Sand-wiches	Carl's Jr.	Sweet & Bold BBQ HB Chicken Ten-der Wrapper	1 wrap	290	13	5	26	16	1	40	910	1 1/2 Starch, 2 Medium-Fat Protein, 1/2 Fat
French Fries	McDonald's	French Fries	Small	230	11	1.8	29	3	3	0	160	2 Starch, 2 Fat
French Fries	Carl's Jr.	French Fries	Small	300	15	2.5	39	3	4	0	600	2 1/2 Starch, 2 1/2 Fat
Sides	Burger King	Apple Slices	1 portion	30	0	0	7	0	n/a	0	0	1/2 Starch
Sides	McDonald's	Apple Slices	1 portion	15	0	0	4	0	0	0	0	Free Food
Sides	Chick-fil-A	Fruit Cup	1 portion	45	0	0	12	0	1	0	0	1 Fruit
Desserts	Burger King	Strawberry Sundae	1 portion	190	4	2.5	35	4	0	15	125	2 Other Carbohydrate, 1 Fat

(table continues on next page)

Healthier Bets

Category	Restaurant Name	Dish Name	Serving Size	Cal.	Total Fat (g)	Sat. Fat (g)	Carb. (g)	Pro. (g)	Fiber (g)	Chol. (mg)	Sodium (mg)	Exchanges/ Choices
Desserts	Dairy Queen	Fudge Bar	1 bar	50	0	0	13	4	6	0	70	1 Other Carbohydrate
Desserts	Kentucky Fried Chicken	Lil' Bucket Strawberry Shortcake Parfait Cup	1 cup	200	7	3.5	35	2	2	20	140	2 Other Carbohydrate, 1 Fat
Desserts	Wendy's	Jr. Original Chocolate Frosty	1 junior size	200	5	3.5	33	5	0	20	95	2 Other Carbohydrate, 1 Fat
Soups	Chick-fil-A	Hearty Breast of Chicken Soup (medium)	1 cup	140	4	1	19	7	2	25	1110	1 Starch, 1 Vegetable, 1 Lean Protein
Soups	Wendy's	Large Chili	1 bowl	310	9	3.5	31	26	10	60	1330	2 Starch, 3 Lean Protein

(table continues on next page)

Healthier Bets

Category	Restaurant Name	Dish Name	Serving Size	Cal.	Total Fat (g)	Sat. Fat (g)	Carb. (g)	Pro. (g)	Fiber (g)	Chol. (mg)	Sodium (mg)	Exchanges/Choices
Kids' Meals	Chick-fil-A	Chick-N-Strips Kids' Meal (2 count)	2 chicken strip pieces	230	11	2	11	23	0	55	550	1 Starch, 3 Lean Protein, 1 Fat
Kids' Meals	Hardee's	Kids' Meal—Chicken Tenders	1 portion	380	18	4	36	19	3	45	1050	2 1/2 Starch, 2 Lean Protein, 2 Fat
Kids' Meals	Dairy Queen	Chicken Strip, Kids'	2 pieces	220	12	2	15	13	2	40	750	1 Starch, 2 Medium-Fat Protein
Kids' Meals	Popeye's Chicken & Biscuits	Get Up & Geaux Kids' Meal	1 meal	260	5	0.5	32	21	3	45	680	2 Starch, 2 1/2 Lean Protein
Kids' Meals	Wendy's	Hamburger, Kids' Meal	1 sandwich	250	10	4	25	15	1	35	540	1 1/2 Starch, 2 Medium-Fat Protein

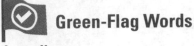 **Green-Flag Words**

Ingredients:

- ► Whole grain

Cooking Methods/Menu Descriptions:

- ► Grilled
- ► Junior
- ► Low-fat
- ► Nonfat
- ► Regular
- ► Roasted
- ► Sautéed
- ► Single
- ► Steamed

 Red-Flag Words

Cooking Methods/Menu Descriptions:

- ► Aioli
- ► Battered
- ► Breaded
- ► Buttered
- ► Creamy
- ► Crispy
- ► Crunchy
- ► Deep-fried
- ► Double
- ► Fried
- ► Melt
- ► Smothered
- ► Stacked

Healthy Eating Tips and Tactics

- ► Plan ahead. If you eat at fast-food restaurants regularly, be sure you have one very healthy order memorized and make it your own personal default meal. Limit "splurges" to no more than once a month.

▶ Make words like "regular," "junior," "small," or "single" part of your menu ordering vocabulary. These help to ensure you get smaller portions.

▶ Avoid meal deals, which can push you to eat larger portions because you can buy more food (most often fried items and drinks) for less. Don't get caught up in this unhealthy mentality.

▶ Try using lower-calorie ketchup, mustard, or barbecue sauce to replace higher-fat mayonnaise or special sauce.

▶ Walk in rather than drive through. If you eat and drive, you'll hardly realize that food has passed your lips.

▶ Order less food to start. Remember, you can go back and get more in a flash.

▶ Try not to look at the pictures on menu boards, which may tempt you to deviate from your healthy eating plan.

▶ Use positive reinforcement words with yourself. If you are tempted to stray from your plan, say things like "I feel best when I choose the healthier option."

▶ Want fries? Go ahead, but split a small or medium order with a friend.

▶ Remove the top of the bun to create an open-faced sandwich. This is an easy way to cut calories without cutting flavor.

▶ If there's enough food for two meals, ask for a takeout container and split the meal in two before you dig in. Take half home for another meal.

Get It Your Way

▶ Avoid the busy times at fast-food restaurants if possible. This way the restaurant will have more time to accommodate your special requests.

▶ Be ready to wait. Fast-food restaurants are not set up for special requests, so limit them to what's reasonable.

▶ Ask for simple changes: leave off the special sauce or mayonnaise, hold the pickles, bacon, or cheese, or hold the salt on the french fries.

▶ If you're at a chicken-focused restaurant, ask to have the skin removed, especially if you can't trust yourself to do it.

▶ Request gravy, butter, or salad dressing on the side.

Tips and Tactics for Gluten-Free Eating

▶ Your best bet here is to check the allergen statement on the website of the fast-food chain you choose to go to. Or call the corporate office to determine what is safe to eat on the menu.

▶ The risk for cross-contamination in fast-food restaurants is high. Employee turnover and lack of training contribute to mistakes in food preparation.

Tips and Tactics to Help Kids Eat Healthy

▶ Opt for a small burger or grilled chicken sandwich as your child's entrée. Similar to your own meal strategy, forgo higher-fat mayonnaise and special sauces in favor of ketchup, mustard, or barbecue sauce on your child's sandwich.

▶ If your child wants chicken nuggets, choose the smallest size possible.

▶ Be smart about portion sizes. Some fast-food restaurants offer bigger-size kids' meal options, which are higher in calories, fat, sodium, and everything else. Order the smallest size available or plan to split the meal.

▶ Be specific when placing your order to ensure your child gets healthier sides, such as fruit and low-fat milk. Otherwise, he or she may end up with fries and a soda, which are the "default" side options at many restaurants.

▶ Choose low-fat milk or water as your child's beverage. Fruit juice made of 100% juice is also an acceptable option, but keep in mind that kids between the ages of 1 and 6 years old should drink no more than 4–6 ounces a day, while older kids should limit juice to 8–12 ounces a day. And children with diabetes won't want to allot so many carb grams for fruit juice.

What's Your Solution?

You are having a busy day at work and don't have time for lunch, but you know you need to eat and can't delay a meal too long. Your co-worker offers to dash over to a fast-food restaurant and bring food back for you. You're not familiar with the restaurant they picked and don't have time to look at the online menu to find out about the healthier options.

Which of the following orders should you ask your co-worker to bring back for you?

a) "Order me the biggest value meal on the menu—I'm really hungry!"
b) "Order me the double burger value meal. Ask them to hold the special sauce."
c) "I'll have a small burger, small french fries, a side salad with light vinaigrette, and a diet coke."
d) "I'd like a grilled chicken sandwich with extra lettuce and tomato. Ask them to hold the special sauce and get me a package of mustard. Also get me a side salad with low-fat vinaigrette dressing and a bottle of water."

See page 221 for answers.

Menu Samplers

Light 'N' Healthy

Menu Samplers Section	Menu Item	Amount	Calories	Fat (g)	% Calories from Fat	Saturated Fat (g)	Chol. (mg)	Sodium (mg)	Carb. (g)	Fiber (g)	Protein (g)	Exchanges/ Choices
Light 'N' Healthy (Women)	Hamburger (single beef patty with ketchup, mustard, pickles, and onion)	1 burger	253	12		4.8	45	573	20	1	16	1 Starch, 2 Medium-Fat Protein
	Fruit and yogurt parfait (with yogurt, berries, and granola)	5 oz	150	2		1	5	70	30	1	4	1 Fruit, 1 Low-Fat Milk
Totals			**403**	**14**	**31**	**6**	**50**	**643**	**50**	**2**	**20**	1 Starch, 1 Fruit, 1 Low-Fat Milk, 2 Medium-Fat Protein

(table continues on next page)

Light 'N' Healthy

Menu Samplers Section	Menu Item	Amount	Calories	Fat (g)	% Calories from Fat	Saturated Fat (g)	Chol. (mg)	Sodium (mg)	Carb. (g)	Fiber (g)	Protein (g)	Exchanges/ Choices
Light 'N' Healthy (Men)	Chili	1 small (about 8 oz)	180	5		2	30	700	20	4	13	1 Starch, 1 Medium-Fat Protein
	Baked potato with cheese and broccoli	1 large	440	14		4	40	510	67	8	16	4 Starch, 1 Vegetable, 2 High-Fat Protein
Totals			620	19	28	6	70	1210	87	12	29	5 Starch, 1 Vegetable, 3 Medium-Fat Protein

(table continues on next page)

Hearty 'N' Healthy

Menu Samplers Section	Menu Item	Amount	Calories	Fat (g)	% Calories from Fat	Saturated Fat (g)	Chol. (mg)	Sodium (mg)	Carb. (g)	Fiber (g)	Protein (g)	Exchanges/ Choices
Hearty 'N' Healthy (Women)	6 piece chicken nugget	1 order	278	18		3.3	41	592	17	1	13	1 Starch, 2 Medium-Fat Protein, 2 1/2 Fat
	Side garden salad (mixed greens and tomato) without croutons or cheese	1 order (2 cups of leafy greens and a few additional veggies)	14	0		0	0	0	3	1	1	1 Vegetable
	Dressing, lite balsamic	1 packet (1.5 oz)	90	8		1	0	620	5	0	0	1 1/2 Fat

(table continues on next page)

Hearty 'N' Healthy

Menu Samplers Section	Menu Item	Amount	Calories	Fat (g)	% Calories from Fat	Saturated Fat (g)	Chol. (mg)	Sodium (mg)	Carb. (g)	Fiber (g)	Protein (g)	Exchanges/ Choices
	Reduced-fat vanilla soft serve cone	1 cone (3.7 oz)	170	5		3	15	70	27	0	5	1 Reduced-Fat Milk, 1 Other Carbohydrate
	Low-fat milk	8 oz	90	0		0	5	125	13	0	9	1 Fat-Free Milk
Totals			642	31	43	7	61	1407	65	2	28	1 Starch, 1 Fat-Free Milk, 1 Reduced-Fat Milk, 1 Other Carbohydrate, 1 Vegetable, 2 Medium-Fat Protein, 4 Fat

(table continues on next page)

Hearty 'N' Healthy

Menu Samplers Section	Menu Item	Amount	Calories	Fat (g)	% Calories from Fat	Saturated Fat (g)	Chol. (mg)	Sodium (mg)	Carb. (g)	Fiber (g)	Protein (g)	Exchanges/ Choices
Hearty 'N' Healthy (Men)	Grilled chicken sandwich	1 sand-wich	460	16		6	90	1030	43	3	35	3 Starch, 4 Lean Protein, 1 Fat
	Apple slices	1 side order	33	0		0	0	0	8	2	0	1 Fruit
	Small french fries	1/2 small order	126	5		1	0	186	19	1.5	1.5	1 Starch, 1 Fat
	Low-fat milk	8 oz	90	0		0	5	125	13	0	9	1 Fat-Free Milk
Totals			**709**	**21**	**27**	**7**	**95**	**1341**	**83**	**7**	**46**	**4 Starch, 1 Fruit, 1 Fat-Free Milk, 4 Lean Protein, 2 Fat**

(table continues on next page)

Lower Carb 'N' Healthy

Menu Samplers Section	Menu Item	Amount	Calories	Fat (g)	% Calories from Fat	Saturated Fat (g)	Chol. (mg)	Sodium (mg)	Carb. (g)	Fiber (g)	Protein (g)	Exchanges/ Choices
Lower Carb 'N' Healthy (Women)	Red beans and rice	1/2 regular order	230	14		4	19	580	23	5	7	1 1/2 Starch, 3 Fat
	Grilled chicken	1 drumstick	90	4		1	60	290	0	0	13	2 Lean Protein
	Mashed potatoes	1 side order	90	3		0.5	0	320	15	1	2	1 Starch, 1/2 Fat
	House side salad	1 side order	15	0		0	0	10	3	1	1	1 Vegetable
Totals			**425**	**21**	**44**	**5.5**	**79**	**1200**	**41**	**7**	**23**	**2 1/2 Starch, 1 Vegetable, 2 Lean Protein, 3 1/2 Fat**

(table continues on next page)

Lower Carb 'N' Healthy

Menu Samplers Section	Menu Item	Amount	Calories	Fat (g)	% Calories from Fat	Saturated Fat (g)	Chol. (mg)	Sodium (mg)	Carb. (g)	Fiber (g)	Protein (g)	Exchanges/ Choices
Lower Carb 'N' Healthy (Men)*	Grilled chicken	1 breast	220	7		2	133	730	0	0	40	5 Lean Protein
	Mashed pota-toes	1 side order	90	3		0.5	0	320	15	1	2	1 Starch, 1/2 Fat
	Coleslaw	1 side order	180	10		1.5	5	150	20	2	1	4 Vegetable, 2 Fat
	Corn	1 side order	100	0		0	0	0	21	2	3	1 1/2 Starch
	BBQ sauce	1 dipping packet	49	0		0	0	180	12	0	0	1 Other Carbohydrate
Totals			639	20	28	4	138	1380	68	5	46	2 1/2 Starch, 4 Vegetable, 1 Other Carbohydrate, 5 Lean Protein, 2 1/2 Fat

*This meal has a slightly higher than recommended cholesterol level due to the chicken.

(i) What's Your Solution? Answers

a) This is an impulsive order, which is easy to turn to if you're hungry and stressed. Take a deep breath, try again, and be specific.

b) This is a healthier option. Requesting your burger without the special sauce will help reduce the calories, fat, and sodium content. (Good thinking!) But unless you specify otherwise, the value meal will come with medium french fries.

c) This is an even healthier option! The small burger and small order of french fries will give you that crunchy oily taste you might be craving, but will keep the portion small. The side salad will provide nutrition and something to chew on to help you feel more full. Use that low-fat dressing sparingly.

d) You're a fast-food ordering pro! Grilled chicken options are often among the healthiest fast-food options, as long as you order them without the sauce to keep the fat and sodium content in check. Bulking up the sandwich with extra vegetables will inch you towards your daily vegetable goal, and water is the healthiest beverage there is.

CHAPTER 14

Sandwiches, Subs, Soups, and Snacks

I f you want to eat a meal fast but don't want a fast-food burger and fries (covered in Chapter 13), then a delicatessen (deli, for short), or sandwich or sub shop may fit the bill. A sandwich, sub, or wrap shop can be the epitome of convenience. The foods are served quickly and are easy to eat even with just one hand.

A few national chains specialize in putting protein, cheese, and/or veggies between some sort of starch. Subway is the most well-known from coast to coast in the U.S. and beyond. You'll also find plenty of independent sandwich and sub shops from Main Streets to malls. You'll also find them in or near coffee shops, bagel spots (where sandwiches will likely be served on a full bagel, bagel thin, or wraps), gas stations, which today may share space with a Subway right off the highway, and airports.

Soups are a common accompaniment to sandwiches, so they're covered in this chapter. Snacks, too, from chips to pretzels and popcorn, are another common sandwich partner. The array and availability of snacks has broadened and many snacks are at the ready to eat or drink (think smoothies) in this category of restaurant.

On the Menu

The number of restaurants in which you can grab a sandwich, wrap, sub, hoagie, grinder, hero—or whatever else you may call them in your part of the country—has multiplied. Among the most popular national chains are

Au Bon Pain, Blimpie, Panera Bread, Schlotzsky's Deli, Subway, and Quiznos. They all offer unique menus focused around soups, breads, and sandwiches or subs. Many small chains are on big growth curves: Charley's, Jason's Deli, Jersey Mike's, Le Pain Quotidien, Potbelly, Rising Roll, and Great Wraps are just a few. Their menus feature unique spins on sandwiches and wraps.

Coffee shops like Starbucks and Dunkin' Donuts have expanded their menus to include the ever-popular sandwich, now often available morning, noon, and night in these establishments. Many of these restaurants have figured out how to fit eggs, cheese, and/or a breakfast meat into a sandwich. You'll find breakfast sandwiches covered in Chapter 11 (page 124).

Though you might think of soups and sandwiches as lighter meals, if you don't order with care, even a half sandwich or 6-inch sub can tip the calorie, fat, carbohydrate, and sodium scale just as easily as a hot meal at a fast-food or family-fare restaurant. Portion control, as always, is a critical skill to use in these restaurants. Even though these meals seem to be light, portions can be large, toppings can be heavy, and meal deals can push the calories even higher. (Keep in mind that meal deals also work in the restaurant's favor—they're upselling and increasing the volume of your meal with chips and drinks at a low cost to them.) Most sub shops offer small subs, such as the 6-inch sub that Subway has made famous. And many of the sandwich shops offer a half-sandwich option you can combine with a cup of soup or a salad to help keep a lid on calories and grams of carbohydrate.

One of the best things about sub or sandwich shops is that your sandwich is usually made to order in front of your eyes. You're in control (don't jump over the counter, just verbalize your desires)! Take advantage of this reality. A few easy changes can have you ordering healthier without compromising taste and satisfaction in no time. If this is how you eat several days a week at lunch or dinner, then these small changes will add up to have a positive impact on your weight (if weight loss is one of your goals) and your glucose control.

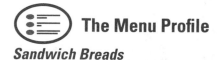 **The Menu Profile**

Sandwich Breads

Healthier breads, even whole-wheat and whole-grain breads that contain a few grams of fiber, are becoming easier to order. When you choose the bread for your sandwich or sub, apply two strategies: 1) choose a smaller portion, like a small roll, 6-inch sub, flatbread, or wrap, and 2) choose higher-fiber options. Avoid large buns or long sub rolls that double the amount of carbohydrate (and fillings) you'll get. Sandwiches on focaccia bread or a muffaletta (a big round sesame loaf, made popular in New Orleans) are often large, usually containing more than 1,000 calories and sometimes even more than 2,000 calories (like the Turkey Muffaletta at Jason's Deli). Definitely opt for a half size, or even a quarter-size, if you choose one of these big bread sandwiches. Schloztsky's Deli has made popular a variation of the muffaletta, which uses a sesame sourdough bun. Fortunately, in their twist on the sandwich, they've made the bun smaller than a traditional muffaletta, and they offer both small and medium sizes. Their small original-style turkey version has 610 calories and 56 grams of carbohydrate. But this is still quite a carbohydrate and calorie load for some.

Wraps can be deceiving, depending on their size. For example, a wrap alone at Subway has 310 calories, 51 grams of carbohydrate, and 1 gram of fiber. Yes, they're large. You'd be better off with the 6-inch cut of their 9-grain wheat bread, which has just 210 calories, 40 grams of carbohydrate, and 4 grams of fiber. On the other hand, Jamba Juice has mini wrap sandwiches, which range from 250–300 calories and 23–30 grams of carbohydrate for the entire sandwich. It's all about the size of the wrap. If you want to go with a wrap, you can peel off some of the wrap as you eat the sandwich to spare carbohydrate grams.

Bagels, too, can vary greatly. For example, a plain bagel at Einstein Bros Bagels has 260 calories and 56 grams of carbohydrate. A better choice is one of their "thintastic" bagels for just 140 calories and 29 grams of carbohydrate. Bagel thins have gone mainstream and are available at both supermarkets and bagel shops for sandwiches all day long.

Finally, skip croissants. Unlike the rest of the bread options discussed above, they're loaded with fat. An average croissant contains 230 calories, 26 grams of carbohydrate, and 12 grams of fat!

Sandwich Fillers

Examples of relatively healthy and available sub and sandwich fillers are turkey, smoked turkey, ham, chicken breast (plain, grilled, or barbecued—unless it's smothered in high-sugar and -sodium sauce), roast beef, and beef brisket.

Make these your go-to sandwich fillers. Many restaurants also offer vegetarian sandwiches and subs, which are a great way to achieve that goal of eating more vegetables. Make sure the sandwiches aren't loaded with cheese, oil, and mayonnaise-based dressings.

There is no need to purchase double meat as some sub shops now offer. Combo or double-meat sandwiches total up to about 6 or more ounces of meat, which is more protein than you need at a meal. A more appropriate serving is 3 ounces of meat, about the size of a deck of cards. If you get more than that, simply take some off or save half for later.

Tuna, chicken, and seafood salads sound healthy, but they've been mixed up with fat-dense mayonnaise and are chock full of fat and calories. If you want one of these pre-mixed spreads, find restaurants that use minimal mayonnaise. Schlotzsky's Deli is one that does a good job with this. A small Homestyle Tuna sandwich there is just 380 calories with 11 grams of fat and 50 grams of carbohydrate. Meanwhile, the Napa Almond Chicken Salad on Sesame Semolina at Panera Bread sounds wholesome, but racks up 700 calories, 27 grams of fat, and 89 grams of carbohydrate!

When it comes to other sandwiches, club sandwiches should be left alone due to the heavy dose of bread (and, therefore, carbohydrate), bacon, and mayonnaise. Watch out as well for the high-fat melts—the tuna melt is the most famous. You might also find cheese melted on chicken or seafood salad or cold cuts. Avoid egg salad, cheeseburgers, burgers loaded with high-fat items, cheese steaks (made famous in Philly), grilled cheese, pimiento cheese, ham salad, and hot dogs.

Several other meat fillings should be put off limits. Among them are bologna, all types of salami, mortadella, pepperoni, sausage and peppers, and steak and cheese. A meatball marinara sub can be an okay choice, assuming it's not loaded with cheese. Some other sandwich fillers to avoid are breaded and fried eggplant, chicken, or veal parmigiana. These options sound healthy, but they are breaded, deep-fried, and then cheese is layered on.

If you are at a traditional delicatessen, you'll find even more unhealthy choices lurking on the menu. Avoid the high-fat meats: regular corned beef (unless they promise it's lean and you've cast your eyes upon it), hot pastrami, beef bologna, salami, knockwurst, hot dogs, liverwurst, and tongue (as well as the mayonnaise-based tuna, chicken, and seafood salads). Delis are known for Reuben sandwiches, which are not a healthy choice. A Reuben consists of bread grilled with butter, corned beef, melted cheese, Thousand Island dressing, and coleslaw or sauerkraut. It's a fat and sodium nightmare!

Sandwich Toppings

Cheese is a frequent sub or sandwich addition. Some restaurants give their nutrition information minus the cheese. (Make sure you read the information given for the way you eat your sandwich.) Keep the cheese to a minimum. Not ordering it at all is best, especially if you're keeping close tabs on your saturated fat and cholesterol counts. Cheese is one of the largest contributors of saturated fat to the American diet.

Do ask your sandwich maker to load on the veggies—lettuce, tomatoes, cucumbers, onions, and peppers. The more the merrier. If you like some zip, have them toss on some hot peppers. Or if you want some creaminess, go with a thin spread of avocado or guacamole. At Jimmy John's, adding avocado spread to a regular sub adds just 10 calories. It's a great way to bump up the flavor! Pickles and olives add flavor but are high in sodium, so use them sparingly and be mindful of your sodium goals.

To moisten your sandwich you have a choice of mustards (Dijon, brown, or yellow), vinegars, or mayonnaise. Some sandwich shops get fancier with honey mustard, mayonnaise blends, and ranch-type dressings. The healthier condiments are mustards (all types) and vinegars (all types). They'll keep your sub or sandwich moist and add minimal calories.

Soups

Healthy soup options are warm and ready in many sandwich shops and delicatessens. Soups can be a wonderful way to squeeze some added fiber and nutrition into your meal, especially when paired with a half sandwich. Plus they're filling. Panera Bread is just one of many restaurants that promote the soup-and-half-sandwich combo. A low-fat garden vegetable soup paired with half of a sandwich of smoked turkey breast on country bread makes a healthy meal with a total of just 320 calories, but it's a bit high in sodium.

When choosing soups, look for options that are broth based (clear, not creamy) and that have vegetables, healthy grains, and/or beans. Healthy options you'll often see are chicken noodle, chicken and rice, chili, split pea, lentil, black bean, or gazpacho (a cold tomato and vegetable–based soup with a kick). Popular healthy options in delicatessens are beet borscht, barley, and matzo ball chicken soups. Avoid creamy soups such as New England clam chowder, creamy broccoli, cream of mushroom, or cream of ... well, just about anything. They're loaded with calories, fat, and sodium.

Sides

The most common sides at sandwich shops are chips and sometimes french fries. Your best bets for a side that comes from a "bag" are baked chips, pretzels, or popcorn, which are typically lower in fat than traditional potato chips. You may not naturally think of popcorn as your go-to accompaniment for a sandwich, but it's a filling and crunchy choice with a bit of fiber.

Sides of fruits and vegetables are rare, but they are slowly becoming more present, albeit mostly on kids' menus. Oftentimes, you can find apples or bananas at the register of sandwich or sub shops. Plan to grab one of these or bring your own fruit to enjoy after your meal or later in the day. Your best bet at getting vegetables in your meal will be in the form of sandwich toppings or as a salad (side or entrée) with light or fat-free dressing. Vinegar-based coleslaw is also an option. Just be sure to avoid mayonnaise-based slaws with too much fat.

Salads

Depending on the restaurant, salads may be a core part of the menu or more of an afterthought. Either way, they can be an ally in helping you to feel full with fewer calories, and they can help you check off a serving of vegetables. Le Pain Quotidien and Panera Bread are two restaurants that have made creative healthful salads part of their core menus. At Le Pain Quotidien, all salads are under 600 calories, including flavorful options such as Smoked Salmon & Roasted Beet and Tuscan White Bean & Prosciutto. At Panera Bread, most salad options are also under 600 calories, except for two: Chicken Cobb with Avocado and Steak & Blue Cheese. If you're craving one of these options, order a half-salad portion, available for all salads at Panera Bread. Remember to choose vinaigrette-based dressings and use them sparingly.

At a traditional delicatessen, salad plates are common. Stick with a chef, turkey, or grilled chicken salad plate. Make sure the grilled chicken salad plate is not just chicken salad mixed up with lots of mayonnaise—just plain unadulterated chicken, as is often the case today. Also, make sure they don't scoop potato or creamy macaroni salad onto the plate. If so, request a trade for more tomatoes, carrots, cucumbers, or other healthy side items. Always ask for salad dressing on the side.

Desserts & Baked Goods

Cookies are the most commonly offered dessert. But be cautious—portions are often large. (Save your calories and carbohydrate grams for a treat much more delectable.) At Au Bon Pain, for example, most of the dessert options range from 300–450 calories. If you opt for dessert, your strategy here is to choose something small—like a mini chocolate chip cookie or brownie bite (160 calories each)—and eat it slowly, savoring each bite. Or you can share an item among several diners. At delicatessens, you may find more dessert options, including cakes. Again, think small and eat mindfully or simply save those calories.

You may be tempted by desserts and baked goods when you stop into your favorite coffee shop for an afternoon pick-me-up, but remember that the calories and grams of carbohydrate in the drink alone can quickly escalate (see Chapter 9 for beverage-choosing strategies). Try not to add a calorie-heavy baked good on top of a high-calorie beverage. Most of the baked goods in the coffee-shop pastry case are at least 300–500 calories. Better options are fruit, yogurt, nuts, or even a small bag of popcorn.

At the mall, you may be tempted to grab a hot pretzel as a quick snack. Remember, even snacks can be customized. At Auntie Anne's, a popular pretzel shop, for example, you can request a pretzel without butter, saving you 30 calories and 4 grams of fat. If you need a dip, opt for a mustard or marinara dip, which are lower in calories and fat than cheese dip. But do keep in mind that Auntie Anne's pretzels are BIG, thus loaded with carbohydrate and calories. Split it or skip it.

Smoothies and Frozen Yogurt

Smoothies and frozen yogurt are popular snack options, thanks, in part, to their healthy halo, which is rarely deserved. If you choose a smoothie, stick with the smallest size available (and that's not really small) and make sure you're able to "afford" the carbohydrate grams and calories just for something to slurp. At Jamba Juice, most smoothies average between 250–300 calories with 60–80 grams of carbohydrate—and that's just for a small size. Jamba Juice does offer a "make it light" option on their classic smoothies. These lighter options have about 35–45% fewer calories and grams of carbohydrate.

We're on round two, or maybe three, of frozen yogurt shops. Are you old enough to remember TCBY? Frozen yogurt shops, such as TCBY, Yogurt Land, Sweet Frog, Pinkberry, and a number of other local independents, have regained popularity for the moment. They often boast about the low-fat, low-calorie frozen yogurt they offer, but these frozen concoctions are a far cry from more nutritious plain fat-free yogurts, including the Greek yogurt that's taken the supermarket shelves by storm. Many frozen yogurt shops also tantalize with you a bunch of add-ons—everything from fruit and granola to chocolate chips and gummy worms. Be savvy about your portion size and add-ons if you choose to have frozen yogurt. Otherwise, a somewhat healthy snack can quickly turn to a high-fat, high-sugar disaster.

Nutrition Snapshot

Health Busters

Category	Restaurant Name	Dish Name	Serving Size	Cal.	Total Fat (g)	Carb. (g)	Sod. (mg)
Soups	Jason's Deli	Broccoli Cheese Soup (bowl)	1 bowl	452	30	27	2035
Soups	Au Bon Pain	Baked Stuffed Potato Soup (large)	1 bowl	510	30	43	1450
Sandwiches	Schlotsky's Deli	Deluxe Original-Style (medium)	1 sandwich	957	46	80	4084
Sandwiches	Jason's Deli	Meataballa	1 sandwich	1160	71	67	2700
Sandwiches	Jason's Deli	The New York Yankee (no dressing)	1 sandwich	1200	71	46	2370
Sandwiches	Panera Bread	Full Steak & White Cheddar on French Baguette	1 panini	970	33	111	1820
Sub Sandwiches	Great Steak	Pastrami, 12"	1 sandwich	1410	80	102	3390
Sub Sandwiches	Subway	Footlong Mega Melt	1 sandwich	1310	79	90	3190
Sub Sandwiches	Great Steak	Chicken Bacon Ranch, 12"	1 sandwich	1390	67	101	1810

(table continues on next page)

Health Busters

Category	Restaurant Name	Dish Name	Serving Size	Cal.	Total Fat (g)	Carb. (g)	Sod. (mg)
Wraps	Jason's Deli	Ranchero Wrap	1 sandwich	680	28	59	2060
Wraps	Jason's Deli	Maverick Wrap (limited availability)	1 sandwich	660	36	43	1240
Wraps	D'Angelo Grilled Sandwiches	Mushroom Swiss Burger Wrap	1 sandwich	810	44	51	800
Sides	Mr Goodcents	Sun Chips Original	1 bag	210	10	27	180
Sides	Mr Goodcents	Fritos Corn Chips	1 bag	320	20	32	320
Sides	Nature's Table	Chipotle Rice Bowl	1 portion	655	21	80	444
Sides	Port of Subs	Potato Salad Regular	1 portion	325	13	52	958
Pasta Salads	Papa Romano's	Pasta Salad Personal	1 portion	449	6	82	269
Pasta Salads	Port of Subs	Caesar Bow Tie Pasta Salad Regular	1 portion	357	18	37	974
Desserts	Panera Bread	Carrot Cake with Walnuts	1 slice	590	24	86	710
Desserts	Au Bon Pain	Lemon Pound Cake	1 slice	490	25	63	480
Desserts	Panera Bread	Double Fudge Brownie with Icing	1 brownie	470	18	76	320
Desserts	Jason's Deli	Classic Strawberry Shortcake	1 piece	630	37	74	550

Healthier Bets

Category	Restaurant Name	Dish Name	Serving Size	Cal.	Total Fat (g)	Sat. Fat (g)	Carb. (g)	Pro. (g)	Fiber (g)	Chol. (mg)	Sodium (mg)	Exchanges/ Choices
Soups	Au Bon Pain	Split Pea with Ham Soup (small)	1 bowl	180	1	0	30	13	11	5	890	1 1/2 Starch, 1 1/2 Lean Protein
Soups	D'Angelo Grilled Sandwiches	Portuguese Kale Soup (large)	1 bowl	190	7	2	24	12	4	15	940	1 Starch, 2 Vegetable, 1 Medium-Fat Protein
Soups	Souplantation	Border Black Bean & Chorizo Soup	1 cup	240	10	3	27	11	6	20	880	1 1/2 Starch, 1 Vegetable, 1 High-Fat Protein
Soups	Au Bon Pain	Red Beans, Italian Sausage, and Rice Soup (small)	1 bowl	200	5	2	30	10	13	10	810	1 1/2 Starch, 1 Medium-Fat Protein

(table continues on next page)

Healthier Bets

Category	Restaurant Name	Dish Name	Serving Size	Cal.	Total Fat (g)	Sat. Fat (g)	Carb. (g)	Pro. (g)	Fiber (g)	Chol. (mg)	Sodium (mg)	Exchanges/ Choices
Sand-wiches	Au Bon Pain	Kids' Grilled Chicken Sandwich on Multigrain Bread	1 sand-wich	240	6	1	28	20	5	40	570	2 Starch, 2 Lean Protein
Sand-wiches	Panera Bread	Half Napa Almond Chicken Salad on Sesame Semolina	1/2 sand-wich	340	13	2	45	15	2	30	600	3 Starch, 1 Medium-Fat Protein, 1 Fat
Sand-wiches	Schlotsky's Deli	Chicken & Pesto (small)	1 sand-wich	384	8	1	51	23	3	48	1259	3 1/2 Starch, 2 Lean Protein, 1/2 Fat
Sand-wiches	Togo's	#27 Avocado & Cucumber (half/mini)	1/2 half/ mini sandwich	280	7	1	48	8	5	0	760	3 Starch, 1 Fat

(table continues on next page)

Healthier Bets

Category	Restaurant Name	Dish Name	Serving Size	Cal.	Total Fat (g)	Sat. Fat (g)	Carb. (g)	Pro. (g)	Fiber (g)	Chol. (mg)	Sodium (mg)	Exchanges/ Choices
Wraps	Roly Poly	Popeye's Tuna (wheat)	1 wrap	303	10	2	31	21	4	49	778	2 Starch, 2 1/2 Lean Protein, 1 Fat
Wraps	Jason's Deli	Savvy Chicken Salad Wrap	1 wrap	354	14	3	45	16	5	28	536	3 Starch, 1 Lean Protein, 1 1/2 Fat
Wraps	Roly Poly	Monster Veggie	1 wrap	285	9	3	27	12	4	22	269	1 1/2 Starch, 1 Vegetable, 1 High-Fat Protein
Wraps	Roly Poly	Italian Veggie	1 wrap	255	8	4	33	14	5	16	386	1 1/2 Starch, 2 Vegetable, 1 High-Fat Protein

(table continues on next page)

Healthier Bets

Category	Restaurant Name	Dish Name	Serving Size	Cal.	Total Fat (g)	Sat. Fat (g)	Carb. (g)	Pro. (g)	Fiber (g)	Chol. (mg)	Sodium (mg)	Exchanges/ Choices
Wraps	Jason's Deli	Spinach Veg- gie Wrap	1 wrap	350	16	5	43	13	8	15	570	2 Starch, 1 Vegetable, 1 High-Fat Protein, 1 Fat
Sub Sand- wiches	Subway	6" Oven Roasted Chicken Breast	1 sand- wich	320	5	1.5	47	23	5	45	610	3 Starch, 3 Lean Protein
Sub Sand- wiches	Subway	6" Roast Beef	1 sard- wich	320	5	1.5	45	24	5	45	700	3 Starch, 2 Lean Protein
Sub Sand- wiches	Subway	6" Oven Roasted Chicken	1 sard- wich	320	5	1.5	47	23	5	25	640	3 Starch, 2 Lean Protein

(table continues on next page)

Healthier Bets

Category	Restaurant Name	Dish Name	Serving Size	Cal.	Total Fat (g)	Sat. Fat (g)	Carb. (g)	Pro. (g)	Fiber (g)	Chol. (mg)	Sodium (mg)	Exchanges/ Choices
Sub Sandwiches	Subway	6" Veggie Delite	1 sandwich	230	2.5	0.5	44	8	5	0	310	2 1/2 Starch, 1/2 Fat
Sub Sandwiches	Blimpie	6" Tuna (regular)	1 sandwich	460	21	3	41	25	2	55	780	3 Starch, 3 1/2 Lean Protein, 2 Fat
Sub Sandwiches	Subway	6" Sweet Onion Chicken Teriyaki	1 sandwich	266	5	1	57	25	5	50	770	4 Starch, 3 Lean Protein
Pasta Entrée	Jason's Deli	"Lighter" Pasta Alfredo (no chicken and no bread)	1 portion	260	19	11	11	8	0	60	680	1/2 Starch, 1 Vegetable, 1 High-Fat Protein, 2 Fat

(table continues on next page)

Healthier Bets

Category	Restaurant Name	Dish Name	Serving Size	Cal.	Total Fat (g)	Sat. Fat (g)	Carb. (g)	Pro. (g)	Fiber (g)	Chol. (mg)	Sodium (mg)	Exchanges/ Choices
Pasta Entrée	Jason's Deli	"Lighter" Zucchini Garden Pasta (no bread)	1 portion	330	26	7	16	9	5	25	640	1/2 Starch, 2 Vegetable, 1 High-Fat Protein, 3 1/2 Fat
Pasta Salads	Port of Subs	California Style Pasta Salad (regular)	1 portion	235	6	1	38	6	2	0	439	2 1/2 Starch, 1 Fat
Kids' Meals	Subway	Roast Beef, Kids'	1 sandwich	200	3	1	30	14	4	25	410	2 Starch, 1 Lean Protein
Kids' Meals	Subway	Turkey Breast, Kids'	1 sandwich	180	2	0.5	30	10	3	10	460	2 Starch, 1/2 Lean Protein

(table continues on next page)

Healthier Bets

Category	Restaurant Name	Dish Name	Serving Size	Cal.	Total Fat (g)	Sat. Fat (g)	Carb. (g)	Pro. (g)	Fiber (g)	Chol. (mg)	Sodium (mg)	Exchanges/ Choices
Desserts	Arby's	Outside-In Cinnamon Bites	1 bite	300	15	4.5	36	5	2	10	480	2 Other Carbohydrate, 3 Fat
Desserts	Au Bon Pain	Chocolate Chip Cookie	1 cookie	280	13	7	40	3	2	30	230	2 1/2 Other Carbohydrate, 2 1/2 Fat
Desserts	Jason's Deli	Low Fat Fruit & Yogurt Parfait Cup	1 parfait	230	4	2	43	9	2	10	135	1 1/2 Fruit, 1/2 Low-Fat Milk, 1 Other Carbohydrate

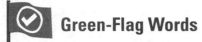 **Green-Flag Words**

Ingredients:

- Chicken—not fried or smothered in BBQ, teriyaki, or other sauce
- Ham
- Lean cuts of meat (roast beef, corned beef)
- Low-fat
- Multi-grain
- Mustard (any type)
- Roast beef
- Turkey, smoked turkey
- Vinegar (any type)
- Whole grain, whole wheat, oat

Cooking Methods/Menu Descriptions:

- Grilled
- Toasted

 Red-Flag Words

Ingredients:

- Aioli (garlic mayonnaise)
- Bacon
- Cheese
- Mayonnaise, mayonnaise-based special sauces
- Pepperoni
- Sausage

Cooking Methods/Menu Descriptions:

- Big
- Cheesy
- Club
- Creamy
- Double
- Grilled (when used to describe a sandwich, this means "buttered")
- Melt

- Parmigiana (eggplant, chicken, veal)
- Smothered
- Stacked
- Triple

Healthy Eating Tips and Tactics

- Complement a sub or sandwich with a side that's healthier than fried snack food, such as potato chips, tortilla chips, and the like. For some crunch, try a side salad, popcorn, baked chips, or pretzels. (Better yet, go for vegetables or fruit, like a side salad or sliced apples.)
- Ask to have large subs cut in two. Pack up half for another day.
- Check out the kids' menu. Many sandwich shops offer smaller sandwiches (like a 3-inch sub) with a side of fruit for kids. This is a perfect small meal for an adult, too.
- Order a cup of broth-based vegetable or bean soup to accompany a sandwich. These types of soup will fill you up but not out.
- Pack a piece of fruit from home to bring to the sub or sandwich shop (or eat it later).

Get It Your Way

- Hold the mayonnaise and oil on sandwiches. Substitute any type of mustard or vinegar.
- Ask the sub maker to go light on the meat and heavy on the lettuce, onions, tomatoes, peppers, and any other vegetables they have.
- Have the sandwich made on a wrap or bagel thin to save carbohydrate grams.
- Skip the cheese. This will save on fat, saturated fat, and calories.
- Spread on slices of avocado or guacamole.
- Say "no" to butter on pretzels and popcorn.

Tips and Tactics for Gluten-Free Eating

- Soups frequently contain gluten from bases, bouillon, broth, or roux or they may contain noodles or barley. Question the ingredients carefully.

▶ Gluten-free sandwiches and subs require a separate preparation area in a restaurant to ensure they are gluten-free. Ask that the preparer change gloves and also grab different utensils before preparing your sandwich on a *clean* surface. In addition, if the servers' gloved hands are going in and out of toppings that are used for both gluten-containing and gluten-free sandwiches, the toppings will be contaminated. Separate ingredients are required.

Tips and Tactics to Help Kids Eat Healthy

▶ Order fruit instead of chips to accompany the meal.

▶ Choose whole-grain bread when possible.

▶ Don't shy away from veggie toppings on kids' sandwiches. This is a great time to introduce a little bit of color and crunch to their meals and subtly point out the value of vegetables. If they don't like them on their sandwich, get veggies like peppers, cucumber, and tomatoes that they can pick up and eat.

▶ Split one 6-inch sandwich among two eaters or order mini-size sandwich portions (3 inches).

What's Your Solution?

Several times a week, you grab lunch at the sub shop near where you work. You typically get a 12-inch Italian sub loaded with salami, pepperoni, ham, and mayonnaise. A bag of potato chips and a 20-ounce bottle of sugar-sweetened soda are your go-to side and beverage. You have just been diagnosed with type 2 diabetes. Though you're tempted to make drastic changes to get some weight off fast, you've been encouraged to make small and hopefully lasting changes to your eating habits. Lunch is a place to start because you eat in these restaurants several days a week.

Which of the following reasonable and realistic healthy changes could you implement for this lunch?

a) Order your usual lunch but ask them to leave off the mayonnaise and cheese.

b)   Skip the mayonnaise and cheese. Bring a piece of fruit with you to eat instead of the chips.

c)   Order a 6-inch Italian sub, minus the mayo, and ask for extra veggies. Order a cup of chicken noodle soup plus a piece of fruit. Have a diet soda to drink.

d)   Switch to a 6-inch ham sub topped with mustard and extra veggies. Order a cup of black bean soup plus a piece of fruit. Have a diet soda or water to drink.

See page 249 for answers.

▥ Menu Samplers

Light 'N' Healthy

Menu Samplers Section	Menu Item	Amount	Calories	Fat (g)	% Calories from Fat	Saturated Fat (g)	Chol. (mg)	Sodium (mg)	Carb. (g)	Fiber (g)	Protein (g)	Exchanges/ Choices
Light 'N' Healthy (Women)	Turkey on whole-wheat sub (with swiss, vegetables, and olive oil blend)	6-inch sub	380	13		4.5	35	690	46	5	22	3 Starch, 1 Vegetable, 2 1/2 Lean Protein, 1 Fat
	Oatmeal raisin cookie	1/2 cookie	153	5		3	17	108	24	1	2	1 1/2 Other Carbohydrate, 1 Fat
Totals			**533**	**18**	**30**	**7.5**	**52**	**798**	**70**	**6**	**24**	**3 Starch, 1 1/2 Other Carbohydrate, 1 Vegetable, 2 1/2 Lean Protein, 2 Fat**

(table continues on next page)

Light 'N' Healthy

Menu Samplers Section	Menu Item	Amount	Calories	Fat (g)	% Calories from Fat	Saturated Fat (g)	Chol. (mg)	Sodium (mg)	Carb. (g)	Fiber (g)	Protein (g)	Exchanges/ Choices
Light 'N' Healthy (Men)	Club sub (with turkey, roast beef, ham, swiss cheese, vegetables, mustard, and light mayo)	6-inch sub	430	15		4.5	60	1040	48	5	27	3 Starch, 1 Vegetable, 3 Lean Protein, 1 Fat
	Baked Lay's potato chips	1/2 snack sized bag (about 1 oz)	130	2		0	0	200	26	0	2	1 1/2 Starch, 1/2 Fat
	Apple	1/2 large or 1 small apple	40	0		0	0	0	10	2	0	1 Fruit
Totals			**600**	**17**	**26**	**4.5**	**60**	**1240**	**84**	**7**	**29**	**4 1/2 Starch, 1 Fruit, 1 Vegetable, 3 Lean Protein, 1 1/2 Fat**

(table continues on next page)

Hearty 'N' Healthy

Menu Samplers Section	Menu Item	Amount	Calories	Fat (g)	% Calories from Fat	Saturated Fat (g)	Chol. (mg)	Sodium (mg)	Carb. (g)	Fiber (g)	Protein (g)	Exchanges/ Choices
Hearty 'N' Healthy (Women)	Almond chicken salad sandwich	1/2 sandwich	340	13		2	35	580	44	2	15	3 Starch, 2 Lean Protein, 1 1/2 Fat
	Baked Lay's potato chips	1/2 snack sized bag (about 1 oz)	130	2		0	0	200	26	0	2	1 1/2 Starch, 1/2 Fat
	Fruit cup	5 oz	60	0		0	0	10	15	2	1	1 Fruit
	Reduced-fat milk	8 oz	120	4.5		3	20	115	12	0	8	1 Reduced-Fat Milk
Totals			**650**	**20**	**28**	**5**	**55**	**905**	**97**	**4**	**26**	**4 1/2 Starch, 1 Fruit, 1 Reduced-Fat Milk, 2 Lean Protein, 2 Fat**

(table continues on next page)

Hearty 'N' Healthy

Menu Samplers Section	Menu Item	Amount	Calories	Fat (g)	% Calories from Fat	Saturated Fat (g)	Chol. (mg)	Sodium (mg)	Carb. (g)	Fiber (g)	Protein (g)	Exchanges/ Choices
Hearty 'N' Healthy (Men)	Asiago steak sandwich	1/2 sandwich	390	17		8	60	650	33	2	25	2 Starch, 3 Medium-Fat Protein
	Salad with apple and chicken	1 small side salad	280	17		3.5	50	330	18	3	16	1 Vegetable, 1 Fruit, 2 Lean Protein, 2 Fat
	Fruit cup	8 oz	90	0		0	0	15	20	3	1	1 Fruit
Totals			**760**	**34**	**40**	**11.5**	**110**	**995**	**71**	**8**	**42**	**2 Starch, 2 Fruit, 1 Vegetable, 5 Medium-Fat Meat, 2 Fat**

(table continues on next page)

Lower Carb 'N' Healthy

Menu Samplers Section	Menu Item	Amount	Calories	Fat (g)	% Calories from Fat	Saturated Fat (g)	Chol. (mg)	Sodium (mg)	Carb. (g)	Fiber (g)	Protein (g)	Exchanges/ Choices
Lower Carb 'N' Healthy (Women)	Chicken Caesar wrap (without dressing)	1 wrap	530	15		13	10	1460	62	3	37	4 Starch, 5 Lean Protein
Totals			**530**	**15**	**25**	**13**	**10**	**1460**	**62**	**3**	**37**	**4 Starch, 5 Lean Protein**

(table continues on next page)

Lower Carb 'N' Healthy

Menu Samplers Section	Menu Item	Amount	Calories	Fat (g)	% Calories from Fat	Saturated Fat (g)	Chol. (mg)	Sodium (mg)	Carb. (g)	Fiber (g)	Protein (g)	Exchanges/ Choices
Lower Carb 'N' Healthy (Men)	Power steak lettuce wraps	1 bowl	210	10		3.5	65	240	7	2	24	1 1/2 Vegeta-ble, 3 Medium-Fat Protein
	Whole-wheat baguette	1/2 of a 1.5 oz baguette	90	1		0	0	200	17	2	3.5	1 Starch
	Margarine	1 teaspoon	34	3.8		0.6	0	0	0	0	0	1/2 Fat
	Black bean soup	1 cup	165	2		0	0	900	35	6	9	2 Starch, 1 Lean Protein
	Low-fat milk	8 oz	120	4.5		3	20	115	12	0	8	1 Low-Fat Milk
Totals			**619**	**21**	**30**	**7**	**85**	**1455**	**71**	**10**	**45**	**3 Starch, 1 Low-Fat Milk, 1 1/2 Vegetable, 4 Medium-Fat Protein**

(i) What's Your Solution? Answers

a) It's a start. This will save you 50–100 calories, mostly from fat.

b) This is good progress. Choosing fruit over chips will save on calories and fat, whereas the added fiber will help you feel more satisfied.

c) Great order! You downsized your sandwich but added a clear-broth soup to help you feel full. The switch to diet soda is a big calorie-saving change alone (it saves about 250 calories!).

d) Now you're talking. Not only did you downsize your sandwich, but you went with a leaner meat. Do keep in mind that if you make all these change at once, it might feel too drastic. Try making changes gradually in a progression of steps.

CHAPTER 15

Salads—From Bar to Entrée and Side

Salads are on the menus of nearly every style of restaurant covered in this book (other than a few ethnic restaurants, such as Chinese and Indian). You'll find salads in restaurants everywhere, from fast food to fine dining, Mexican to Middle Eastern, sandwich and sub shops to steakhouses, and beyond. Then you'll find restaurants predicated on and dedicated to delivering those leafy greens and their accessories to you within a wrap, in a bowl, on a plate, or on full display at their salad bar, from which you assemble your salad (and sometimes soup, bread, and more). To name a few small growing salad chains capturing the lunch and/or dinner crowd, there's Chop't, Sweet Green, and Souplantation & Sweet Tomatoes.

As you work to eat healthier and make vegetables a focal point on your plate or bowl, mastering the art of ordering salads in restaurants will be a key to your success. After all, the word "salad" brings to mind visions of healthy, low-calorie lettuce, spinach, tomatoes, and bell peppers in a rainbow of colors. While salads inherently possess a halo of health, beware; their healthfulness can quickly be unraveled by dressings and toppings loaded with fat (sometimes healthy and sometimes not) and sodium.

Restaurants have upped their creativity with a wider gamut of salad ingredients. You can find many flavorful, filling, and healthy salads that are a far cry from a bowl of iceberg lettuce topped with tomatoes, cucumbers, and a few shreds of carrots.

The types of salads and toppings on menus vary depending on the style of restaurant. This chapter shows you how to enjoy healthful and satisfying salads, whether it be a salad you make on a trip to a salad bar, an entrée salad you order as your main course, or a side salad that starts or accompanies your meal. The restaurant-specific chapters in Sections 2 and 3 cover the salads popular at those respective types of restaurants.

On the Menu

How many times have you used or heard these words: "You guys go have your burgers and fries; I'll just take a trip to the salad bar," or "I'm watching my waistline. I'll just have the Cobb salad." Unfortunately, the well-intended decision to order a salad can sometimes result in a shockingly high-fat, high-calorie meal if you don't practice care and caution.

Salad bars had their heyday back in the late 1990s and early 2000s, when they were popular in steakhouses, fast-food establishments, cafeterias, and supermarkets. But concerns rose about the hygiene of salad bars and their upkeep was labor intensive. Their popularity waned. They still make an appearance, at some steakhouses and seafood and family restaurants, as part of those large troughs that stock a wide array of foods and provide you with a refillable plate and endless trips back. Beware; danger lurks.

Salad bars can still be found, in supermarkets as well as in hospital, employee, and university cafeterias. Some salad bars feature standard salad fixings with a few extras, whereas others are stocked for a feeding frenzy with raw vegetables, cheese, legumes, canned fruit, pasta salad, tuna and chicken salad, fruit ambrosia, baked goods, puddings, and more.

Last, and perhaps most hazardous, is the array of salad dressings waiting for you with a large ladle (generally a 2-tablespoon serving) at the end of the bar. American favorites—blue cheese and thousand island dressings—contain upward of 70 calories per tablespoon. And most people, after piling the "vegetables" high, are likely to pour at least a few tablespoons of dressing on an entrée salad. You do the math. Under the guise of a "healthy" food choice, the salad bar can actually be higher in fat and calories than a meal containing a sandwich and fries.

As salad bars have become less common, entrée salads, packaged or plated, have become more popular. Whether it's a popular Cobb, chef, or Caesar salad or an ethnic-inspired one, such as Southwestern or Greek salad, you can order an entrée salad at many types of restaurants and even bagel and coffee shops.

In the fast-food category, Wendy's led the pack with their introduction of entrée salads in the early 2000s. Others followed suit. Today, most fast-food chains offer garden salads, side salads, and three to five different entrée salads. Entrée salads are also common at family-style and soup 'n' sandwich restaurants. Think about Ruby Tuesday, Panera Bread, Au Bon Pain, and Applebee's. Of course, side salads are available at all of these restaurants, too. Although side salads were once a simple bowl of greens with tomatoes, cucumbers, and onion, some restaurants have elevated the side salad to include a number of other toppings, such as crispy noodles, garbanzo beans (also known as chickpeas), or feta cheese.

There are lots of salad landmines, but if you are strategic about your salad toppings, dressing, and portions, salads can be a definite winner, outshining most other foods on the menu. An entrée salad or a trip to a salad bar can be a nutritionally complete lunch or dinner, and a side garden salad can add a vegetable serving to your meal and help you limit higher-fat items that usually accompany sandwiches or burgers—namely, potato chips or french fries.

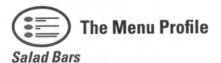 # The Menu Profile

Salad Bars

Because the slew of items you may find on a large salad bar can overload your sensory and visual system, you'll need a dose of willpower (or "won't power") when you approach the salad bar. If you are extremely hungry, unleashing yourself at the salad bar can be disastrous. If your "won't power" just doesn't hold up around a tempting salad bar, stay at your table and order from the menu. In some lower-priced steakhouses, where the salad bar should more appropriately be called a food bar, you might be better off ordering a small steak, baked potato, vegetables, and a side salad, than risking a trip to the salad bar.

Rather than choosing with your eyes and taste buds, make decisions with your nutrition and health goals in mind. Think about what foods you really need to eat and in what quantities. If you are unfamiliar with a particular salad bar, cast a glance at the lineup before you even pick up a plate. Then, once you've prioritized your choices, grab a small plate (not the large one) to automatically build in some portion control. Finally, limit yourself to just one trip.

Nutritionally speaking, salad bars have a number of offerings that can fit into your diabetes eating plan, including plenty of healthy carbohydrate with lots of fiber and minimal fat. The best salad bar strategy is to load up on the veggies—greens, tomatoes, cucumbers, bell peppers, onions, mushrooms, raw broccoli, carrots, and the like. Vegetables give you plenty of crunch and volume with few calories. Table 15.1, *Salad Bar Calorie Counter* (page 257), divides common salad bar items into categories based on their calorie content. Review this to learn what to take lots of and what to take less of when you reach the salad bar.

If you wish to add some lower-calorie sources of protein, choose from plain tuna (not tuna salad), cubed ham (not ham salad), hard-boiled eggs (whole or chopped), feta cheese, and cottage cheese (though, most likely, it won't be low fat). Two of these choices—ham and feta cheese—are high in sodium. Try to minimize high-fat items. Tuna, chicken, and seafood salad sound healthy but they're mixed with mayonnaise and are loaded with fat, so steer clear. You'll also want to avoid chunks of cheese and pepperoni, which contain more calories from fat than protein.

From a sodium standpoint, salad bars can range from great to disaster land. Again, it's a matter of which foods you choose to eat and how you dress them up. Vegetables are extremely low in sodium, but salad mix-ins, such as macaroni salad, coleslaw, ham, olives, pickles, and heavily seasoned croutons, can max out the sodium count.

The bigger the salad bar, the more mixed higher-calorie "salads" you'll see on it, such as pasta salad, potato salad, coleslaw, marinated mushrooms or vegetables, and others. Some of these are decent choices and others should be left in the serving bowl. Marinated beets, marinated mixed vegetables or mushrooms, three-bean salad, vinegar-based coleslaw, and mixed fruit salad are moderately healthy choices, though they are not low in sodium. Take only small quantities of these options (about 1/4–1/2 cup), especially if you need to closely monitor your calories, fat, and sodium.

Another group of foods that can add on calories are the so-called "salad bar accessories." These little temptations include nuts, raisins, seeds, Chinese noodles, croutons, olives, and bacon bits. And don't forget the sides: crackers, pita pockets, garlic bread, and fresh baked bread. Granted, most people add these accessories and sides to their plate in small quantities, but a small amount of these foods can rack up calories. Your strategy should be to try a little bit of this but skip a whole lot of that.

Entrée Salads

Keep four key strategies in mind when you order and eat an entrée salad: 1) make sure low-calorie options form the base of your salad, 2) limit high-fat toppings, 3) be savvy about salad dressings you use, and 4) control your portions.

First, when you peruse a menu for an entrée salad, make sure (ask questions if necessary) that the featured ingredients of the salad are leaner items, such as grilled chicken, salmon, shrimp, ham, smoked turkey, beans, or the like. And make sure the base of the salad is well padded with a load of veggies— lots of greens, cucumbers, tomatoes, carrots, or other options from the lower-calorie section of *Salad Bar Calorie Counter* (Table 15.1, page 257). Finally, don't forget about the accessories. Is your salad of choice topped off with unnecessary sources of excess carbohydrate and fat like fried tortilla strips, cheese, or bacon bits? If so, it's time to be creative. If you think the basic salad is a healthy choice and there are one or two ingredients that aren't healthy, ask that they be left in the kitchen or sprinkled on sparingly. Or ask that they be replaced with a healthier ingredient or topping you see on another salad on the menu.

Take, for example, the ever-popular Cobb salad, which features chopped greens, tomatoes, grilled chicken, hard boiled eggs, avocado, blue cheese, and bacon. The last three ingredients of this salad are high in fat and can send the calorie count soaring, but the avocado is at least healthy. You can certainly ask that your salad be served without those ingredients, but then it wouldn't be a Cobb salad anymore. So try these tips: request that they only put half the amount of those ingredients on your salad or choose the two ingredients that are healthiest, like avocado versus bacon, or that you like best and skip the third ingredient. You'll still get the flavor, but with fewer calories and fat. Moderation is the key here.

The classic Caesar is another example of a sabotaged salad. The romaine lettuce and pieces of grilled chicken, salmon, or shrimp are not the issue. It's the Parmesan cheese and creamy Caesar dressing frequently used today that send calories skyrocketing. (To set the facts straight, true Caesar dressing is not creamy. It's an olive oil–based dressing with lemon juice or vinegar.) For example, the Grilled Chicken Caesar Salad at Applebee's has 800 calories—more than half of which are from the dressing! Order it without the dressing and the salad nets only 370 calories. Is the dressing really worth it? Or do you need all of it? No matter what salad you order, request the dressing on the side so you can be in control of the quantity. Also ask to get some vinegar or lemon juice to dilute your dressing of choice and use less of the high-fat stuff. See *The Lowdown on Salad Dressings* below for more suggestions to whittle down the calories.

Last but not least, controlling the portion size of your entrée salad is an important strategy. As portions have grown, even salads have become large enough for two. Many dressed salads at family restaurants now top the 1,000-calorie mark. Consider sharing entrée salads or order a half-size salad, if that's an option. Or request a take-home container and eat half now, then save half for a second meal.

Side Salads

Side salads are a common item on many menus. A typical side salad has lettuce, tomato, cucumber, and onion. The toppings vary depending on the style of the restaurant. A family-style restaurant may add croutons, cheese, and bacon. An Italian restaurant may add a few beans or even fried pasta noodles. A Greek restaurant may add a bit of feta cheese. At Middle Eastern restaurants, fried pita chips and fresh herbs are common. Clearly, a side or garden salad when paired with a sandwich instead of french fries improves the healthfulness of a meal. But be sure to read the menu or ask your server to specify what's on the salad to avoid any unexpected surprises. And, as always, watch the dressing.

The Lowdown on Salad Dressings

By far the biggest culprit in adding abundant, hidden, and possibly unhealthy calories to salads is their crowning touch—salad dressing. Check out the nutrition numbers for salad dressings in this chapter's *Health Busters* and *Healthier Bets* (page 260).

Most restaurants, cafeterias, and even supermarket salad bars pour regular commercial salad dressing—the same dressings you find on the supermarket shelves—from oil-based Italian and balsamic vinaigrette to the creamier French, honey mustard, Thousand Island, and blue cheese. Use the nutrition facts on salad dressings in supermarkets to educate yourself on their nutrition counts. Very few large chain restaurants make their salad dressing from scratch. Conversely, you may find made-from-scratch dressings in independently owned family, fine dining, and upscale ethnic restaurants. In most restaurants, particularly sit-down ones, request olive oil, and one of a variety of vinegars they likely have on their kitchen shelves, on the side. Request the addition of fresh ground pepper (when available) and you've got the healthiest salad dressing in town.

Most oil-based commercial salad dressings contain one healthy oil—either soybean or cottonseed—or a combination of the two, which contains mainly polyunsatured fats. Some salad dressings contain canola or olive oil, which ups the monounsaturated fats. Regular salad dressings served in restaurants ring in at 60–80 calories per level tablespoon, but most people aren't leveling or limiting themselves to a tablespoon, they're heaping. In addition to calories, creamy dressings may contain mayonnaise, sour cream, and/or cheese, all of which can add saturated fat and/or cholesterol.

These days, it's common to find at least one low-fat, reduced-calorie, or fat-free salad dressing available in large chain restaurants, especially in fast-food restaurants. Lighter dressings range from 15–30 calories per tablespoon. That's half (or less than half) the calories of regular dressing. These lower-calorie and lower-fat salad dressings, however, can deliver even more sodium and carbohydrate than regular salad dressings. That's because if you take the fat out, you've got to replace the taste and mouth feel with something. The "something" ends up being carbohydrate-based and high-sodium ingredients. Four tablespoons (a quarter of a cup or the common serving in a package of fast-food salad dressing) of either a regular or reduced-calorie dressing can provide in the range of 500 milligrams of sodium. And some of the fat-free salad dressings are even higher in sodium.

But this does not mean you need to eat your salads undressed. There are lots of healthier options. But if you are used to seeing enough dressing to swim in when you finish a salad, then learning to enjoy salads with less dressing is a great move in the right direction.

Tips to Dress with Less

Putting one or more of these tips into action can help you cut the calories, total fat, saturated fat (depending on the dressing), and sodium. Any reduction will be significant because of the high calorie level of salad dressings. You'll come to realize that using less dressing helps you enjoy the various tastes of the vegetables and accessories more.

▶ Always order dressing on the side. This puts you, rather than the cook or your server, in control.

▶ Drizzle rather than pour. If you want to use your favorite dressing, fine. Just pour less and spread it out. When you get a large packet of salad dressing from a fast-food restaurant, drizzle slowly and gingerly. Mix up your salad in between drizzles to see if your salad is sufficiently coated.

▶ Instead of drizzling your dressing, you could try dipping your fork in the dressing before you use it to pick up your food. This ensures you get a taste of dressing with each bite, while using less overall.

▶ Use half the amount of your favorite dressing and thin it with vinegar, lemon juice, or water.

▶ Think about simply using olive oil and vinegar. This is the healthiest salad dressing combo because it has healthy oils with no sodium.

Table 15.1 Salad Bar Calorie Counter

	Serving Size	Calories	Examples
Low-Calorie Vegetables (mainly raw)	1 cup	25 (approx.)	▶ Broccoli ▶ Cabbage (red or green) ▶ Cauliflower ▶ Celery ▶ Cucumbers ▶ Endive ▶ Radicchio, red cabbage ▶ Lettuce (all types) ▶ Onions, raw (all types) ▶ Peppers (all types) ▶ Radishes ▶ Sauerkraut (high in sodium) ▶ Spinach ▶ Sprouts (all types) ▶ Summer squash, raw ▶ Watercress ▶ Zucchini, raw
Higher-Calorie Vegetables	1/2 cup	25 (approx.)	▶ Artichoke hearts, canned (not marinated in oil) ▶ Beets, canned (plain, not pickled) ▶ Carrots, raw ▶ Tomatoes, raw

(table continues on next page)

Table 15.1 Salad Bar Calorie Counter (continued)

	Serving Size	Calories	Examples
Starches	1/2 cup	60–100	▶ Bread (1 slice or 1 oz) ▶ Chickpeas (garbanzo beans) ▶ Crackers (4–6 pieces) ▶ Croutons (commercial) ▶ Green peas ▶ Kidney beans ▶ Pita pocket (1/2 of 6–8")
Lean Sources of Protein	1 oz	40–80	▶ Cottage cheese ▶ Egg (hard boiled) ▶ Feta cheese ▶ Ham ▶ Plain tuna
Higher-Fat Sources of Protein	1 oz	100	▶ Cheese ▶ Pepperoni
Salad Bar Mixtures	1/4 cup	35–50	▶ Fruit salad ▶ Gelatin with fruit ▶ Marinated artichoke hearts ▶ Marinated assorted vegetables ▶ Marinated mushrooms ▶ Marinated/pickled beets ▶ Pasta salad, oil-based ▶ Three-bean salad
Higher-Calorie Mixtures	1/4 cup	50–80	▶ Chicken salad ▶ Corn relish ▶ Fruit ambrosia ▶ Macaroni salad ▶ Pasta salad, mayonnaise-based ▶ Potato salad ▶ Seafood salad ▶ Tuna salad

(table continues on next page)

Table 15.1 Salad Bar Calorie Counter *(continued)*

	Serving Size	Calories	Examples
Salad Bar "Accessories"	1 Tbsp	2–5	Pickles
		2–5	Hot Pepper
		10	Raisins
		20	Chinese noodles
		27	Bacon bits
		47	Sunflower seeds
		50	Olives, green or black
		50	Peanuts
		52	Sesame seeds

Nutrition Snapshot

Health Busters

Category	Restaurant Name	Dish Name	Serving Size	Cal.	Total Fat (g)	Carb. (g)	Sod. (mg)
Fast-Food Entrée Salads	Carl's Jr.	Taco with Ground Beef	1 salad	920	57	69	1720
Fast-Food Entrée Salads	Carl's Jr.	Taco with Chicken	1 salad	780	44	66	1710
Fast-Food Entrée Salads	Wendy's	Spicy Chicken Caesar	1 salad	770	49	42	1810
Fast-Food Entrée Salads	Burger King	Garden Fresh Chicken Apple & Cranberry with Tendercrisp and Dressing	1 salad	700	41	54	1090
Fast-Food Entrée Salads	Wendy's	BLT Cobb	1 salad	660	46	14	1840
Sandwich Shop Entrée Salads	Jason's Deli	Taco with Chili (no salsa)	1 salad	1310	78	110	1510
Sandwich Shop Entrée Salads	Jason's Deli	Taco Salad SW Chicken Chili (no salsa)	1 salad	1220	70	115	1410
Sandwich Shop Entrée Salads	Au Bon Pain	Turkey Apple Brie	1 salad	660	38	59	1270
Sandwich Shop Entrée Salads	Panera Bread	Full Chicken Caesar	1 salad	510	29	29	820
Family Restaurant Entrée Salads	Boston Market	Oriental Chicken (regular)	1 salad	1380	99	91	1430

(table continues on next page)

Health Busters

Category	Restaurant Name	Dish Name	Serving Size	Cal.	Total Fat (g)	Carb. (g)	Sod. (mg)
Family Restaurant Entrée Salads	Outback Steakhouse	Aussie Chicken Cobb Crispy w/ Honey Mustard Dressing	1 salad	1302	99	64	2119
Family Restaurant Entrée Salads	Chili's	Quesadilla Explosion	1 salad	1300	86	75	2070
Family Restaurant Entrée Salads	Boston Market	Santa Fe Chicken (regular)	1 salad	1290	92	59	3550
Family Restaurant Entrée Salads	Boston Market	Santa Fe Chicken (half)	1/2 salad	990	72	53	2570
Family Restaurant Entrée Salads	Boston Market	Bruschetta Chicken (half)	1/2 salad	740	44	45	2090
Family Restaurant Entrée Salads	Boston Market	Santa Fe Chicken (half, without dressing)	1/2 salad	810	54	49	1920
Salad Dressings	T.G.I. Friday's	Honey Mustard	4 Tbsp/2 oz	310	29	12	460
Salad Dressings	T.G.I. Friday's	Thousand Island	4 Tbsp/2 oz	310	30	9	510
Salad Dressings	T.G.I. Friday's	Balsamic Vinaigrette	4 Tbsp/2 oz	300	31	7	380
Salad Dressings	T.G.I. Friday's	Bleu Cheese	4 Tbsp/2 oz	320	34	2	500

Note: Salads contain no dressing unless noted.

Healthier Bets

Category	Restaurant Name	Dish Name	Serving Size	Cal.	Total Fat (g)	Sat. Fat (g)	Carb. (g)	Pro. (g)	Fiber (g)	Chol. (mg)	Sodium (mg)	Exchanges/ Choices
Fast-Food Entrée Salads	McDonald's	Premium Southwest with Grilled Chicken	1 salad	290	8	2.5	28	27	7	70	650	1 Starch, 2 Vegetable, 3 1/2 Lean Protein
Fast-Food Entrée Salads	Carl's Jr.	Original Grilled Chicken	1 salad	270	9	3	23	25	4	70	800	1/2 Starch, 3 Vegetable, 3 Lean Protein
Fast-Food Entrée Salads	Jack in the Box	Grilled Chicken	1 salad	240	8	3.5	15	28	5	70	650	1/2 Starch, 2 Vegetable, 3 1/2 Lean Protein
Fast-Food Entrée Salads	McDonald's	Premium Bacon Ranch with Grilled Chicken	1 salad	230	9	4	10	30	4	85	700	2 Vegetable, 4 Lean Protein

(table continues on next page)

Healthier Bets

Category	Restaurant Name	Dish Name	Serving Size	Cal.	Total Fat (g)	Sat. Fat (g)	Carb. (g)	Pro. (g)	Fiber (g)	Chol. (mg)	Sodium (mg)	Exchanges/ Choices
Fast-Food Entrée Salads	McDonald's	Premium Caesar with Grilled Chicken	1 salad	190	5	3	10	27	4	70	580	2 Vegetable, 3 1/2 Lean Protein
Fast-Food Entrée Salads	Wendy's	Apple Pecan Chicken	1/2 salad	340	18	4.5	29	18	4	60	700	1 Fruit, 2 Vegetable, 2 1/2 Lean Protein, 2 Fat
Fast-Food Entrée Salads	Wendy's	BLT Cobb	1/2 salad	330	23	8	7	23	2	155	920	1 1/2 Vegetable, 3 Medium-Fat Protein, 1 1/2 Fat
Sandwich Shop Entrée Salads	Au Bon Pain	Tuna Garden	1 salad	270	13	2	19	21	5	45	530	1 Starch, 1 Vegetable, 3 Lean Protein, 1 Fat

(table continues on next page)

Healthier Bets

Category	Restaurant Name	Dish Name	Serving Size	Cal.	Total Fat (g)	Sat. Fat (g)	Carb. (g)	Pro. (g)	Fiber (g)	Chol. (mg)	Sodium (mg)	Exchanges/Choices
Sandwich Shop Entrée Salads	Jason's Deli	"Lighter" Nutty Mixed Up (no dressing)	1 salad	240	6	3	30	17	3	45	430	1 1/2 Fruit, 1 1/2 Vegetable, 2 1/2 Lean Protein
Sandwich Shop Entrée Salads	Au Bon Pain	Thai Peanut Chicken	1 salad	200	5	1	18	22	4	40	300	1 Starch, 1 Vegetable, 2 1/2 Lean Protein
Sandwich Shop Entrée Salads	Au Bon Pain	Mandarin Sesame Chicken	1 salad	310	11	2	31	20	4	35	440	1 Starch, 3 Vegetable, 2 1/2 Lean Protein, 1 Fat
Sandwich Shop Entrée Salads	Jason's Deli	Nutty Mixed Up (no chicken)	1 salad	310	12	6	47	9	5	30	380	2 Fruit, 3 Vegetable, 2 1/2 Fat

(table continues on next page)

Healthier Bets

Category	Restaurant Name	Dish Name	Serving Size	Cal.	Total Fat (g)	Sat. Fat (g)	Carb. (g)	Pro. (g)	Fiber (g)	Chol. (mg)	Sodium (mg)	Exchanges/ Choices
Sandwich Shop Entrée Salads	Togo's	Santa Fe Chicken	1/2 salad	180	8	2	16	14	5	30	480	1 Starch, 2 Lean Protein, 1/2 Fat
Sandwich Shop Entrée Salads	Au Bon Pain	Caesar Asiago	1 salad	220	12	6	18	11	3	25	470	1 Starch, 2 Vegetable, 2 Fat
Sandwich Shop Entrée Salads	Togo's	Farmer's Market	1 salad	160	6	2.5	20	7	5	10	550	1/2 Starch, 2 Vegetable, 1/2 High-Fat Protein, 1 Fat
Sandwich Shop Entrée Salads	Jason's Deli	"Lighter" Nutty Mixed Up (no chicken)	1 salad	170	6	3	29	4	3	10	170	1 1/2 Fruit, 1 Vegetable, 1 1/2 Fat

(table continues on next page)

Healthier Bets

Category	Restaurant Name	Dish Name	Serving Size	Cal.	Total Fat (g)	Sat. Fat (g)	Carb. (g)	Pro. (g)	Fiber (g)	Chol. (mg)	Sodium (mg)	Exchanges/ Choices
Sandwich Shop Entrée Salads	Jason's Deli	Three Bean (side item)	1 portion	360	12	1	37	20	11	0	500	2 1/2 Starch, 2 Lean Protein, 1 1/2 Fat
Sandwich Shop Entrée Salads	Panera Bread	Full Classic Café	1 salad	170	11	1.5	18	2	4	0	280	3 Vegetable, 3 Fat
Sandwich Shop Side Salads	Au Bon Pain	Caesar Asiago (side)	1 salad	110	6	3	9	6	2	15	240	1/2 Starch, 1 Vegetable, 1 Fat
Sandwich Shop Side Salads	Au Bon Pain	Side Garden	1 salad	60	2	0	11	2	2	0	85	2 Vegetable
Sandwich Shop Side Salads	Togo's	Santa Fe Chicken	1/2 salad	180	8	2	16	14	5	30	480	1 Starch, 2 Lean Protein, 1/2 Fat

(table continues on next page)

Healthier Bets

Category	Restaurant Name	Dish Name	Serving Size	Cal.	Total Fat (g)	Sat. Fat (g)	Carb. (g)	Pro. (g)	Fiber (g)	Chol. (mg)	Sodium (mg)	Exchanges/ Choices
Sandwich Shop Side Salads	Togo's	Chicken Caesar	1/2 salad	110	3.5	1	9	12	2	25	340	1/2 Starch, 1 1/2 Lean Protein
Family Restaurant Entrée Salads	Friendly's	Garden w/ Thousand Island Dressing	1 salad	250	19	3	18	2	2	10	520	1/2 Starch, 2 Vegetable, 3 1/2 Fat
Family Restaurant Entrée Salads	Friendly's	Garden w/ Ranch Dressing	1 salad	220	18	3	12	5	2	20	480	2 Vegetable, 3 1/2 Fat
Family Restaurant Entrée Salads	Bob Evans	Specialty Garden (no dressing)	1 salad	123	7	3	10	6	2	16	337	2 Vegetable, 1 1/2 Fat
Family Restaurant Entrée Salads	Friendly's	Garden w/ Fat-Free Italian Dressing	1 salad	90	1	0	18	2	2	0	520	1/2 Starch, 2 Vegetable

(table continues on next page)

Healthier Bets

Category	Restaurant Name	Dish Name	Serving Size	Cal.	Total Fat (g)	Sat. Fat (g)	Carb. (g)	Pro. (g)	Fiber (g)	Chol. (mg)	Sodium (mg)	Exchanges/ Choices
Family Restaurant Entrée Salads	Friendly's	Side Garden	1 side salad	60	1	0	10	2	2	0	100	2 Vegetable
Family Restaurant Entrée Salads	Boston Market	Southwest Santa Fe	1/2 salad	370	23	5	25	18	3	40	620	1 Starch, 2 Vegetable, 2 1/2 Medium-Fat Protein, 1 1/2 Fat
Family Restaurant Entrée Salads	Boston Market	Mediter-ranean	1/2 salad	320	22	5	14	18	1	45	595	3 Vegetable, 2 1/2 Medium-Fat Protein, 1 Fat
Salad Dressings	T.G.I. Friday's	Low Fat Balsamic Vinai-grette	4 Tbsp/ 2 oz	80	3	0	15	0	0	n/a	290	1 Starch

Note: Salads contain no dressing unless noted.

Get It Your Way

► Replace fried items with grilled items. Instead of fried chicken, for example, request that grilled chicken top your salad. Or skip a crispy onion topping in favor of grilled or raw onions.

► Say "no, thank you" to bacon, cheese, sour cream, and other high-fat toppings. If you are craving bacon, ask for nuts, which have all of the crunch, but are a healthier source of fat. If you want the creaminess of sour cream, try sliced avocado or guacamole (if served), which are also healthy sources of fat.

► Ask for higher-fat (bacon, cheese, etc.) or higher-carbohydrate items (such as croutons) to be used sparingly. You'll get all the flavor and texture, but in lesser amounts.

► Request the salad dressing on the side. Thin it with lemon juice (slices of limes or oranges work too), vinegar, or water.

► Scan the menu for other favorite vegetables that are not on the salad you plan to order. You can ask that these be added to your salad for more flavor and bulk.

Tips and Tactics for Gluten-Free Eating

► Request that croutons or any other bread products be left off your salad. Bacon bits may contain gluten. A separate preparation area for your salad is ideal.

► If a salad typically includes croutons and the same person is preparing the gluten-free version of the salad, ask that they change gloves before preparing your salad.

► Avoid salad bars. It's likely that not all of the ingredients are gluten-free. The scoops used for the various toppings don't always stay where they belong, so they may become contaminated.

► Ask for salad dressing such as olive oil and balsamic or red wine vinegar or lemon to be served on the side or bring your own salad dressing.

Tips and Tactics to Help Kids Eat Healthy

► Set an example. Kids are more likely to eat what they see a parent eating. If salads are a regular part of your meal, your child will be more likely to eat them.

▶ Think positively. Sure, salads may not be "kid food," but your child doesn't necessarily know that. Give your child lots of opportunities to try salads—you may be surprised by the results. Get an extra side plate and share your salad. Ask your child what vegetables from your salad they'd like to try. This is a good way to expose them to new or different ingredients.

▶ Use dressing as dip. It's no secret that kids like to dip and dunk.

▶ Let your child be the chef. Kids who make their own meals are more likely to eat them. Have your child join you on a trip to the salad bar, letting him or her make a salad, with some guidance from you, of course.

? What's Your Solution?

You're at a business lunch in a local family restaurant. Your colleagues all opt for burgers and sandwiches, but you're working hard to manage your weight, blood glucose, and blood pressure. You're determined to order a salad for a lighter lunch. Still, you don't want to seem like you're being virtuous by ordering something healthy while everyone else indulges.

Which of the following could you order to meet your healthy eating goals without feeling awkward?

a) Order a Crispy Chicken Salad that comes with bacon, cheese, tomatoes, cucumber, and ranch dressing. It's a salad, but the toppings are similar to what your colleagues are getting on their sandwiches and burgers, so you won't feel out of place.

b) Order a Crispy Chicken Salad, but without the cheese and request the dressing on the side.

c) Order a Southwest Grilled Chicken salad, which comes with fried tortilla strips, grilled vegetables, black beans, avocado, cheese, and a spicy ranch dressing.

d) Order a Southwest Grilled Chicken salad, without the fried tortilla strips and cheese. Plus, request a vinaigrette dressing and slices of fresh lime on the side, in place of the spicy ranch dressing.

See page 277 for answers.

▦ Menu Samplers

Light 'N' Healthy

Menu Samplers Section	Menu Item	Amount	Calories	Fat (g)	% Calories from Fat	Saturated Fat (g)	Chol. (mg)	Sodium (mg)	Carb. (g)	Fiber (g)	Protein (g)	Exchanges/Choices
Light 'N' Healthy (Women)	Taco salad (romaine, black beans, chicken, and fresh tomato salsa)	2.5 oz lettuce, 2 oz black beans, 2 oz chicken, 4 oz brown rice, 3.5 oz fresh salsa	380	10		1.5	63	955	49	10	25	3 Starch, 1 Vegetable, 2 Medium-Fat Protein
	Chipotle vinaigrette	1 oz	107	7		1.25	0	425	9	0	0	1/2 Other Carbohydrate, 1 1/2 Fat
Totals			**487**	**17**	**31**	**3**	**63**	**1380**	**58**	**10**	**25**	**3 Starch, 1/2 Other Carbohydrate, 1 Vegetable, 2 Medium-Fat Protein, 1 1/2 Fat**

(table continues on next page)

Light 'N' Healthy

Menu Samplers Section	Menu Item	Amount	Calories	Fat (g)	% Calories from Fat	Saturated Fat (g)	Chol. (mg)	Sodium (mg)	Carb. (g)	Fiber (g)	Protein (g)	Exchanges/ Choices
Light 'N' Healthy (Men)	Grilled chicken salad (includes grilled chicken, 3 cups of veggies, cheese, and bacon)	1 salad (10 oz)	230	9		4	80	700	10	4	30	2 Vegetable, 4 Lean Protein
	Ranch dressing	2 oz	170	15		2.5	15	530	9	0	1	1/2 Other Carbo-hydrate, 3 Fat
	Fruit smoothie	12 oz	210	0.5		0	5	50	47	3	3	2 Fruit, 1 Fat-Free Milk
	Apple slices	1 side order	33	0		0	0	0	8	2	0	1/2 Fruit
Totals			**643**	**25**	**35**	**6.5**	**100**	**1280**	**74**	**9**	**34**	**2 1/2 Fruit, 1 Fat-Free Milk, 1/2 Other Carbo-hydrate, 2 Vegetable, 4 Lean Protein, 3 Fat**

(table continues on next page)

Hearty 'N' Healthy

Menu Samplers Section	Menu Item	Amount	Calories	Fat (g)	% Calories from Fat	Saturated Fat (g)	Chol. (mg)	Sodium (mg)	Carb. (g)	Fiber (g)	Protein (g)	Exchanges/ Choices
Hearty 'N' Healthy (Women)	Chicken Caesar salad	1 entrée salad	440	26		7	125	60	19	3	34	1/2 Starch, 2 Vegetable, 5 Lean Protein, 2 Fat
	Whole-wheat baguette	1.5 oz baguette	180	2		0	0	400	32	4	7	2 Starch
Totals			620	28	41	7	125	460	51	7	41	2 1/2 Starch, 2 Vegetable, 5 Lean Protein, 2 Fat

(table continues on next page)

Hearty 'N' Healthy

Menu Samplers Section	Menu Item	Amount	Calories	Fat (g)	% Calories from Fat	Saturated Fat (g)	Chol. (mg)	Sodium (mg)	Carb. (g)	Fiber (g)	Protein (g)	Exchanges/ Choices
Hearty 'N' Healthy (Men)	Grilled chicken Cobb salad	1 entrée salad	580	17		13	75	850	17	7	53	3 Vegetable, 7 Medium-Fat Protein
	Low-fat balsamic dressing	2 oz	80	3		0	15	290	15	0	0	1 Other Carbohydrate, 1/2 Fat
	Sweet potato fries	1/2 side order	120	8		4.5	-	115	10	3	1	1 Starch, 1 1/2 Fat
	Dinner roll	2 oz	178	4		1	8	230	30	1	4	2 Starch, 1 Fat
Totals			**958**	**32**	**30**	**18.5**	**98**	**1485**	**72**	**11**	**58**	**3 Starch, 1 Other Carbohydrate, 3 Vegetable, 7 Medium-Fat Protein, 3 Fat**

(table continues on next page)

Lower Carb 'N' Healthy

Menu Samplers Section	Menu Item	Amount	Calories	Fat (g)	% Calories from Fat	Saturated Fat (g)	Chol. (mg)	Sodium (mg)	Carb. (g)	Fiber (g)	Protein (g)	Exchanges/ Choices
Lower Carb 'N' Healthy (Women)	Asian sesame chicken salad (romaine, chicken, wonton slices, sesame dressing)	1 entrée salad	417	22		3	78	499	25	3	31	1/2 Starch, 2 Vegetable, 4 Lean Protein, 3 Fat
	Baked Lay's potato chips	1/2 snack-sized bag (about 1 oz)	130	2		0	0	200	26	0	2	1 1/2 Starch, 1/2 Fat
Totals			**547**	**24**	**39**	**3**	**78**	**699**	**51**	**3**	**33**	**2 Starch, 2 Vegetable, 4 Lean Protein, 3 1/2 Fat**

(table continues on next page)

Lower Carb 'N' Healthy

Menu Samplers Section	Menu Item	Amount	Calories	Fat (g)	% Calories from Fat	Saturated Fat (g)	Chol. (mg)	Sodium (mg)	Carb. (g)	Fiber (g)	Protein (g)	Exchanges/ Choices
Lower Carb 'N' Healthy (Men)	Steakhouse salad	1 entrée salad	517	31		10	52	724	25	10	25	5 Vegetable, 3 Medium-Fat Protein, 3 Fat
	Baked potato	1/2 potato	128	0.2		0	0	14	29.2	3	3.5	2 Starch
Totals			**645**	**31**	**43**	**10**	**52**	**738**	**54**	**13**	**29**	2 Starch, 5 Vegetable, 3 Medium-Fat Protein, 3 Fat

What's Your Solution? Answers

a) Even though this is a salad, it likely contains more than 1,000 calories and loaded with fat. You'd have been better off choosing a simple sandwich or burger, and ordering a side salad.

b) These changes are a step in the right direction and will save you 100–300 calories. Make the salad even healthier by requesting grilled chicken and asking for only half the bacon.

c) Because this salad has grilled chicken and no bacon, it automatically has fewer calories and less fat than the Crispy Chicken Salad. If you're self-conscious about ordering a salad, choose the healthiest one possible so you don't have to request a lot of changes.

d) Now this is a great salad! It's loaded with lots of satisfying flavors and crunch without a ton of fat. Your colleagues may be tempted to change their order to mimic yours.

CHAPTER 16

Going Upscale—Fine Dining

Today, upscale restaurants serve quite a range of cuisines, from continental American to nearly any type of ethnic cuisine to a fusion of two or many cuisines. The age of the celebrity chef and TV food shows, as well as the availability of and the push to use locally grown and sourced foods, have upped the ante on fine dining. No matter what type of cuisine you choose, your expectations for the dining experience in an upscale restaurant are different than your expectations of a fast-food spot or family-style eatery. You expect starched linen, a water glass that is kept full, and an informed waitperson who will fully describe the menu offerings and respond to your requests and desires. Unlike less formal spots, you usually plan to linger over your meal in upscale restaurant, to enjoy each and every morsel, and soak in the ambiance and moments of relaxation.

Dining at an upscale restaurant is likely not something you do every day, unless you're lucky enough to be a restaurant critic! Chances are, when you dine upscale you're celebrating a special occasion, at a business meeting or on a business trip, or on vacation. Maybe you've read great reviews about the restaurant and booked your reservation months in advance. Whatever the case, the uniqueness and specialness of an upscale meal can make it more challenging to engage your willpower. The skills and strategies discussed in Chapter 4 (page 29) will help you make healthy choices as you enjoy these one-of-a-kind meals.

The types and serving sizes of foods served at fine dining establishments differ greatly between restaurants, making it difficult to estimate portions and provide details on nutrition counts. Nutrition information at upscale restaurants is rarely made available. However, by becoming savvy about menu lingo, being an informed restaurant patron (as informed as possible), and implementing healthy eating strategies, you can have a healthy, yet very satisfying, upscale dining experience. For dining upscale for ethnic cuisines, from Italian to Middle Eastern and beyond, see the cuisine-specific chapters in Section 3.

On the Menu

Today, upscale restaurants offer a wider gamut of foods than ever before. Fine dining has evolved from standard American fare to menus filled with a fusion of different cuisines. The menu could be a blend of French and Vietnamese food or a hybrid of Chinese and Mexican cuisines, to name just two possibilities. Fine dining menus expose us to foods, cooking styles, and culinary techniques from around the world and often showcase exciting chef creations. It's an exciting time to dine upscale!

The restaurant you choose may be one of many successful upscale establishments owned and operated by a celebrity chef who splits his or her time between the kitchen and the TV studio. From Bobby Flay to Tom Colicchio, celebrity chefs are more popular than ever, and opportunities abound to taste their craft firsthand in restaurants across the country. Many fine-dining restaurants in major U.S. cities are part of larger restaurant groups with several sister restaurants around town or in different cities. Typically, each of these restaurants has a unique menu, theme, and/or blend of cuisines, but the quality of the dining experience is ensured by an entrepreneurial chef or restaurant group.

In fine dining today, restaurants are trending toward serving organic and/or locally grown produce and promoting sustainable agriculture. Alice Waters, owner of Chez Panisse in Berkeley, California, is a long-time leader and promoter of this movement. More recently, other chefs and restaurateurs have followed suit—from celebrity chef Jamie Oliver to award-winning chef José Andrés in Washington, D.C., and a quickly growing list of others often catapulted to stardom by *Top Chef, Chopped,* and other TV shows. Depending on the restaurant's priorities and local climate, the definition of "local food" varies. It can mean the food comes from across the state, around the corner, or even from the restaurant's own rooftop garden. More and more, you'll find the name and location of the farm where certain foods in the dish were grown or raised on menus.

Local doesn't necessarily mean organic, however. When pressed, most chefs at fine dining restaurants will choose local over organic because of their trust in and relationship with local farmers and because local produce is often fresher and, therefore, more flavorful. Several of the changes that have happened in fine dining serve not only the eco-conscious diner, but the health-conscious one as well. A wider variety of foods and tastes means a wider array of nutrients to feed our bodies. Recently, the popularity of healthy whole grains has soared, like quinoa, millet, freekah, farro, amaranth, and buckwheat. These once only saw the inside of a food co-op store, but are now gracing the tables of upscale restaurants across the country (and hopefully your dining table as well). Vegetables are also enjoying a march to the center of the plate. As more of the population looks to limit meat (think of "meatless Mondays" and flexitarian and vegetarian eating plans), restaurants are responding by celebrating the humble vegetable as a main course option, or at least as a creative appetizer or side dish. Kale salads are ubiquitous, roasted vegetable salads are considered the new power lunch, and cauliflower steaks are snagging orders away from filet mignon and lamb chops.

Choosing these healthier whole grains and vegetable-centric entrées can be a good way to manage your health and blood glucose during a special meal, especially when you choose these healthier menu options over carbohydrate sources that contain added fats or sugars.

Another trend in fine dining is the prevalence of tapas, or small plates. As the tapas concept takes the upscale dining world by storm, portion sizes are skewing in favor of the health-conscious diner, at least at the restaurants that are adopting the trend. Tapas originated as a way for the Spanish to eat standing up while keeping the flies out of their wine (they used the small plates of food to cover their wine glasses). Today, you'll find small plates on the menus of restaurants serving all types of cuisines. Depending on the style of restaurant, you may see these dishes described as "small plates" or "bites" or as part of a sharing menu. When the menu is inspired by tastes from around the world, you may see other words used to describe little dishes, including "mezze," at Middle Eastern restaurants, "dim sum," in Asian settings, and "antojitos," in Latin American restaurants. No matter what they are called, small plates are a great option that can fit into your healthy eating strategy.

They are perfect for sharing, and they allow you to enjoy the tastes of many foods but in small quantities. Since Spanish cuisine inspired the small plate trend, it makes sense to also follow the Spanish culture's method of ordering: take your time. Rather than ordering the count of dishes suggested by your server at once, choose just one or two small plates at a time. Take the time to truly taste the food and enjoy good conversation. If you're still hungry, go ahead and order one or two more, but try to balance your food groups and choose a variety of foods. Always consider your level of fullness (that's your stomach, not your eyes) before ordering more.

One trend at upscale restaurants that generally doesn't work in the health-conscious diner's favor is that of the tasting menu. At some restaurants, the tasting menu may be an option in addition to the regular menu. Some examples of this are pre-theatre or fixed-price menus that allows you to choose from a quickly prepared appetizer, entrée, and dessert. Other restaurants—and these are few and far between—have a tasting menu that consists of a chef-determined seven- or twelve-course meal. The downside to any predetermined, chef-chosen meal is that you have little to no control over the meal. While these outings can certainly be a palate-pleasing extravaganza, you're generally better off dining at a restaurant where you have more control over the food you're served. Fortunately, at the majority of upscale restaurants, the chefs are more than willing to handle your special requests with aplomb, so don't hesitate to ask them to prepare your meal exactly how you want it.

Several factors—the foods placed on the table without being requested (bread and butter), the length of the meal, the portion sizes served, the elaborate preparations, and the availability of higher-fat foods, alcohol, and tempting desserts—can make upscale dining more difficult for people with diabetes. You can find more information on the pitfalls of restaurant meals in Chapter 3 (page 21), but the skills and strategies for healthier restaurant eating discussed in Chapter 4 (page 29) apply to all kinds of restaurants, including fine dining restaurants. Use them to your advantage. You should have a game plan in mind, practice portion control from the get-go, make special requests, and know when you've had enough. One strategy that is especially helpful in fine dining restaurants is to focus on the pleasure of the special occasion and/or enjoyable environment. Luxuriate in the ambiance; it helps take the importance off the food and place it on the surroundings.

The Menu Profile

Drinks

The first question your server will ask at a fine dining restaurant is: "What can I bring you to drink?" An expectation may be that diners will order a mixed drink before dinner, wine with dinner, and/or a cordial to top off the meal. A liberal flow of alcohol can tally up to hundreds of calories. If you plan to drink alcohol, figure out a plan that works best for you. Is a glass of wine before dinner sufficient, or are you better off ordering a club soda with lime before your meal and then a glass of wine with your meal? Gather more tips and tactics in Chapter 5 (page 44) and Chapter 9 (page 87).

Appetizers

Once your beverage order is in, you may be greeted with a small tastebud teaser and/or a basket of bread and butter or the signature items served in that restaurant. These items are often hard to resist. Set a limit with yourself. If the bread is to die for, allow yourself one piece, preferably without butter. If you can take or leave the items on the table, leave them and bank your calories and grams of carbohydrate for a wonderful starch or dessert.

Appetizers are often laden with fat, but there are usually a few healthy choices. When it comes to appetizers, look for an unadulterated, unfried seafood or vegetable option—marinated ceviche, a shrimp cocktail, or blanched asparagus—then share it. Keep an open mind and be creative with the menu. You can combine an appetizer, salad, and soup, for example, to create a portion-controlled meal.

Soups and Salads

Soups, if there are healthy choices such as broth- or vegetable-based, tomato, or bean soup, can be nutritious and filling. They're usually served by the bowl, which presents another opportunity to split the serving down the middle. Don't hesitate to ask the kitchen to split it for you. You should stay away from creamy soups and bisques due to their high fat content. If any item is not well explained on the menu, ask questions. The ingredients and preparations that appear on some upscale menus today can challenge even the culinary gurus among us.

Opt for a salad rather than an appetizer or soup. Look for salads containing healthy greens and low-calorie vegetables. Try salads with interesting and unique ingredients, such as kale, endive, arugula, jicama, radicchio, beets, pears, apples, nuts, and so on. Be cautious about salad dressing. Get the vinaigrette, another oil-based dressing, or request olive oil and vinegar on the side. The good news is you don't run into nearly as many creamy dressings because the chefs at upscale restaurants want their vegetables to shine. Plus, dressings are generally home-made. Be on guard against high-fat salad toppings, such as bacon, croutons, and cheeses (blue, feta, goat, or Parmesan). Simply ask that high-fat ingredients be left off or used sparingly.

Entrées

On to the entrée, which may, depending on the style of the restaurant, include a large amount of protein. Will it be chicken, duck, lamb, or shrimp? Or perhaps one of the adventurous cuts of meat, such as cheek, liver, tongue, pork belly, or marrow, that seem to be taking the culinary world by storm? No matter which entrée you choose, you'll likely be served a cooked portion weighing at least 6–8 ounces. Yes, that's about double what you need. So, be ready to practice portion control and menu creativity. Split or share complementary dishes to minimize the amount of protein you eat. You could also request that half be put in a takeout container, or you could leave a few bites on your plate.

Think about choosing low-fat fish, shellfish, or chicken as your entrée—as long as these options aren't deep-fried or covered with loads of butter or cream before they reach your table. Consider the description of Chicken Kiev: a breast of chicken filled with herb butter and garlic and topped with butter sauce. Now, compare this with the description of a chicken and vegetable sauté: diced chicken breast sautéed in olive oil with sun-dried tomatoes, herbs, and asparagus. Neither dish is fat-free, but the latter is certainly a lower-fat choice. Some seafood medleys, such as cioppino and bouillabaisse, offer healthfully prepared fish in a light broth. Additionally, preparations of fish that keep the amount of fat low (e.g., grilling or poaching) are healthy choices. You still need to be mindful of portion with these dishes, but their fat content is tame compared to family-style American meals and portions are typically much smaller. Another trend in upscale dining is to serve an entire fish, head and all, rather than just a fillet. If this is the case with a dish you order, be prepared to share.

Seafood and chicken are often healthier choices, but unadulterated beef, lamb, or veal might be wiser bets if the seafood or chicken is loaded with fat during preparation. If you order meat, stick with a small cut—"petite," "queen," "filet mignon," and "8-ounce" are descriptions of small servings. You can even split these as there's often enough for two. Better yet, search for dishes that mix protein with starches or vegetables. That way you'll end up with smaller amounts of protein. Next, choose leaner cuts of meat. Filet mignon (also called tenderloin) and sirloin are leaner cuts than rib eye, porterhouse, T-bone, or prime rib. Veal is often breaded and sautéed prior to cooking, but if you spot a broiled veal chop on the menu and you like veal, you can consider this choice, but you should also consider splitting it. The portion will be large. Lamb, depending on the cut, can be high in fat, but it is most often broiled or grilled, which doesn't add much fat. If there's fat to trim once the meat arrives, do so. Loin lamb chops are the lamb choice with the lowest fat content. Duck, skin and all, is quite high in fat. However, today, sliced duck breast is served, rather than the half duck of yesteryear. Sliced duck is quite lean and the fatty skin is gone. Often light fruit sauces or glazes are used on duck breast. Be careful of these, they can ramp up the carbohydrate grams. Order them on the side and use a small amount for flavor boosts.

Many upscale restaurants now offer vegetarian entrées. Survey these options. They're a good way to cut back on the protein. There might be pasta dishes, Chinese stir-fries, or grilled vegetable platters. Be careful that vegetarian entrées don't come loaded with fat, cheese, or a double dose of carbohydrate. Be creative and design your own vegetarian meal by ordering à la carte appetizers, soups, salads, and side items, and skipping the entrée. Or consider splitting one vegetarian entrée and one protein-dense entrée between two or even three people. Keep that strategy of ordering fewer dishes than the number of people at the table in mind. Enjoy the tastes and control portions with one strategy.

Side Dishes

A starch is usually, but not always, included with entrées or available à la carte. Again, it's a good idea to search for unadulterated starches (starches with no or minimal added fats). Healthy starch choices include baked potatoes, red potatoes, rice, couscous, or any new, interesting grain that you'd like to be introduced to—millet, freekah, or quinoa. If you believe fat will be added to the starch you choose, ask to have it left off or on the side. If you order a baked potato, ask that the butter and sour cream be served on the side. Your entrée may also include a side of vegetables. Ask how these are prepared if it's not clear. Make sure that cream, cheese, sour cream, and hollandaise sauces are left in the kitchen. Steamed vegetables are the healthiest choices; sautéed, grilled, and roasted vegetables likely have some oil added. If vegetables don't come with your entrée, order them à la carte. But consider the preparation method.

Desserts

Upscale restaurants cry out: "Have some dessert! It's a special occasion." Needless to say, these desserts are often decadent and the carbohydrate count can range from 50–100 grams and beyond, making glucose control a challenge. If you want to save your calories and carbohydrate grams earlier in the meal and splurge on dessert, remember that a taste or two of a sweet may be all you need to satisfy that sweet tooth. To limit your bites, share a dessert with several dining partners. In upscale restaurants serving lighter cuisine, fruit might be found on the dessert menu. Often the offering is berries with crème fraîche and liqueur. Hold the crème fraîche, but let them pour a few drizzles of the liqueur—it's fat-free (and relatively low in calories). See Chapter 8 (page 78) for additional tips on navigating the dessert menu.

 Green-Flag Words

Ingredients:

- Amaranth, barley, couscous, freekah, farro, millet, polenta, quinoa, cracked wheat, wheat berries, other whole grains
- Balsamic, raspberry, or any type of vinegar
- Chipotle peppers or sauces
- Herbs and spices
- Leafy green vegetables (kale, spinach, collards)
- Vinaigrette dressing (made with a combination of various oils, vinegars, and herbs)
- Onion, garlic, shallots
- Rice (brown, wild, risotto)
- Roasted peppers
- Sun-dried tomatoes
- Mustards

► Olives, olive oil
► Salsa (fruit or vegetable based)

Cooking Methods/Menu Descriptions:

► Au jus (with juice of meat)
► Au poivre (heavily peppered)
► Blackened
► Cajun
► En brochette (on skewer)
► En papillote (in parchment package)
► Fruit sauce
► Grilled, grilled on mesquite or hickory chips
► Marinated
► Mustard sauce (make sure it's not a cream sauce)
► Petite or queen size
► Poached
► Roasted
► Steamed
► Tomato, garlic, or herb sauce
► Wine sauce (red or white; make sure it's not a cream sauce)

⊗ Red-Flag Words

Ingredients:

► Bacon
► Butter, drawn butter, cream, beurre blanc, brown butter, béchamel (white sauce), béarnaise (brown sauce)
► Cheese (blue, goat, mozzarella, feta, Parmesan)
► Hollandaise, rémoulade, mornay sauce (other white sauces and mayonnaise-based sauces)
► Melted cheese
► Nuts (small amounts are alright)
► Pancetta
► Pistachio, orange, herb, garlic butter
► Sausage
► Sour cream, crème fraiche, whipped cream

Cooking Methods/Menu Descriptions:

- ▶ Au gratin
- ▶ Casserole (usually has butter, cream, and/or cheese and breadcrumb topping)
- ▶ Cheese sauce
- ▶ Creamy mushroom sauce
- ▶ Garlic and herbed cream sauce
- ▶ Served in pastry shell
- ▶ Stroganoff
- ▶ Stuffed with seasoned breadcrumbs
- ▶ Wellington
- ▶ Wrapped in bacon, phyllo dough, or puff pastry

At the Table:

- ▶ Butter
- ▶ Extra-high-fat sauces
- ▶ Olive oil
- ▶ Salad dressing
- ▶ Sour cream

Healthy Eating Tips and Tactics

- ▶ Have a plan. Peruse the menu and read online reviews from other diners before you even set foot in the restaurant. It's easier to make decisions when you're not hungry, and reviews from other diners can clue you in on preparation details that you may not hear from the wait staff (a reviewer might let you know if a certain dish is too salty or too greasy, for example).
- ▶ Observe portion sizes before you order as you eye others being served appetizers, main entrees, and more.
- ▶ Talk to your waitperson. Ask them what they think the healthiest, yet tastiest, dish is. They not only are familiar with every item on the menu, but they have the benefit of seeing all the items as they are being prepared and have likely tasted nearly every dish. They may even be able to make off-menu recommendations—delicious and healthy items that the chef prepares for the staff, but doesn't feature on the menu.

▶ Follow the strategy that food critics use: enjoy your meal in moderation. Relish the experience by taking a bite of this and a taste of that. Now is not the time to join the clean-plate club.

▶ Request that the chef use less oil, butter, or cream when preparing your dish. Chefs appreciate a challenge and will often come up with a new way to flavor your meal, such as with a special vinaigrette that they may whip up just for you.

▶ Fill up on vegetables before your entrée arrives. Upscale restaurants are really doing fabulous things with vegetables these days. Choose a vegetable-centric appetizer, soup, or salad to enjoy before your entrée. A healthy starter will help fill you up so that you're less tempted to polish off every last bite of your entrée or dessert.

▶ Soak in your surroundings. Enjoy conversation with your dining companions. Order one course at a time and relish the taste of every single bite.

Get It Your Way

▶ Talk to your waitperson about how the dish is prepared. He or she will likely be well versed in discussing all the main ingredients and preparation methods. Use the information provided to customize your order healthfully.

▶ Ask for your entrée to be split in the kitchen so that you and your dining companion can both enjoy a smaller amount of it.

▶ Request that less oil, butter, cream, or cheese be used in the preparation of your dish or ask that high-fat ingredients be served on the side so you can control the amount that goes on your dish.

▶ Request a healthy preparation method, when possible. For example, if the entrée you want is typically fried, ask if they can grill it or broil it instead.

▶ Make small substitutions to what you order. Choose healthier salad dressings, ask for sauces on the side, pick steamed rather than sautéed vegetables, ask for your entrée to be grilled not fried. You get the picture. Lots of little tweaks can add up to a big nutritional difference.

Tips and Tactics for Gluten-Free Eating

▶ You may have better luck eating gluten-free in more expensive restaurants, as the staff may be more attentive to your gluten-free dining requests and willing to tackle bigger challenges in the kitchen.
Be sure to ask the usual questions before you order *and* once your
meal is served. You may want to call ahead to ask some questions.
See Chapter 6 (page 56) for some examples of the kinds of questions you should ask.

Tips and Tactics to Help Kids Eat Healthy

▶ Upscale restaurants aren't usually kid-friendly places, thus you won't
often find kids' menus. So it's the perfect time to expose your child to a
variety of foods that may be new or different and prepared to perfection.

▶ Share dishes with your child. This will allow both of you to enjoy a few
tastes of a variety of options.

▶ Talk to your child about the menu. Discuss where the food comes
from, how it was prepared, and what it tastes like. Kids who are knowledgeable about food and have the vocabulary to describe various
tastes and textures are more likely to make healthier food choices no
matter where they eat.

▶ Think of fine dining restaurants as a training ground to teach your
children about table manners and healthy eating behaviors that can
last them a lifetime.

(?) What's Your Solution?

It's your wedding anniversary and you and your spouse have reservations at a
highly reviewed traditional French restaurant. You rarely go to such an expensive restaurant and you want to thoroughly enjoy this dining experience.

*How can you celebrate, enjoying this restaurant's offerings to the fullest, and still
honor your healthy eating goals?*

a) Read the menu online (if available) and check out online reviews
from other diners before you head to the restaurant. Pick out a

few options that you think you'd like to try, discuss them with your spouse, and, together, evaluate how these could fit into your healthy eating plan.

b) Engage your spouse in sharing an appetizer, entrée, and/or dessert with you. How romantic!

c) Customize your order. For example, if you plan to order the traditional French onion soup, ask them to skip the bread and put very little cheese on it. For your salad, request the dressing on the side. If you want a steak, order the petite portion, request that they hold the herb butter. Skip the mashed potatoes and order the side of barley and herbs you spotted served with another dish. Say yes to the garden-fresh green beans that come with your dish.

d) All of the above.

See page 297 for answers.

Menu Samplers

Light 'N' Healthy

Menu Samplers Section	Menu Item	Amount	Calories	Fat (g)	% Calories from Fat	Saturated Fat (g)	Chol. (mg)	Sodium (mg)	Carb. (g)	Fiber (g)	Protein (g)	Exchanges/Choices
Light 'N' Healthy (Women)	Braised lamb (leg and shoulder)	1/2 entrée (3 oz cooked)	190	7.5		3	92	660	0	0	29	4 Lean Protein
	Jasmine rice	3/4 cup	210	3.75		0	0	549	40	1	4	3 Starch, 1/2 Fat
	Roasted butternut squash	1 cup	82	0		0	0	8	22	2	2	1 1/2 Starch
	Mixed berries	1 cup	70	0		0	0	0	17	5	0	1 Fruit
Totals			**552**	**11**	**18**	**3**	**92**	**1217**	**79**	**8**	**35**	**4 1/2 Starch, 1 Fruit, 4 Lean Protein, 1/2 Fat**

(table continues on next page)

Light 'N' Healthy

Menu Samplers Section	Menu Item	Amount	Calories	Fat (g)	% Calories from Fat	Saturated Fat (g)	Chol. (mg)	Sodium (mg)	Carb. (g)	Fiber (g)	Protein (g)	Exchanges/Choices
Light 'N' Healthy (Men)	Mussels in red, white, and garlic sauce	1/2 entrée (3 oz)	146	4		1	48	314	6	0	20	3 Lean Protein
	Linguine with red sauce	1/2 entrée (3 oz)	310	4		1	0	670	55	5	23	4 Starch, 2 Lean Protein
	Mixed greens side salad	1 cup	8	0		0	0	12	1	0	0	1/2 Vegetable
	Oil and vinegar dressing	1 Tbsp olive oil	120	14		2	0	0	0	0	0	3 Fat
	Fruit tart	1 mini (individual)	220	9		3.5	5	370	31	1	1	1 Fruit, 1 Other Carbohydrate, 2 Fat
Totals			**804**	**31**	**35**	**7.5**	**53**	**1366**	**93**	**6**	**44**	**4 Starch, 1 Fruit, 1 Other Carbohydrate, 1/2 Vegetable, 5 Lean Protein, 3 Fat**

(table continues on next page)

Hearty 'N' Healthy

Menu Samplers Section	Menu Item	Amount	Calories	Fat (g)	% Calories from Fat	Saturated Fat (g)	Chol. (mg)	Sodium (mg)	Carb. (g)	Fiber (g)	Protein (g)	Exchanges/ Choices
Hearty 'N' Healthy (Women)*	Roast duck breast	4 oz	227	13		0	101	73	0	0	27	4 Lean Protein, 1 Fat
	Rice pilaf	1/2 cup	180	3		0	0	650	34	1	4	2 Starch
	Sautéed spinach with garlic	3 oz	45	3		1	0	320	4	2	3	1 Vegetable, 1 Fat
	Whole-wheat roll	2 rolls (1 oz each)	148	2		0	0	280	27	5	6	2 Starch
	Chocolate mousse	1/2 small portion	150	11		7	60	25	13	1	2	1 Other Carbohydrate, 2 Fat
Totals			750	32	38	8	161	1348	78	9	42	4 Starch, 1 Other Carbohydrate, 1 Vegetable, 4 Lean Protein, 4 Fat

*This meal has a slightly higher than recommended cholesterol level due to the duck.

(table continues on next page)

Hearty 'N' Healthy

Menu Samplers Section	Menu Item	Amount	Calories	Fat (g)	% Calories from Fat	Saturated Fat (g)	Chol. (mg)	Sodium (mg)	Carb. (g)	Fiber (g)	Protein (g)	Exchanges/Choices
Hearty 'N' Healthy (Men)*	Sirloin steak	4 oz cooked with 1/8 inch fat	275	16		6	85	663	0	0	31	4 Medium-Fat Protein
	Baked potato	1 medium	256	1		0	0	28	58	6	7	4 Starch
	Sour cream	1 Tbsp	26	2.5		1.6	5	6	0	0	0.5	1/2 Fat
	Grilled asparagus	5 spears	78	5		0	0	418	5	3	3	1 Vegetable, 1 Fat
	Beet, goat cheese, and spinach salad	1 oz goat cheese, 1 cup salad	130	9		6	22	285	7	2	8	1 Vegetable, 1 High-Fat Protein
	Oil and vinegar dressing	1 Tbsp olive oil	120	14		2	0	0	0	0	0	3 Fat
Totals			885	47.5	48	16	112	1400	70	11	50	4 Starch, 2 Vegetable, 5 Medium-Fat Protein, 4 1/2 Fat

*This meal has a slightly higher than recommended cholesterol level due to the steak and goat cheese.

(table continues on next page)

Lower Carb 'N' Healthy

Menu Samplers Section	Menu Item	Amount	Calories	Fat (g)	% Calories from Fat	Saturated Fat (g)	Chol. (mg)	Sodium (mg)	Carb. (g)	Fiber (g)	Protein (g)	Exchanges/ Choices
Lower Carb 'N' Healthy (Women)	Gnocchi	1/2 cup	159	0		0	0	503	36	0	4	2 Starch
	Sautéed mushrooms	2 oz	47	1		0	0	415	10	2	2	2 Vegetable
	Roasted chicken breast	3 oz (without skin)	142	3		1	73	164	0	0	26	3 1/2 Lean Protein
	Arugula greens salad with walnuts	1 cup greens, 1/2 oz walnuts	98	9		1	0	5	3	1	2	1 Vegetable, 2 Fat
	Oil and vinegar dressing	1 Tbsp olive oil	120	14		2	0	0	0	0	0	3 Fat
Totals			**566**	**27**	**43**	**4**	**73**	**1087**	**49**	**3**	**34**	**2 Starch, 3 Vegetable, 3 1/2 Lean Protein, 5 Fat**

(table continues on next page)

Lower Carb 'N' Healthy

Menu Samplers Section	Menu Item	Amount	Calories	Fat (g)	% Calories from Fat	Saturated Fat (g)	Chol. (mg)	Sodium (mg)	Carb. (g)	Fiber (g)	Protein (g)	Exchanges/Choices
Lower Carb 'N' Healthy (Men)	Black pepper crusted pork tenderloin	4 oz	185	5		2	80	63	0	0	32	4 Lean Protein
	Braised collard greens	3 oz	35	0		0	0	200	7	3	3	1 1/2 Vegetable
	Steamed carrots	1/2 cup	55	4		0	0	87	9	4	1	1 Vegetable, 1 Fat
	Rustic mashed potatoes	1/2 cup	160	8		1.5	0	400	20	1	2	1 1/2 Starch, 1 Fat
	Whole-wheat roll	2 rolls (1 oz each)	148	2		0	0	280	27	5	6	2 Starch
	Apple pie	1/2 slice	215	10		4	10	230	15	2	2	1 Other Carbohydrate, 2 Fat
Totals			**798**	**29**	**33**	**7.5**	**90**	**1260**	**78**	**15**	**46**	**3 1/2 Starch, 1 Other Carbohydrate, 2 1/2 Vegetable, 4 Lean Protein, 4 Fat**

(i) What's Your Solution? Answers

a) Excellent strategy. Having a plan in advance is one of the best ways to make smart choices. And talking about it with your spouse increases your accountability and the likelihood of success.

b) Sharing is a smart way to feel satisfied. You get to experience lots of flavors and textures while limiting your portion sizes. Given the number of courses you are ordering, this is still likely to be a lot of food, so consider leaving some food on your plate or taking some home.

c) Customization is key, especially at French restaurants that are notorious for high-fat ingredients. Asking your waitperson for additional ways to customize your order is another great way to make your meal even healthier.

d) Yes, yes, and yes! Combining all these strategies together will help ensure that you have a delicious, satisfying meal that controls portions, calories, and your blood glucose level. After all, you are not just celebrating your anniversary, you're also celebrating each other, and your health is a key part of that.

CHAPTER 17

Seafood

Seafood, from finfish to shellfish, is a menu option in many restaurants. Several large chains specialize in seafood. The best known and largest seafood chains are Bonefish Grill, Joe's Crab Shack, Legal Seafood, and Red Lobster. You'll also find plenty of individually owned and operated seafood restaurants scattered throughout the country (though they're more abundant on our east and west coasts, where fresh seafood is most plentiful).

You'll also find seafood served fast, from fried fish sandwiches in fast-food spots, including the ones covered in Chapter 13 (page 190), to the seafood served in a few fast-food chains dedicated to seafood, such as Captain D's and Long John Silver's. You'll find these restaurants covered in this chapter. Seafood and tuna salad are frequently stuffed into subs, sandwiches, and increasingly in hard and soft tacos. Sandwiches and subs are covered in Chapter 14 (page 222). Fish and shellfish dishes are served in most family-style restaurants covered in Chapter 12 (page 156).

Seafood is frequently found on the menus of upscale restaurants (covered in Chapter 16, page 278), with offerings including fried calamari, ceviche, slowly simmered mussels, and a variety of fillets prepared on the grill. Seafood is also served aplenty in ethnic restaurants, from Asian cuisines to Mexican. Check out the cuisine-specific chapters in Section 3 for more information on the seafood offerings at ethnic restaurants.

🍴 On the Menu

On the health spectrum, seafood dishes range from being prepared very healthfully—using methods such as steaming, poaching, or grilling—to being soaked in fat and carbohydrate when they are battered or breaded and fried. Consider the huge nutritional differences between grilled swordfish and fried clams that then may be dunked in mayonnaise-based tartar sauce. Granted, the portion size of the swordfish dish is likely big enough for two. But overall, grilled swordfish, with its high omega-3 fat content, is much healthier than clams that have been breaded and deep-fried.

Due to the increased demand for healthfully prepared finfish and shellfish, tasty cooking methods have evolved to please the nutrition-conscious. Seafood can be grilled on charcoal or flavored wood chips, lightly pan-fried, seasoned with different combinations of spices, topped with a variety of wine- or mustard-based sauces, or paired with a variety of fruit or vegetable salsas. Seafood dishes featuring these preparation methods are usually healthy options. And sushi, which may contain raw or cooked seafood (or even no seafood at all), has become increasingly popular in recent years.

Health Benefits of Seafood

Seafood (shellfish and finfish) has earned a gold star for health, largely because of the high amount of omega-3 polyunsaturated fatty acids some of it provides. An increase in omega-3 consumption has been shown to benefit cholesterol levels and to help reduce the risk of heart disease. According to the *Dietary Guidelines for Americans*, common seafood varieties that rank among the highest in omega-3 fatty acid content are different types of salmon (Atlantic, chinook, coho, pink, and sockeye), anchovies, herring, shad, mackerel (Atlantic and Pacific, not King), tuna (bluefin, albacore, and canned white albacore), sardines (Atlantic and Pacific), oysters (Pacific), freshwater trout, blue mussels, and squid.

A bonus incentive to eat more seafood is that when you eat fish, you not only gain the health benefits from the fish, but the fish you eat is likely replacing (or actually displacing) the fatty red meat and full-fat dairy foods, most often cheese, that you may have eaten. You're eating a lower-fat food with healthier fats and fewer calories! This is one reason why choosing to eat fish has been shown to help people eat less saturated fat.

When it comes to seafood, especially fish, the bottom line is to eat more of it as long as it's prepared healthfully and served in reasonable portions. Health authorities recommend eating two or more servings of fish each week to gain the health benefits of this type of food. According to the *Dietary Guidelines for Americans,* this means that most people should eat a total of at least 8 ounces of fish (two 4-ounce cooked servings) per week. Pregnant women, however, should aim for no more than 12 ounces of fish per week due to potential health concerns (see *The Safety of Seafood* below).

Yet, even with all this positive news about seafood, Americans haven't increased seafood consumption much. According to the *Dietary Guidelines for Americans,* the mean intake of seafood in the United States is about 3.5 ounces per week. One more concern is that Americans eat a limited variety of fish: the five most popular fish we eat are canned tuna, shrimp, pollock, salmon, and cod. So, think about eating seafood more often and branching out to include different varieties of omega-3–rich seafood.

The Safety of Seafood

From time to time you may hear a warning to eat less fish due to potential unhealthy contaminants in seafood; people talk about mercury, polychlorinated biphenyls, and other contaminants. The bottom line for most people is that the benefits of fish, as noted above, outweigh the risks. Plus, there are ways to minimize your risk of consuming contaminants. According to the Environmental Protection Agency (EPA), shark, swordfish, king mackerel, and tilefish are among the varieties of fish that can be high in mercury. These fish should be avoided by pregnant women and young children. While this recommendation may scare pregnant women away from eating all types of fish, the *Dietary Guidelines for Americans* recommend that pregnant women eat up to 12 ounces of cooked seafood per week. This is because of the health benefits of fish, particularly the benefits that omega-3s may provide to the developing child's brain.

If you're looking for seafood options that are low in mercury, five of the most commonly eaten low-mercury varieties, according to the EPA, are shrimp, canned light tuna, salmon, pollock, and catfish. If mercury is still a concern to you, visit the EPA's Fish Advisory Website at www.epa.gov/ost/fish for a listing of the mercury levels in fish. Another good resource to check in on seafood sustainability is the Monterey Bay Aquarium Seafood

Watch program, which assesses how fisheries and farmed seafood impact the environment and provides recommendations. You can visit their website at http://www.seafoodwatch.org/cr/seafoodwatch.aspx. Other tips for minimizing contaminants in the seafood you eat: Check local advisories about contaminants in fish caught in your area and remove the skin and surface fat, where some contaminants concentrate.

Another safety concern relates to eating raw seafood. Since the early 2000s, when an FDA regulation went into effect, restaurants serving raw seafood (or undercooked animal foods) are required to provide both a disclosure and reminder about this on their menu. The consumer advisory is intended to inform consumers, especially susceptible populations (the elderly, children, pregnant mothers, people who have an immune deficiency disease), about the increased risk of foodborne illness that comes from eating these foods. If you believe it's safe for you, go ahead and enjoy raw fish. But make sure that the raw bar, sushi counter, or restaurant you choose sells a lot of raw fish. That generally indicates that they get fresh fish regularly and use what they get quickly. Look at the fish, if possible, to make sure it looks and smells fresh. If in doubt, don't eat it. Anyone who has a compromised immune system, including pregnant women, infants, young children, and older adults, should avoid eating raw seafood. Read more about eating sushi and sashimi in Chapter 23 on Japanese food (page 475).

The Menu Profile

Fish and seafood are naturally low in total and saturated fat and low in calories as long as they are not fried. All seafood, exclusive of how it is prepared, ranges from about 30–60 calories per ounce (cooked). Check out *Health Busters* and *Healthier Bets* on page 306, later in this chapter, to see the nutrition numbers for commonly served seafood dishes. Cod, scallops, and monkfish are on the low-calorie side, whereas swordfish, salmon, and bluefish are on the higher-calorie side of the range due to their slightly high fat content (mostly omega-3s). Most flatfish, such as flounder, sole, and halibut, are lower in calories and fat compared to most cuts of red meats and some poultry.

One point of frequent misinformation is the belief that seafood is, in general, lower in dietary cholesterol than red meat and poultry. The reality is, the cholesterol numbers for most finfish are in the same ballpark as the numbers for red meat and poultry—around 45–75 milligrams (mg) of cholesterol per 3-ounce (oz) cooked portion. And in fact, some shellfish, namely shrimp (165 mg per 3 oz) and calamari (255 mg per 3 oz), is quite high in dietary cholesterol. To see the cholesterol content of some seafood dishes, check out *Healthier Bets* on page 309.

Fish is fairly low in sodium prior to preparation, which is another health benefit. To maintain this health benefit, choose low-sodium preparations. A few items, such as surimi (imitation crab), crab, lobster, shrimp, mussels, and oysters, have a slightly higher sodium count.

The nutritional virtues of fish and seafood are lost in most chain seafood restaurants because their favorite preparation method is battering or breading and deep-frying seafood. After fish and seafood have been battered and fried, you may wonder where the fish is. When you read the nutrition numbers, there's not much left that resembles the health benefits and nutritional value of fish. Additionally, fried fish is often surrounded by high-fat plate fillers—hush puppies, french fries, or coleslaw drenched in a mayonnaise-based dressing. Thus, the once-healthy seafood is now part of a fat- and calorie-dense meal.

Appetizers

If you're at a family-style or upscale restaurant specializing in seafood, your dining partner may choose to fill up on a high-fat cup of New England clam chowder or fried calamari or shrimp. Your best bet is to start with a healthy appetizer from the raw bar, where almost all the items are very low in fat and served with low-calorie sauces, such as a tomato-based cocktail sauce or a broth-based garlic sauce. Healthy options to look for include oysters on the half shell, tuna tartar or carpaccio, yellowtail sashimi, mussels steeped in garlic wine sauce, shrimp cocktail, or mixed shellfish ceviche.

Of course, no matter where you are, be wary of anything fried. For example, Joe's Crab Shack's Great Balls of Fire appetizer features lean crab, but it's loaded with cream cheese, battered, and then deep fried, bringing the calorie total to over 1,000 with 71 grams of fat and 77 grams of carbohydrate! The Singapore Calamari at Bonefish Grill has similar nutritional values. If the only seafood appetizers available are fried, you'd be better off avoiding them altogether.

Soups and Salads

Clam chowder is typical in many seafood restaurants, whether family style or upscale. New England clam chowder has a base of milk and/or cream, whereas Manhattan clam chowder has a tomato base, which would be healthier. But you don't see Manhattan chowder served nearly as much as New England chowder. Another popular menu option in seafood-specialty restaurants is bouillabaisse, a fish stew featuring at least three kinds of fish and often some shellfish in a tomato base with traditional Provençal herbs. This can be a hearty, filling dish that is high in protein and relatively low in fat. Just be mindful of the portion size, which can often be quite large.

Salads featuring a variety of seafood are also common at seafood restaurants. Several options are available, from a Caesar salad topped with salmon to a Niçoise salad, typically featuring grilled tuna, hard boiled eggs, green beans, potatoes, olives, and tomatoes. A salad with lots of crunchy vegetables and grilled seafood is certainly a very healthy option. But be sure to use dressing sparingly, limit high-fat toppings, and be mindful of portions. See Chapter 15 (page 250) for more tips on eating healthy restaurant salads.

Sandwiches and Tacos

The fried fish sandwich, served with hush puppies or french fries, is a staple in many restaurants, especially fast-food restaurants. Generally speaking, these sandwiches feature more breading, fat, and bread than they do fish. To add insult to injury, sometimes more fat is added on top in the form of cheese and/or mayonnaise-based sauces, like tartar sauce. Granted, you can ask for these additions to be left off your sandwich, but you're still eating a piece of fried fish. Family-style or seafood-specialty restaurants will likely allow you to customize your fish sandwich order to include a grilled fillet, rather than the fried version.

Fish tacos are growing in popularity, not just at restaurants and bars, but also at food trucks and the beachside stands that dot the coasts. Usually these tacos feature a white, flaky fish, such as mahi mahi or tilapia. But any type of seafood can be used. Shrimp, salmon, halibut, and tuna frequently make an appearance. Sometimes the fish is grilled or fried. Opt for grilled fish, when possible, to keep the fat level down. Taco toppings vary, but guacamole, sour cream (you should opt for guacamole but hold the sour cream), and some type of slaw, either a cabbage or mango slaw, or lettuce or cabbage typically finishes off the tacos. Fish tacos, especially soft tacos with fish that's not fried, can be a healthy choice. Do be aware of a few extra carbohydrate grams in salsa and sauces, especially those made with fruits.

Surimi, Sashimi, and Sushi

Surimi is the crabmeat look-alike that is substituted for or used in combination with crabmeat in sushi (California rolls and others), seafood salads, and casseroles. You'll typically find this ingredient in moderately priced restaurants. Surimi is most often made from pollock, which gets a good health rating for its omega-3 fatty acid content with minimal mercury. However, it's a bit higher in sodium than other finfish due to processing. It also contains a bit of sugar (it even tastes a bit sweet) and thus carbohydrate. Surimi is much less expensive and more available than crabmeat. If you spot a menu listing for "seafood" salad rather than crabmeat salad, it will likely contain surimi.

Sashimi, which is raw fish sliced into thin pieces, and sushi, which is a roll made with fish (cooked or raw), vegetables, avocado, and/or other ingredients and then rolled up with seaweed and a sweetened vinegar rice, have gained considerable popularity in the United States. Sushi can be a healthy option, but as always, preparation impacts everything. Sushi sometimes contains, or is topped with, mayonnaise-based sauces or cream cheese, and certain rolls feature tempura-battered and fried seafood, like shrimp or softshell crab. For detailed information about sushi and sashimi, check out Chapter 23 (page 475).

Entrées

There are many varieties of finfish served in seafood and upscale restaurants today, which makes this a great time to be adventurous and broaden your seafood horizons. Explore the tastes of the creative low-fat and low-calorie preparation methods used by many chefs today. Consider, for example, trying poached salmon, steamed halibut and vegetables, barbecued shrimp, mesquite-grilled tuna, swordfish kebabs, braised monkfish with wine sauce, or blackened mahi mahi. Make sure you ask about any marinades, sauces, or toppings that might add grams of carbohydrate to the dish you choose. It's not unusual for sauces and toppings to contain some sugar, juice, and/or cornstarch.

It's best to stay away from the classic fish 'n' chips entrée—fried fish and potatoes—due to its high fat and calorie content. Another popular menu item is the crab cake. Be sure to ask about the preparation style: some crabcakes contain more breading than crabmeat or the converse, while others can have a large dollop of tartar sauce slopped on top before it's put on the bread or roll. Crabcakes can be broiled, grilled, pan-fried, or deep-fried. Make sure the description of your dish matches your healthy eating criteria before you order or you're able to get it your way.

As always, you'll need dodge the fat. You'll often see healthy options stuffed with unhealthy ingredients or doused in cream or butter sauce. It's best to avoid these dishes due to the high fat and calorie content. So, learn to be an avid fat detective.

Finally, don't forget the healthy restaurant eating strategy of practicing portion control from the start. Think about sharing an entrée. Often you'll get 8–10 ounces of cooked fish when you order from a seafood restaurant. Split the portion with your dining partner or put half into a take-home container before you dig in. Order an extra side of vegetables so you can fill yourself up for fewer calories and less fat.

Nutrition Snapshot

Health Busters

Category	Restaurant Name	Dish Name	Serving Size	Cal.	Total Fat (g)	Carb. (g)	Sod. (mg)
Appetizers	Red Lobster	Batterfried Crawfish (appetizer)	1 portion	1190	69	104	2740
Appetizers	Red Lobster	Parrot Isle Jumbo Coconut Shrimp (appetizer)	1 portion	530	36	34	1110
Appetizers	Joe's Crab Shack	Crazy Good Crab Dip	1 portion	1270	87	92	3430
Appetizers	Joe's Crab Shack	Calamari, Fried	1 portion	900	58	61	1070
Soups	Outback Steakhouse	Clam Chowder Soup (bowl)	1 bowl	564	41	23	2275
Soups	Red Lobster	Creamy Potato Bacon Soup (bowl)	1 bowl	450	30	37	1580
Soups	Ninety Nine Restaurant	Maine Lobster Bisque (crock)	1 crock	700	53	39	1550
Salads	Applebee's	Clam Chowder (bowl)	1 bowl	370	26	22	1050

(table continues on next page)

Health Busters

Category	Restaurant Name	Dish Name	Serving Size	Cal.	Total Fat (g)	Carb. (g)	Sod. (mg)
Salads	Applebee's	Grilled Shrimp on Spinach Salad (regular, without dressing)	1 salad	630	46	20	1660
Salads	Applebee's	Grilled Shrimp on Spinach Salad (half, without dressing)	1/2 salad	400	30	12	1120
Seafood Entrées	Red Lobster	Walleye, Beer Battered	1 portion	700	42	24	1200
Seafood Entrées	Red Lobster	Walleye, Fried	1 portion	600	29	35	990
Seafood Entrées	Red Lobster	Seaside Shrimp Trio	1 portion	1010	55	65	3940
Seafood Entrées	Ruby Tuesday	Lobster Carbonara	1 portion	1406	95	80	3796
Seafood Entrées	Joe's Crab Shack	Seafood Fun-Do	1 portion	1310	69	127	3190
Seafood Entrées	Joe's Crab Shack	Fried Oysters	1 portion	1060	64	104	2510
Seafood Entrées	Captain D's	1/2 lb Clams	1 portion	770	47	64	1450
Sandwiches	Applebee's	Blackened Tilapia Sandwich	1 sandwich	740	42	54	1800

(table continues on next page)

Health Busters

Category	Restaurant Name	Dish Name	Serving Size	Cal.	Total Fat (g)	Carb. (g)	Sod. (mg)
Sandwiches	Long John Silver's	Ultimate Alaskan Pollock Sandwich	1 sandwich	530	27	50	1500
Sandwiches	Joe's Crab Shack	Crab Cake Sandwich	1 sandwich	810	61	40	1490
Sandwiches	Captain D's	Classic Fish Sandwich	1 sandwich	744	41	63	1478
Sides	Applebee's	Chili Cheese Fries (side)	1 portion	590	32	60	1510
Kids Meals	Joe's Crab Shack	Captain's Catch (kids)	1 portion	1060	70	78	1860
Kids Meals	Ruby Tuesday	Kid Fried Shrimp	1 portion	444	23	41	1817
Kids Meals	Joe's Crab Shack	Kids' Mini Beach Burgers	1 portion	760	41	68	870
Kids Meals	The Fish House	Child's Fish Sandwich	1 portion	489	28	55	547
Desserts	Joe's Crab Shack	Chocolate Shack Attack	1 portion	1530	63	225	1660
Desserts	Captain D's	Pecan Pie	1 slice	470	26	56	270

Healthier Bets

Category	Restaurant Name	Dish Name	Serving Size	Cal.	Total Fat (g)	Sat. Fat (g)	Carb. (g)	Pro. (g)	Fiber (g)	Chol. (mg)	Sodium (mg)	Exchanges/ Choices
Appetizers	Captain D's	Crab Cake	1 portion	174	11	5	12	7	1	2	467	1 Starch, 1/2 Lean Protein, 1 1/2 Fat
Appetizers	Red Lobster	Pan-Seared Crab Cakes	1 portion	280	14	2.5	13	26	n/a	n/a	1110	1 Starch, 3 Lean Protein, 1 1/2 Fat
Soups	Red Lobster	Manhattan Clam Chowder	1 bowl	160	2	1	25	10	n/a	n/a	1420	1 Starch, 2 Vegetable, 1 Lean Protein
Salads	Applebee's	Grilled Shrimp on Spinach (half, without dressing)	1/2 salad	400	30	6	12	28	5	n/a	1120	2 Vegetable, 4 Lean Meat, 4 Fat

(table continues on next page)

Healthier Bets

Category	Restaurant Name	Dish Name	Serving Size	Cal.	Total Fat (g)	Sat. Fat (g)	Carb. (g)	Pro. (g)	Fiber (g)	Chol. (mg)	Sodium (mg)	Exchanges/ Choices
Seafood Entrées	Long John Silver's	Grilled Pacific Salmon	2 fillets	150	5	1	2	24	0	50	440	3 1/2 Lean Protein
Seafood Entrées	Captain D's	Grilled Salmon	1 serving	241	11	3	1	31	0	86	392	4 1/2 Lean Protein
Seafood Entrées	Long John Silver's	Grilled Tilapia	1 filet	110	2.5	1	1	22	0	55	250	3 Lean Protein
Seafood Entrées	Captain D's	Catfish	1 piece	105	6	2	6	7	0	0	233	1/2 Starch, 1 Medium-Fat Protein
Seafood Entrées	Captain D's	Seasoned Tilapia	1 piece	130	3	2	1	24	0	0	520	3 Lean Protein
Seafood Entrées	Captain D's	Shrimp Skewers	6 shrimp	50	0	0	0	11	0	0	390	1 1/2 Lean Protein
Seafood Entrées	Captain D's	Grilled Shrimp	1 serving	95	4	0	3	10	0	72	571	2 Lean Protein

(table continues on next page)

Healthier Bets

Category	Restaurant Name	Dish Name	Serving Size	Cal.	Total Fat (g)	Sat. Fat (g)	Carb. (g)	Pro. (g)	Fiber (g)	Chol. (mg)	Sodium (mg)	Exchanges/ Choices
Seafood Entrées	Captain D's	Scampi Shrimp	4 shrimp	28	0	0	0	4	0	0	120	1/2 Lean Protein
Sandwiches	Captain D's	Wild Alaskan Salmon Sandwich	1 sandwich	520	18	2	48	42	0	5	980	3 Starch, 5 Lean Protein, 1 Fat
Kids' Meals	The Fish House	Child's Fish Sandwich	1 portion	489	28	7	55	21	1	39	547	3 1/2 Starch, 2 Lean Protein, 4 Fat
Kids' Meals	Red Lobster	Popcorn Shrimp (kids)	1 portion	140	7	0.5	13	7	n/a	n/a	530	1 Starch, 1 Lean Protein, 1/2 Fat
Kids' Meals	Joe's Crab Shack	Kids' Snow Crab	1 portion	90	1	0	7	13	1	35	350	1/2 Starch, 1 1/2 Lean Protein
Side Salads	Joe's Crab Shack	Caesar Side Salad	1 salad	220	18	4.5	8	6	2	15	540	2 Vegetable, 4 Fat
Side Salads	Joe's Crab Shack	House Side Salad (no dressing)	1 salad	120	7	3	10	6	2	15	250	2 Vegetable, 1 1/2 Fat

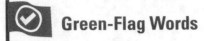 **Green-Flag Words**

Ingredients:

- All finfish and shellfish (raw and cooked)
- All herbs, spices, garlic, and seasonings
- Pickled ginger
- Vegetables (all types)
- Wasabi

Cooking Methods/Menu Descriptions

- Barbecued
- Blackened
- Broiled
- Cajun style
- En papillote (steamed in a package)
- Kebabs
- Marinated
- Mesquite-grilled or grilled
- Seared
- Served with tomato or fruit salsa
- Steamed
- Stir-fried (be aware of increased sodium)
- Teriyaki (be aware of increased sodium)
- White or red clam sauce

At the Table:

- Cocktail sauce
- Soy sauce (ask for low-sodium variety)

Red-Flag Words

Ingredients:

- Bacon, sausage
- Breadcrumbs (usually means sautéed or fried)
- Cheese
- Coconut (as in coconut shrimp)

- ▶ Drawn butter
- ▶ Stuffing

Cooking Methods/Menu Descriptions:

- ▶ Breaded and fried, battered and fried
- ▶ Casserole
- ▶ Coconut crusted
- ▶ Cream or cheese sauce
- ▶ Creamy chowder or bisque
- ▶ Fish 'n' chips
- ▶ Fried, deep-fried
- ▶ Hush puppies
- ▶ Lobster or seafood pie
- ▶ Newburg or Thermidor

At the Table:

- ▶ Mayonnaise-based sauces
- ▶ Oyster crackers
- ▶ Rolls and butter
- ▶ Tartar sauce

🍎 Healthy Eating Tips and Tactics

- ▶ Try the catch of the day to broaden your seafood horizons. Just double-check that the preparation method meets your criteria.
- ▶ Avoid fish that is battered and fried, slathered in butter, or covered in cream sauce.
- ▶ Lemon is plentiful and a perfect flavor complement to most seafood. Use it to add flavor without calories.
- ▶ Enjoy a salad or something from the raw bar while everyone else is eating their high-fat appetizers. Then order an appetizer as your main course to help control portion size.
- ▶ Split an entrée with your dining companion, or request a take-home container to pack up half of your meal before you dig in. When using these portion-control tactics, remember that you are not eating less than you need; the restaurant is giving you double what you need.

👍 Get It Your Way

▶ At many seafood restaurants, french fries or hush puppies are the default side. Substitute a baked potato or rice to cut back on fat. Or better yet, go for a side salad or cooked vegetables, such as a steamed vegetable medley or green beans.

▶ Swap out your sauces. Ask for cocktail sauce or lemon wedges instead of tartar sauce or other mayonnaise-based sauces.

▶ Avoid fried fish. But if you're craving a bit of crunch, request that your fish be topped with a few breadcrumbs and then broiled.

▶ Watch out for creamy salad dressings and coleslaw. Swap these out in favor of a garden salad served with a vinaigrette dressing on the side.

Tips and Tactics for Gluten-Free Eating

▶ Seafood is naturally gluten-free, but preparation methods may add or contaminate your entrée with gluten. Be sure to discuss the preparation method with your waitperson to make sure your dish won't be contaminated.

▶ Imitation crabmeat (surimi) may contain gluten. Crab cakes or fishcakes are usually prepared with breadcrumbs, so they likely contain gluten.

▶ Request that your meal be batter and breading free. Request clean cooking surfaces (not shared surfaces), such as grills, pots, or pans, for the preparation of your dish.

▶ Ask if there is a dedicated fryer for gluten-free foods.

🧒 Tips and Tactics to Help Kids Eat Healthy

▶ If your child is new to fish, you may want to start out with a milder white fish, such as tilapia or halibut.

▶ Use your child's favorite sauces as a way to make fish taste more familiar. For example, grilled salmon glazed with a light soy-based sauce can make a fish that is new to your child seem more appealing. Or let them dip the fish in a bit of ketchup.

▶ Most of the fish options on kids' menus are fried. Split an adult seafood entrée with your child or ask if the restaurant can serve your child a half-size portion (may be called a lunch portion) of a healthier entrée.

► Be smart about side dishes. There is no reason why your child should grow up believing that french fries are the only side dish available. Flip this notion on its head and teach your child to treat veggies as the default side instead of fries.

(?) What's Your Solution?

A fried fish sandwich with hush puppies is always irresistible to you. It makes you feel like you're on vacation at a sunny coastal town. On occasion, you treat yourself to this dish at a seafood restaurant near your home. But you're working hard to lose a few pounds and control your lipids and you know that this meal is loaded with fat and carbohydrate.

What can you do to change your habits without feeling like you're missing out on this vacation-like meal?

    a)   Order the tartar sauce on the side.

    b)   Order the fish grilled without any sauce. Request a few extra lemon wedges. Share a few hush puppies with your dining partner.

    c)   Order the fish grilled with cocktail sauce, instead of tartar sauce. Get a side salad, instead of the hush puppies.

    d)   Order a salad topped with grilled fish. Drizzle it with lemon juice or a vinaigrette dressing. Order the hush puppies to share with your dining partner.

See page 323 for answers.

Menu Samplers

Light 'N' Healthy

Menu Samplers Section	Menu Item	Amount	Calories	Fat (g)	% Calories from Fat	Saturated Fat (g)	Chol. (mg)	Sodium (mg)	Carb. (g)	Fiber (g)	Protein (g)	Exchanges/ Choices
Light 'N' Healthy (Women)*	Shrimp cocktail	3 oz	120	1		0	179	805	9	0	19	1/2 Other Carbohydrate, 3 Lean Protein
	Cocktail sauce	1 oz	90	5		1	8	204	6	0	0	1/2 Other Carbohydrate, 1 Fat
	Bar harbor salad (romaine, dried fruit, blue cheese, pecans)	1 side salad	160	6		1	29	35	29	2	3	1 Fruit, 2 Vegetable, 1 Fat

*Total cholesterol levels are higher than recommended due to cholesterol count in shrimp.

(table continues on next page)

Light 'N' Healthy

Menu Samplers Section	Menu Item	Amount	Calories	Fat (g)	% Calories from Fat	Saturated Fat (g)	Chol. (mg)	Sodium (mg)	Carb. (g)	Fiber (g)	Protein (g)	Exchanges/ Choices
	Oil and vinegar dressing	1 Tbsp olive oil	120	14		2	0	0	0	0	0	3 Fat
Totals			**490**	**26**	**47**	**4**	**216**	**1044**	**44**	**2**	**22**	**1 Fruit, 1 Other Carbo-hydrate, 2 Vegetable, 3 Lean Protein, 5 Fat**
Light 'N' Healthy (Men)	Steamed snow crab legs	1 pound	180	2		0	16	950	0	0	40	6 Lean Protein
	Cheddar biscuit	1 biscuit	150	8		2	40	350	16	0	3	1 Starch, 1 1/2 Fat
	Corn on the cob	2 ears of corn	300	6		2	0	4	51	14	10	3 1/2 Starch, 1 Fat

(table continues on next page)

Light 'N' Healthy

Menu Samplers Section	Menu Item	Amount	Calories	Fat (g)	% Calories from Fat	Saturated Fat (g)	Chol. (mg)	Sodium (mg)	Carb. (g)	Fiber (g)	Protein (g)	Exchanges/ Choices
	House salad (greens and 1—3 additional vegetables) without croutons and cheese	2 cups	16	0		0	0	0	3	1	1	1 Vegetable
	Oil and vinegar dressing	1 Tbsp olive oil	120	14		2	0	0	0	0	0	3 Fat
Totals			**766**	**30**	**35**	**6**	**56**	**1304**	**70**	**15**	**54**	**4 1/2 Starch, 1 Vegetable, 6 Lean Protein, 5 1/2 Fat**

(table continues on next page)

Hearty 'N' Healthy

Menu Samplers Section	Menu Item	Amount	Calories	Fat (g)	% Calories from Fat	Saturated Fat (g)	Chol. (mg)	Sodium (mg)	Carb. (g)	Fiber (g)	Protein (g)	Exchanges/ Choices
Hearty 'N' Healthy (Women)	Baked spicy catfish	4 oz fillet	190	9		1.5	100	150	0	0	28	4 Lean Protein
	French fries	4 oz	440	2		1.5	0	770	53	1	5	4 Starch
	Coleslaw	6 oz	200	15		2.5	10	250	13	1	1	1/2 Other Carbohydrate, 1 Vegetable, 3 Fat
	Vegetable medley	1 cup	50	2		0.5	0	350	8	3	1	2 Vegetable
Total			**880**	**28**	**29**	**6**	**110**	**1520**	**74**	**5**	**35**	**4 Starch, 1/2 Other Carbohydrate, 3 Vegetable, 4 Lean Protein, 3 Fat**

(table continues on next page)

Hearty 'N' Healthy

Menu Samplers Section	Menu Item	Amount	Calories	Fat (g)	% Calories from Fat	Saturated Fat (g)	Chol. (mg)	Sodium (mg)	Carb. (g)	Fiber (g)	Protein (g)	Exchanges/ Choices
Hearty 'N' Healthy (Men)	Fried clams appetizer	1/2 order (4 oz)	385	23		4	15	650	32	3	11	2 Lean Protein, 4 Fat
	Cocktail sauce	1 oz	27	0		0	0	200	6	0	0	1/2 Other Carbohydrate
	Broccoli with lemon	1 cup	55	0.5		0	0	64	12	5	4	2 Vegetable
	Jasmine rice	1 cup	180	3		0.5	10	550	34	5	4	2 Starch, 1/2 Fat
	Broiled bay scallops	3 oz	95	1		0	45	200	0	0	20	3 Lean Protein
Totals			**742**	**28**	**34**	**4.5**	**70**	**1664**	**84**	**13**	**39**	**2 Starch, 1/2 Other Carbohydrate, 2 Vegetable, 5 Lean Protein, 4 1/2 Fat**

(table continues on next page)

Lower Carb 'N' Healthy

Menu Samplers Section	Menu Item	Amount	Calories	Fat (g)	% Calories from Fat	Saturated Fat (g)	Chol. (mg)	Sodium (mg)	Carb. (g)	Fiber (g)	Protein (g)	Exchanges/ Choices
Lower Carb 'N' Healthy (Women)*	Crab cakes	2 (3-oz) cakes	280	14		2.5	220	1100	13	0	26	1 Starch, 3 1/2 Lean Protein, 1 Fat
	Coleslaw	3 oz	100	7		1	5	125	7	1	0	1 Vegetable, 1 Fat
	Boiled red potatoes	1 cup	170	7		4	10	500	25	3	3	1 1/2 Starch, 1 Fat
Totals			**550**	**28**	**46**	**7.5**	**235**	**1725**	**45**	**4**	**29**	**2 1/2 Starch, 1 Vegetable, 3 1/2 Lean Protein, 3 Fat**

*Total cholesterol levels are higher than recommended due to crab in crab cakes.

(table continues on next page)

Lower Carb 'N' Healthy

Menu Samplers Section	Menu Item	Amount	Calories	Fat (g)	% Calories from Fat	Saturated Fat (g)	Chol. (mg)	Sodium (mg)	Carb. (g)	Fiber (g)	Protein (g)	Exchanges/ Choices
Lower Carb 'N' Healthy (Men)*	Steamed lobster	1 1/4 pounds	540	15		2	175	1350	0	0	60	8 Lean Protein
	Corn on the cob	1 ear of corn	150	3		1	0	2	26	7	5	2 Starch, 1/2 Fat
	House salad (greens and 1–3 additional vegetables) without croutons and cheese	2 cups	16	0		0	0	0	3	1	1	1 Vegetable
	Oil and vinegar dressing	1 Tbsp olive oil	120	14		2	0	0	0	0	0	3 Fat
Totals			826	32	35	5	175	1352	29	8	66	2 Starch, 1 Vegetable, 8 Lean Protein, 3 1/2 Fat

*Total cholesterol levels are higher than recommended due to the lobster.

(i) What's Your Solution? Answers

a) This is a step in the right direction. Two tablespoons of tartar sauce have about 60 calories, 75% of which come from fat.

b) This is an even better option. Grilling is one of the healthiest methods to prepare fish. It will save you calories and grams of fat and carbohydrate.

c) The healthy changes you made to the sandwich are great. Cocktail sauce is lower in fat and calories than tartar sauce, yet it is still full of flavor. Choosing a salad over the hush puppies is another smart way to save on calories, fat, and carbohydrate.

d) An entrée salad with grilled fish is a smart way to get the flavor of a coastal vacation while taking good care of your health. Sharing an order of hush puppies can make you feel like you're indulging without allowing you to overdo it on calories, fat, and carbohydrate.

SECTION 3

Ethnic Fare

CHAPTER 18

Mexican

Mexican food is among America's top three favorite foods and is available in restaurants from California to Maine and everywhere in between. Variety abounds! Types of Mexican eateries range from independent and authentic to the more typical moderately priced sit-down chains, such as Chevys, Don Pablos, Chi-Chi's, Pepe's, and On the Border Mexican Grill & Cantina. You'll also see upscale sit-down Mexican restaurants. These days, most Mexican restaurants are boasting about the freshness of their food.

Then there are fast-food Mexican restaurants, with Taco Bell leading the pack. And depending on where you live, you may also find other chains: Del Taco, El Pollo Loco, or Taco John's.

Finally, there is a newer breed of so-called "fast casual" Mexican chains growing in popularity, including Baja Fresh, Chipotle, Qdoba Mexican Grill, Moe's Southwest Grill, and Rubios Fresh Mexican Grill. Yes, these are in the walk-up-and-order genre of restaurants where you'll pick your own fixings from a fixings bar or you'll instruct the server on how to assemble your menu item. These restaurants are great for healthier eating because you can pile on the healthier items and avoid the unhealthy ones.

On the Menu

Mexican food in the United States has a rich history. Historically, most Mexican restaurants served a sub-cuisine known as Tex-Mex—an Americanized version of a few items from Mexico's diverse culinary landscape. Tex-Mex dishes include nachos, tacos, burritos, and chimichangas. But over the past decade or so, things have changed. Traditional Mexican herbs and spices are now more readily available in the U.S. and chefs are increasingly exploring and using these bold flavors. Plus, Mexican Americans, who make up a large and growing percentage of the U.S. population and now live all over the country, have influenced menus and helped to shape a new culinary landscape that embraces the complexities of Mexico's various regional cuisines.

The result is a wide variety of Mexican restaurants, which, naturally, offer diverse menus. Specific dishes may vary, but Mexican cuisine typically features five essential ingredients: rice, corn, beans, tomatoes, and a wide array of chilies. The good news is that these ingredients are healthy, at least before being prepared. They are all high in vitamins and minerals and low in fat. Plus, spicy toppings—red or green salsa, pico de gallo, and chilies—can increase your vegetable count and add zip for nearly zero calories.

There's even more good news: in Mexican cuisine, there's minimal focus on animal protein compared to a typical American meal. Compare the small quantity of protein, 1–2 ounces, in one enchilada to the familiar 8- or 10-ounce (or more) steak served in most steakhouses. This has its roots in the old Mexican practice of making a small amount of meat feed many mouths (a common thread in many ethnic cuisines). Soft tacos filled with beans and vegetables, chicken enchiladas, grilled fajitas, and fresh salads are just a few of the healthier dishes you can choose from. But don't get carried away. The health attributes of traditional Mexican ingredients can be quickly squashed if the ingredients are fried, refried, or smothered with cheese or sour cream, as they often are in Mexican cuisine. Think of dishes such as loaded nachos, quesadillas, chimichangas, and Mexican salads served in the fried tortilla bowl. You should probably pass on these high-fat and calorie-rich dishes.

Fat is clearly the villain in Mexican cuisine. There are many fried items on Mexican menus, and many Mexican recipes traditionally call for the use of lard or animal fat drippings. Animal fat contains cholesterol and saturated fat. Due to pressure to improve the healthiness of their foods, large restaurant chains have switched to using healthier liquid oils.

Mexican food can also be high in sodium. Salt is used in many recipes and sauces, and a lot of the prep work, such as spicing the meats, is done in advance. This makes it difficult to request that salt be omitted. However, if you order a dish such as grilled chicken, fish, or beef in an upscale Mexican restaurant, you might be successful with a hold-the-salt request, as these restaurants often cook from scratch. Chips, salsa, and large amounts of cheese can also contribute to raising the sodium level of a dish or meal. Due to its zesty taste, green or red salsa can be used to add punch to salads or chicken and fish dishes. Tomato-based salsa is fine to use in small amounts, like 2 tablespoons, without counting.

Portion sizes can be quite large and your carbohydrate count can escalate quickly with tortillas, beans, rice, and those hard-to-resist chips. The best healthy eating strategies to use at Mexican restaurants include watching your portions, saying no to high-fat toppings, such as cheese and sour cream, and avoiding anything deep-fried.

The Menu Profile

Drinks

If you are in a sit-down restaurant, your server will likely try to entice you with a knock-you-on-your-behind margarita. Beware! Margaritas are often served in super-sized portions and are quite calorie-dense. One 8-ounce Margarita can run 500 calories. This drink isn't just loaded with a high dose of tequila, it also typically contains a hefty dose of simple syrup (aka sugar water) and lime juice. If the drink is created from scratch by a bartender rather than from a sugar-dense mix, request that it be made without the simple syrup to save some calories and carbohydrate. Skip the frozen fruit margaritas, which are loaded with even more carbohydrate. If you're watching your blood pressure, don't order salt on the rim. If you choose to have an alcoholic beverage, a healthier bet is a light beer or a glass of wine.

Several nonalcoholic beverages are also available in Mexican restaurants. If you're at a traditional Mexican restaurant, horchata may be on the menu. This is a cinnamon-rice milk that can have up to 1/4 cup of sugar per serving. Yikes! You may also find a variety of fruit-based drinks; licuados (smoothies) and aqua frescas (fruit juice blends) are popular. It's best to avoid all of these high-sugar beverages. Learn more about all kinds of beverages in Chapter 9 (page 87.)

Appetizers

The first foods to greet you in a sit-down Mexican restaurant are usually chips and salsa. It's easy to empty the basket before you know it and have it quickly refilled. Remember, tortilla chips are deep-fried and often salted (to boost the number of margaritas or beers you'll sip). Exercise the utmost willpower by promising yourself that you'll limit the number of chips you eat. Easier yet, ask the waitperson not to bring you chips and salsa.

Salsa is the winning half of the chips-and-salsa partnership. Salsa, either red or green, is usually made with tomatoes, onions, garlic, chilies, cilantro, and salt. It has almost no fat and very few calories. Best yet, it's a topping with plenty of pizzazz and flavor. Request extra salsa to use on the salads or entrées you order. Most restaurants will gladly oblige. Pico de gallo, often found on Mexican menus, is basically just chopped tomatoes, onions, and cilantro and can be used similarly to salsa. Guacamole is the other common partner to chips. Guacamole has a healthy mix of ingredients, but it is high in fat and calories. Yes, there's a good bit of fat in avocados, albeit a good bit of the healthy monounsaturated fat. Limit the amount of guacamole you eat so you don't overdo it on calories and fat before your meal even arrives.

Beyond chips and dips, Mexican appetizers offer a few healthy choices, but there are also many high-fat, fried items. The healthier choices are soups and salads or ceviche, a raw fish appetizer popular at upscale restaurants. Empanadas, savory turnovers filled with meat or vegetables, can be an acceptable appetizer option when they are baked instead of fried. The appetizers to avoid or limit are nachos, chili con queso, queso fundido, flautas, and quesadillas, which often combine at least two high-fat foods and often have more calories than any other foods on the menu. If your dining partners order high-fat appetizers, start with a cup of soup or salad.

Soups and Salads

Five types of soups or stews are frequent finds at Mexican restaurants: chili, tortilla soup, black bean soup, sopa de fideo, and posole. They're all typically broth or tomato-based soups, making them healthier choices than the cream-based soups. These soups often feature fiber-rich beans, which makes them healthy and filling. Mexican soups are certainly a better option than chips or most other appetizers you'll find on the menu; however they can be high in sodium. Also be mindful of portion sizes. Servings are generally quite large, even when split, so you'll want to keep a close eye on your overall food intake.

A variety of salads are available. Don't fall into the trap of thinking that a salad is always healthy. Take the Quesadilla Explosion Salad at Chili's, which will set you back 1440 calories. You are better off ordering the Grilled Chicken Salad from the lighter choices menu at Chili's, which has a much more respectable 440 calories. Always ask that the tortilla shell in which some Mexican restaurants serve their salads be left in the kitchen. At Qdoba, the crunchy tortilla bowl will cost you 465 calories, 22 grams of fat, 48 grams of carbohydrate, and 525 milligrams of sodium before you even put anything in it!

At fast casual restaurants like Qdobo or Chipotle, a salad can be one of the healthier options on the menu if you order with care and specificity. That's in part because the salads at these restaurants are relatively small. At this breed of restaurants, take advantage of watching your salad being made. Choose exactly what you want on it and control how much of each ingredient is being loaded on by speaking up. These restaurants can be a great place to grab a healthy salad. Consider a salad at Chipotle. If you start with lettuce, chicken, black beans, fajita vegetables, and fresh tomato salsa, you have a very healthy meal with 350 calories, 9 grams of fat, and 32 grams of carbohydrate. The only downside is the sodium count at just over 1200 milligrams. You may be tempted to add more toppings to your salad, but think twice. Little changes can make a big difference. For example, if you add sour cream, cheese, and guacamole, the salad skyrockets to 735 calories, 42 grams of fat, 42 grams of carbohydrate, and 1875 milligrams of sodium.

At traditional or fine dining Mexican restaurants, salads likely aren't a major focus of the menu. You may find a salad composed of greens, jicama, avocado, and lime. Or you may find a Nopalitos salad: a popular Mexican salad made with strips of the prickly pear cactus. These are all healthy options and can be a great low-calorie way to start your meal. Refer to Chapter 15 (page 250) for more tips on ordering a healthy salad.

Entrées

Mexican entrées frequently include beans, tortillas (corn or flour), lettuce, tomatoes, onions, and chilies. All are healthy ingredients. Keep them in mind as you decide what to order. On the flip side, many high-fat and high-calorie ingredients are also found in Mexican entrées—cheese, sour cream, avocado, and chorizo (Mexican sausage). You'll want to watch out for these items no matter what you order.

Chicken, beef, fish, or vegetarian soft tacos are often your best option for an entrée. Chipotle now offers a vegan option (spiced and shredded tofu), which they call sofritas. Carnitas—a shredded and seasoned pork—can be a good taco filling as well, but it's often a bit higher in fat and sodium than other protein options. Enchiladas can be good choices too, as long as they aren't stuffed or topped with loads of cheese and sour cream. Burritos can be good choices as well, but beware of the portion sizes. Some restaurants brag about serving burritos as big as your head. For example, at Taco Bell, the Steak Burrito Supreme has 400 calories, while the Steak Cantina Burrito has 750 calories. What's the difference? Mostly the serving size. The Cantina Burrito is nearly twice the size of the Burrito Supreme, plus it adds rice and guacamole. Rather than ordering something as big as your head, use your head to choose a smaller version of a dish or plan to share or take home half of a large meal.

Chimichangas are similar to burritos but they are deep-fried and doused in cheese. Avoid these. And don't be deceived by quesadillas' flat profile. They are loaded with cheese, often making them among the highest calorie options on Mexican menus. The quesadilla options at Taco Bell and Qdoba are both around 950 calories!

Fajitas are a healthy option, and you can choose from chicken, shrimp, beef, or a combination of meats as fillings. One order often is enough for two, so definitely plan to share or take home half. Another ordering trick with fajitas is to request extra vegetables and less meat. This is a great way to get in an extra serving of vegetables.

If you're worried that all of the entrées on a particular menu will break the calorie bank, you can create your own entrée by ordering à la carte. The ability to order à la carte is a big perk of Mexican restaurants. A bowl of chili con carne (hold the cheese, but load on the onions) is a good choice to pair with a side salad. A single chicken enchilada or bean burrito, paired with a dinner salad, will enable you to avoid the high-fat accompaniments of Mexican cuisine. Steer clear of combination plates unless you plan to share, as they offer too much food and too many foods that should be avoided.

At upscale Mexican restaurants, you'll often find a grilled steak, chicken, or fish dish served with a sauce, such as a complex mole (pronounced mō-lay). There are dozens of mole variations that differ based on region and family recipes, but each kind of mole typically has at least 20 different ingredients, often including chocolate, nuts, and various spices. Moles are very flavorful and are a healthier choice than any cheese- or cream-based topping.

You'll also find a wider variety of vegetables, beyond the fajita-style blend, at upscale Mexican restaurants; look for delectable mushrooms, squashes, and jicama. Fruit is often used more frequently in these restaurants too, often in toppings such as mango- and papaya-based salsas and garnishes. Finally, herbs, such as garlic and cilantro, are heavily used, offering lots of flavor for next to no calories.

Of course, along with Mexican dinners—whether at fast-food or fine dining restaurants—come starches, namely Mexican rice and beans. Beans (usually pinto, kidney, or black beans) are high in vitamins, minerals, and soluble fiber, which means that they may allow your blood glucose to rise a bit more slowly and perhaps not as high. This makes them a great carbohydrate side to accompany your meal. However, if the beans are fried in lard, just say no. While many traditional Mexican restaurants still use lard, most fast-food and fast casual restaurants use a healthier vegetable oil. Either way, it's a better idea to skip the refried beans and order a side of black beans, instead.

Desserts

The list of desserts in Mexican restaurants often involves fried dough. For example, sopapillas and churros are both deep-fried dough topped off with a heavy dose of something sugary: honey, sugar, or chocolate. They are decadent, high-fat, high-sugar disasters and they should be avoided. Flan, an egg custard with caramel topping, is another familiar Mexican dessert and is not a bad choice, but it should be avoided if you're watching your cholesterol numbers. Another decent choice is the pastel de tres leches, a traditional sponge cake that is soaked in three types of milk. It's best to skip the fried ice cream, which often is a bowl of ice cream topped with fried coconut and chocolate. Think about splitting whatever dessert you order to minimize your carbohydrate and fat intake. If you want something nearly calorie-free to top off your meal, opt for a flavorful cup of Mexican coffee.

Nutrition Snapshot

Health Busters

Category	Restaurant Name	Dish Name	Serving Size	Cal.	Total Fat (g)	Carb. (g)	Sod. (mg)
Nachos	Baja Fresh Mexican Grill	Charbroiled Steak Nachos (with jack and cheddar cheese, black or pinto beans, guacamole, pico de gallo, and sour cream)	1 portion	2120	118	163	2990
Nachos	Baja Fresh Mexican Grill	Charbroiled Chicken Nachos (with jack and cheddar cheese, black or pinto beans, guacamole, pico de gallo, and sour cream)	1 portion	2020	110	164	2980
Nachos	Baja Fresh Mexican Grill	Savory Pork Carnitas Nachos (with jack and cheddar cheese, black or pinto beans, guacamole, pico de gallo, and sour cream)	1 portion	2060	117	166	3120
Nachos	Chevys	Nachos Grande	1 portion	1910	106	165	2630
Nachos	La Salsa Fresh Mexican Grill	Nachos, Chicken (black)	1 portion	1600	83	148	2510
Nachos	Taco Bueno	Beef Mucho Nachos	1 portion	1567	97	127	4105

(table continues on next page)

Health Busters

Category	Restaurant Name	Dish Name	Serving Size	Cal.	Total Fat (g)	Carb. (g)	Sod. (mg)
Nachos	Taco Cabana	Super Beef Nachos w/Shredded Cheese (ground)	1 portion	1770	114	109	2360
Chile Con Quesos	On The Border Mexican Grill & Cantina	Empanadas—Beef w/Chile Con Queso	1 portion	620	46	33	870
Chile Con Quesos	On The Border Mexican Grill & Cantina	Empanadas—Ground Beef w/Chile Con Queso	1 portion	620	46	33	870
Chile Con Quesos	On The Border Mexican Grill & Cantina	Empanadas—Chicken w/Chile Con Queso	1 portion	620	46	32	830
Tortilla Chips	La Salsa Fresh Mexican Grill	Guacamole, Salsa and Chips	1 portion	970	55	103	1600
Tortilla Chips	On The Border Mexican Grill & Cantina	Chips and Salsa	1 portion	430	22	52	460
Tortilla Chips	Taco Bueno	Mexidips & Chips	1 portion	1086	62	105	1862

(table continues on next page)

Health Busters

Category	Restaurant Name	Dish Name	Serving Size	Cal.	Total Fat (g)	Carb. (g)	Sod. (mg)
Salad Entrées	Baja Fresh Mexican Grill	Charbroiled Steak Tostada Salad	1 salad	1230	63	98	2380
Salad Entrées	Baja Fresh Mexican Grill	Savory Pork Carnitas Tostada Salad	1 salad	1180	62	100	2520
Salad Entrées	Baja Fresh Mexican Grill	Charbroiled Shrimp Tostada Salad	1 salad	1120	55	99	2460
Salad Entrées	Chevys	Tostada Salad w/o Dressing, Steak	1 salad	1560	100	91	2220
Salad Entrées	Chevys	Tostada Salad w/o Dressing, Chicken	1 salad	1500	91	91	2410
Salad Entrées	Chevys	Tostada Salad w/o Dressing, Carnitas	1 salad	1530	98	93	2550
Salad Entrées	Don Pablo's	Taco Salad (Beef) with Fried Tortilla Shell (no dressing)	1 salad	1380	73	102	2593
Tacos	Don Pablo's	Fried Fish Tacos	1 portion	1018	56	77	2326
Tacos	Don Pablo's	Buffalo Chicken Taco Trio	1 portion	1037	57	94	3156
Tacos	La Salsa Fresh Mexican Grill	Mexico City Taco Platter (pinto beans)	1 portion	1040	39	119	2140

(table continues on next page)

Health Busters

Category	Restaurant Name	Dish Name	Serving Size	Cal.	Total Fat (g)	Carb. (g)	Sod. (mg)
Tacos	On The Border Mexican Grill & Cantina	Dos XX Fish Tacos	1 portion	1400	82	124	2610
Tacos	On The Border Mexican Grill & Cantina	Dos XX & Reg Fish Tacos w/Creamy Red Chile Sauce	1 portion	1950	121	158	3540
Tacos	Rubio's Fresh Mexican Grill	Cabo Plate Shrimp Burrito & The Original Fish Taco	1 portion	1230	49	152	3110
Quesadillas	Don Pablo's	Chicken Quesadilla & Side Salad Combo	1 portion	946	56	75	1516
Quesadillas	Taco Del Mar	Ground Beef Quesadilla Platter	1 portion	1250	57	136	2880
Quesadillas	Taco Del Mar	Pork Quesadilla Platter	1 portion	1180	50	134	2870
Burritos	Rubio's Fresh Mexican Grill	Cabo Plate Shrimp Burrito & The Original Fish Taco	1 portion	1230	49	152	3110
Burritos	Taco Time	Crispy Chicken Ranchero	1 portion	600	31	51	1250

(table continues on next page)

Health Busters

Category	Restaurant Name	Dish Name	Serving Size	Cal.	Total Fat (g)	Carb. (g)	Sod. (mg)
Fajitas	Baja Fresh Mexican Grill	Breaded Fish w/Flour Tortillas Fajitas (with grilled veggies, rice, black or pinto beans, guacamole, pico de gallo, sour cream)	1 portion	1340	45	172	3020
Fajitas	Baja Fresh Mexican Grill	Breaded Fish w/Mixed Tortillas Fajitas (with grilled veggies, rice, black or pinto beans, guacamole, pico de gallo, sour cream)	1 portion	1260	43	162	2740
Fajitas	Baja Fresh Mexican Grill	Steak w/Flour Tortillas Fajitas (with grilled veggies, rice, black or pinto beans, guacamole, pico de gallo, sour cream]	1 portion	1240	45	149	3440
Enchiladas	Taco Cabana	Enchilada Plate	1 portion	1270	66	115	2800
Enchiladas	Don Pablo's	Steak & Enchiladas	1 portion	1331	101	20	3144
Enchiladas	On The Border Mexican Grill & Cantina	Shrimp & Lump Crab Enchiladas	1 portion	1180	56	128	1740
Chimichangas	Don Pablo's	Chimichanga, Spicy Beef De Oro	1 portion	1358	79	89	2509

(table continues on next page)

Health Busters

Category	Restaurant Name	Dish Name	Serving Size	Cal.	Total Fat (g)	Carb. (g)	Sod. (mg)
Chimichangas	On The Border Mexican Grill & Cantina	Classic Chimichanga Ground Beef (without sauce)	1 portion	1420	90	105	2440
Guacamoles	Chevys	Guac-My-Way	1 portion	730	52	63	1140
Guacamoles	On The Border Mexican Grill & Cantina	Guacamole Live (without chips)	1 portion	570	50	34	2330
Desserts	Don Pablo's	Sopapillas	1 portion	1208	61	154	1324
Desserts	On The Border Mexican Grill & Cantina	Sopapillas - Two w/Honey	1 portion	620	17	119	410
Desserts	Chevys	Chevys Flan	1 portion	760	22	123	240
Desserts	Chevys	Deep Fried Ice Cream	1 portion	1060	65	103	590
Desserts	Taco Cabana	Tres Leches Cake	1 portion	510	31	52	330
Desserts	Don Pablo's	Child Fried Ice Cream	1 portion	448	11	78	350

Healthier Bets

Category	Restaurant Name	Dish Name	Serving Size	Cal.	Total Fat (g)	Sat. Fat (g)	Carb. (g)	Pro. (g)	Fiber (g)	Chol. (mg)	Sodium (mg)	Exchanges/ Choices
Salad Entrées	El Pollo Loco	Loco Side	1 bowl	210	18	3.5	8	3	2	15	260	1 1/2 Vegetable, 1/2 High-Fat Protein, 3 Fat
Salad Entrées	Rubio's Fresh Mexican Grill	Balsamic & Roasted Veggie with Chicken	1 salad	310	11	3.5	29	20	7	40	950	1 Starch, 3 Vegetable, 2 1/2 Lean Protein, 1 Fat
Salad Entrées	Chipotle Mexican Grill	Steak Bowl (black beans, cilantro-lime rice, and green tomatillo salsa)	1 bowl	455	11	2.5	51	40	12	65	950	3 Starch, 4 Lean Protein
Salad Entrées	El Pollo Loco	Grilled Chicken (no dressing)	1 bowl	230	7	2	18	25	3	75	520	1 Starch, 1 Vegetable, 3 Lean Protein

(table continues on next page)

Healthier Bets

Category	Restaurant Name	Dish Name	Serving Size	Cal.	Total Fat (g)	Sat. Fat (g)	Carb. (g)	Pro. (g)	Fiber (g)	Chol. (mg)	Sodium (mg)	Exchanges/ Choices
Salad Entrées	Chevys	Mixed Greens Side Salad (no dressing)	1 salad	150	5	1	23	4	4	0	200	1 Starch, 1 Vegetable, 1 Fat
Tacos	Chipotle Mexican Grill	Steak Tacos (3 crispy taco shells, green tomatillo salsa, and cheese)	1 portion	420	15.5	5	32	37	4	n/a	840	2 Starch, 5 Lean Protein, 1 Fat
Tacos	Chipotle Mexican Grill	Chicken Tacos (3 crispy taco shells, green tomatillo salsa, and cheese)	1 portion	420	15.5	5	31	39	4	n/a	540	2 Starch, 5 Lean Protein, 1 Fat
Tacos	Don Pablo's	Beef Taco	1 portion	260	13	6	16	18	3	50	940	1 Starch, 2 Medium-Fat Protein, 1/2 Fat

(table continues on next page)

Healthier Bets

Category	Restaurant Name	Dish Name	Serving Size	Cal.	Total Fat (g)	Sat. Fat (g)	Carb. (g)	Pro. (g)	Fiber (g)	Chol. (mg)	Sodium (mg)	Exchanges/ Choices
Tacos	La Salsa Fresh Mexican Grill	Mexico City Taco, Steak	1 portion	190	5	1	27	11	2	10	440	2 Starch, 1 Lean Protein
Tacos	On The Border Mexican Grill & Cantina	Mexican Plate—Soft Chicken Taco	1 portion	270	11	5	23	19	1	35	540	1 1/2 Starch, 2 Lean Protein, 1 Fat
Tacos	Taco Cabana	Beef Street Tacos (3)	1 portion	290	6	1	46	18	4	n/a	n/a	3 Starch, 1 1/2 Lean Protein
Tacos	Taco Del Mar	Veggie Taco—Rice & Refried Beans	1 portion	250	8	3	38	9	4	195	580	2 1/2 Starch, 1 Fat
Quesadillas	Taco Bueno	Mini Cheese Quesadilla (1)	1 portion	274	15	n/a	23	11	1	35	487	1 1/2 Starch, 1 1/2 High-Fat Protein

(table continues on next page)

Healthier Bets

Category	Restaurant Name	Dish Name	Serving Size	Cal.	Total Fat (g)	Sat. Fat (g)	Carb. (g)	Pro. (g)	Fiber (g)	Chol. (mg)	Sodium (mg)	Exchanges/ Choices
Quesadillas	Taco Del Mar	Quesadilla Kid's (1)	1 portion	290	13	6	35	11	2	38	365	2 Starch, 1 1/2 High-Fat Protein
Quesadillas	Del Taco	Kid's Quesadilla (2 pack)	1 portion	280	13	7	28	12	3	30	435	2 Starch, 1 1/2 High-Fat Protein
Quesadillas	Taco Bueno	Kids Cheese Quesadilla (1)	1 portion	219	11	n/a	23	8	1	15	413	1 1/2 Starch, 1 High-Fat Protein
Burrito Bowls	Taco Time	Crisp Chicken	1 burrito	380	17	6	33	22	2	15	382	2 Starch, 3 Lean Protein, 2 Fat
Burrito Bowls	Moe's Southwest Grill	Moo Moo Mr. Cow (with chicken, black beans, and 8-inch flour tortilla)	1 burrito	266	10	5	27	17	3	n/a	n/a	2 Starch, 2 Lean Protein, 1/2 Fat

(table continues on next page)

Healthier Bets

Category	Restaurant Name	Dish Name	Serving Size	Cal.	Total Fat (g)	Sat. Fat (g)	Carb. (g)	Pro. (g)	Fiber (g)	Chol. (mg)	Sodium (mg)	Exchanges/ Choices
Burrito Bowls	Moe's Southwest Grill	Moo Moo Mr. Cow (with steak, black beans, and 8-inch flour tortilla)	1 burrito	259	10	4	27	15	3	76	885	2 Starch, 2 Lean Protein, 1/2 Fat
Burrito Bowls	Moe's Southwest Grill	Moo Moo Mr. Cow (with pork, black beans, and 8-inch flour tortilla)	1 burrito	258	10	4	27	15	3	120	860	2 Starch, 2 Lean Protein, 1/2 Fat
Fajitas	Chevys	Chicken & Steak Fajita	1 fajita	450	22	9	13	48	3	n/a	n/a	1 Starch, 7 Lean Protein, 1 Fat
Fajitas	Don Pablo's	Lunch Sized Steak Fajita	1 portion	336	17	5	18	30	2	n/a	90	1 Starch, 3 1/2 Medium- Fat Protein

(table continues on next page)

Healthier Bets

Category	Restaurant Name	Dish Name	Serving Size	Cal.	Total Fat (g)	Sat. Fat (g)	Carb. (g)	Pro. (g)	Fiber (g)	Chol. (mg)	Sodium (mg)	Exchanges/ Choices
Fajitas	Chevys	Original Chicken Fajita	1 fajita	390	13	5	13	51	3	30	570	1 Starch, 7 Lean Protein
Enchiladas	Chevys	Salsa Chicken Enchilada	1 enchilada	210	11	4	17	12	2	15	610	1 Starch, 1 1/2 Medium-Fat Protein, 1/2 Fat
Enchiladas	Chevys	Enchilada, Chicken	1 enchilada	210	11	4	17	12	2	40	640	1 Starch, 1 1/2 Medium-Fat Protein, 1/2 Fat
Enchiladas	On The Border Mexican Grill & Cantina	Enchilada, Green Chile Chicken	1 enchilada	190	9	4	15	11	1	15	530	1 Starch, 1 1/2 Medium-Fat Protein

(table continues on next page)

Healthier Bets

Category	Restaurant Name	Dish Name	Serving Size	Cal.	Total Fat (g)	Sat. Fat (g)	Carb. (g)	Pro. (g)	Fiber (g)	Chol. (mg)	Sodium (mg)	Exchanges/ Choices
Guacamoles	On The Border Mexican Grill & Cantina	Side Guacamole	1 portion	50	5	1	3	1	3	n/a	n/a	1 Fat
Guacamoles	On The Border Mexican Grill & Cantina	Guacamole (without chips)	1 portion	260	23	5	16	6	13	65	230	1 Starch, 4 Fat
Mexican Entrées	Taco Bell	Chalupa Supreme— Steak	1 chalupa	340	18	4	29	14	3	35	170	2 Starch, 1 1/2 High-Fat Protein, 1 Fat
Mexican Entrées	Taco Bell	Chalupa Supreme— Chicken	1 chalupa	350	18	4	29	17	3	5	260	2 Starch, 2 Medium-Fat Protein, 1 Fat

(table continues on next page)

Healthier Bets

Category	Restaurant Name	Dish Name	Serving Size	Cal.	Total Fat (g)	Sat. Fat (g)	Carb. (g)	Pro. (g)	Fiber (g)	Chol. (mg)	Sodium (mg)	Exchanges/Choices
Mexican Entrées	Taco Cabana	Bean & Cheese Chalupa	1 chalupa	290	17	7	23	11	5	n/a	0	1 1/2 Starch, 1 High-Fat Protein, 1 1/2 Fat
Mexican Entrées	Taco Bell	Gordita Supreme Beef	1 gordita	300	14	5	31	13	4	0	105	2 Starch, 1 1/2 Medium-Fat Protein, 1 Fat
Desserts	El Pollo Loco	Vanilla Small Cone	1 small cone	320	8	5	53	8	0	0	105	3 1/2 Other Carbohydrate, 1 1/2 Fat
Desserts	Taco John's	Apple Grande	1 portion	260	11	3	39	5	2	0	90	2 1/2 Other Carbohydrate, 2 Fat
Desserts	Taco Bell	Cinnamon Twists	1 portion	170	7	0	26	1	1	n/a	n/a	1 1/2 Other Carbohydrate, 1 1/2 Fat
Desserts	Taco Del Mar	Cookie—Chocolate Chip	1 cookie	170	7	4	24	2	1	n/a	n/a	1 1/2 Other Carbohydrate, 1 1/2 Fat

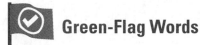 ## Green-Flag Words

Ingredients:

- ▶ Avocado
- ▶ Black beans, pinto beans
- ▶ Chilies
- ▶ Enchilada sauce
- ▶ Lettuce, tomatoes, onions
- ▶ Mole sauce
- ▶ Salsa (green or red)
- ▶ Shredded spicy chicken, beef, or ground beef
- ▶ Soft tortilla (corn or flour)

Cooking Methods/Menu Descriptions:

- ▶ Burritos
- ▶ Fajitas (best to share)
- ▶ Grilled
- ▶ Guacamole
- ▶ Marinated
- ▶ Served with spicy tomato sauce
- ▶ Simmered
- ▶ Soft tacos
- ▶ Wrapped in a soft tortilla
- ▶ Arroz con pollo
- ▶ Tamales
- ▶ Tostadas

At the Table:

- ▶ Salsa

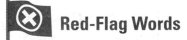 ## Red-Flag Words

Ingredients:

- ▶ Bacon
- ▶ Black olives
- ▶ Cheese (any style: topped, stuffed, covered, shredded)

- ▶ Chorizo (Mexican sausage)
- ▶ Sour cream

Cooking Methods/Menu Descriptions:

- ▶ Cheese quesadillas
- ▶ Cheese sauce
- ▶ Chili con queso
- ▶ Chimichangas
- ▶ Cream sauce
- ▶ Crispy
- ▶ Fried or deep-fried
- ▶ Layered with refried beans
- ▶ Nachos with cheese
- ▶ Queso fundido
- ▶ Served in a tortilla shell
- ▶ Served over tortilla or nacho chips
- ▶ Tacos

At the Table:

- ▶ Sour cream
- ▶ Tortilla chips

Healthy Eating Tips and Tactics

- ▶ Avoid the chips on the table. They can be addicting, especially when your waitperson is adept at refilling a bottomless basket. Before you know it, you can easily eat more than 500 calories. Avoid them altogether by asking your server not to bring them. Or if your dining partner(s) isn't game for that plan, just put a small portion of chips on your plate. Then work to keep the basket out of arm's reach.
- ▶ Choose grilled items when you can. Most Mexican restaurants have healthier grilled items, including fajitas and fish, chicken, or beef dishes. Add flavor to these dishes with salsas and grilled vegetables.
- ▶ Take advantage of ordering à la carte. Choose from appetizers and side dishes to control your portions and make your own healthy, balanced meal.

- Be careful with guacamole. It's certainly healthier than a cheese dip, but its calories can add up quickly.
- Drink wisely. A typical margarita is loaded with sugar and calories, and drinking alcohol has a tendency to make people worry less about eating a healthy meal. Choose sparkling water with fresh lime instead. If you want alcohol, a light beer or skinny margarita, available in some restaurants, is a better choice.

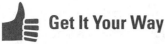

Get It Your Way

- Choose soft tacos instead of hard tacos. Choose corn tortillas instead of flour tortillas because corn is a whole grain.
- Hold the guacamole, cheese, and sour cream or ask for them on the side.
- Request that the kitchen avoid topping your dish with cheese. Or at least ask them to only give you a light helping.
- Substitute black beans (if available) for refried beans to limit fat.
- Ask for extra salsa, tomatoes, lettuce, and onion to use as low-calorie, flavorful toppings.
- Order salads without the fried tortilla shell or fried tortilla strips. You can replace the fried tortilla with a warmed, soft tortilla if you want to.

Tips and Tactics to Help Kids Eat Healthy

- Avoid the chips. If chips are the first thing to hit the table, your child will likely fill up on them and be less interested in the healthier options that are to come. Remember, you're the parent. It's your job to make these executive decisions.
- Order à la carte. Sometimes, kids' meals aren't available at Mexican restaurants. This is a good thing! Go to the à la carte section of the menu and get creative. Choose a soft taco, a side order of rice and beans, and perhaps some guacamole for a colorful, flavorful, nourishing meal.
- Share a small portion. If a healthy food is new to your child, give them just a small portion to taste so they aren't overwhelmed. For example, order black beans for yourself, then share just a few beans with your

child so they can experience the flavor without feeling pressured to eat the whole dish if they don't like it.

▶ Be bold. Sometimes kids like a little kick with their meal! Order a variety of salsas, ranging from mild to medium, and let your child experiment by using them as dips or toppings. You know they love dipping.

Tips and Tactics for Gluten-Free Eating

▶ Many traditional Mexican foods prepared from scratch are gluten-free. Ask about the preparation of mole sauce, enchiladas, and cheese sauces to make sure they are not contaminated by gluten.

▶ Flour tortillas and dishes made with flour tortillas such as burritos, chimichangas, and quesadillas, are not gluten-free. Many other Mexican dishes are deep-fried and contain wheat flour.

▶ Ask if the restaurant makes their corn tortilla chips on site or orders them from a food vendor. Corn tortillas fried at the restaurant in dedicated fryers are gluten-free. If provided by a vendor, ask your sever if the package says "gluten-free" or not.

▶ Rice, beans, salsas, guacamole, and fresh meats and poultry are gluten-free but some seasonings may not be gluten-free. Tamales made from corn are typically gluten-free, but double-check the ingredients and preparation methods with staff.

What's Your Solution?

Every Friday, you and your co-workers grab lunch at a fast casual Mexican restaurant. You normally order a burrito filled with steak, rice, cheese, sour cream, and salsa, along with a side of chips and guacamole. But you know this isn't the best way to manage your waistline and your glucose levels. You're ready to commit to a change.

How could you change your order to still get all the flavor of your favorite burrito, but with fewer fat grams and calories?

a) Order the burrito, but request that they just use half the amount of cheese and sour cream.

b) Order the burrito with brown rice instead of white rice (if available). Ask for half the amount of cheese. Instead of ordering a side of chips and guacamole, skip the chips and put the guacamole directly in the burrito. Skip the sour cream.

c) Order the burrito exactly how you like it. But take half home.

d) Order two soft tacos filled with steak, black beans, salsa, and a sprinkle of cheese. Ask for the sour cream on the side. Share the chips and guacamole with a co-worker.

See page 360 for answers.

Menu Samplers

Light 'N' Healthy

Menu Samplers Section	Menu Item	Amount	Calories	Fat (g)	% Calories from Fat	Saturated Fat (g)	Chol. (mg)	Sodium (mg)	Carb. (g)	Fiber (g)	Protein (g)	Exchanges/ Choices
Light 'N' Healthy (Women)	Loaded nachos (cheese, ground beef, onion, jala-peños, shredded lettuce, salsa)	1 medium order (8 oz)	445	23		4.5	30	640	44	7	14	2 Starch, 1 Vegetable, 2 Medium-Fat Protein, 3 Fat
Totals			**445**	**23**	**47**	**4.5**	**30**	**640**	**44**	**7**	**14**	2 Starch, 1 Vegetable, 2 Medium-Fat Protein, 3 Fat

(table continues on next page)

Light 'N' Healthy

Menu Samplers Section	Menu Item	Amount	Calories	Fat (g)	% Calories from Fat	Saturated Fat (g)	Chol. (mg)	Sodium (mg)	Carb.(g)	Fiber (g)	Protein (g)	Exchanges/ Choices
Light 'N' Healthy (Men)	Chicken quesa- dilla with shred- ded lettuce and salsa	1 quesa- dilla made with 2 tortillas	555	29		13	100	1080	40	3	32	2 1/2 Starch, 1 Vegetable, 4 Lean Protein, 3 Fat
	Cilantro lime rice	3/4 cup	143	2		0.5	0	285	29	1	3	2 Starch
Totals			**698**	**31**	**40**	**13.5**	**100**	**1365**	**69**	**4**	**35**	4 1/2 Starch, 1 Vegetable, 4 Lean Protein, 3 Fat

(table continues on next page)

Hearty 'N' Healthy

Menu Samplers Section	Menu Item	Amount	Calories	Fat (g)	% Calories from Fat	Saturated Fat (g)	Chol. (mg)	Sodium (mg)	Carb. (g)	Fiber (g)	Protein (g)	Exchanges/ Choices
Hearty 'N' Healthy (Women)	Steak fajita salad (steak, beans, rice, cheese, lettuce, sour cream, tortilla strips, and salsa)	16 oz salad	690	30	39	4	60	1100	72	8	32	4 Starch, 2 Vegetable, 4 Lean Protein, 3 1/2 Fat
Totals			**690**	**30**	**39**	**4**	**60**	**1100**	**72**	**8**	**32**	**4 Starch, 2 Vegetable, 4 Lean Protein, 3 1/2 Fat**

(table continues on next page)

Hearty 'N' Healthy

Menu Samplers Section	Menu Item	Amount	Calories	Fat (g)	% Calories from Fat	Saturated Fat (g)	Chol. (mg)	Sodium (mg)	Carb. (g)	Fiber (g)	Protein (g)	Exchanges/ Choices
Hearty 'N' Healthy (Men)	Fish tacos (fish, rice, grilled vegetables, lettuce, and pico de gallo)	3 tacos	594	12		3	42	900	90	6	27	5 Starch, 2 Vegetable, 4 Lean Protein
	Refried beans and cheese	1 side (3 oz)	200	9		3	5	250	22	13	10	1 Starch, 1 Lean Protein, 1 Fat
Totals			794	21	24	6	47	1150	112	19	37	6 Starch, 2 Vegetable, 5 Lean Protein, 1 Fat

(table continues on next page)

Lower Carb 'N' Healthy

Menu Samplers Section	Menu Item	Amount	Calories	Fat (g)	% Calories from Fat	Saturated Fat (g)	Chol. (mg)	Sodium (mg)	Carb. (g)	Fiber (g)	Protein (g)	Exchanges/ Choices
Lower Carb 'N' Healthy (Women)	Pork black bean burrito (rice, black beans, seasoned pork, cheese blend, salsa, shredded lettuce, and flour tortilla)	8 oz	505	14		4.5	32	1120	62	8	22	3 Starch, 1 Other Carbohydrate, 3 Medium-Fat Protein
Totals			**505**	**14**	**25**	**4.5**	**32**	**1120**	**62**	**8**	**22**	**3 Starch, 1 Other Carbohydrate, 3 Medium-Fat Protein**

(table continues on next page)

Lower Carb 'N' Healthy

Menu Samplers Section	Menu Item	Amount	Calories	Fat (g)	% Calories from Fat	Saturated Fat (g)	Chol. (mg)	Sodium (mg)	Carb. (g)	Fiber (g)	Protein (g)	Exchanges/ Choices
Lower Carb 'N' Healthy (Men)	Beef burrito (ground beef, cheese, taco sauce in a flour tortilla)	8 oz	420	19		8	85	1060	24	2	29	1 1/2 Starch, 3 Medium-Fat Protein, 1 Fat
	Chips with corn, pepper, and tomato salsa	4 oz	280	12		1	0	200	48	6	4	2 Starch, 2 Vegetable, 2 Fat
Totals			700	31	40	9	85	1260	72	8	33	3 1/2 Starch, 2 Vegetable, 3 Medium-Fat Protein, 3 Fat

Mexican Menu Lingo

▶ **Arróz:** the Spanish word for rice. Mexican rice is made from long-grain white rice with sautéed tomatoes, onions, and garlic added for flavor.

▶ **Burrito:** a wheat-flour tortilla (soft, not fried) filled with chicken, beef, cheese, and/or beans and served rolled up. Some quick-serve restaurants have begun to serve tortilla-free burritos. It's just the burrito fixings in a bowl.

▶ **Carne:** the Spanish word for meat.

▶ **Carnitas:** a Mexican version of pulled pork, in which the pork is slowly cooked then shredded and spiced.

▶ **Cerveza:** the Spanish word for beer.

▶ **Ceviche:** raw seafood (usually shrimp or scallops) marinated or "cooked" in lime or lemon juice for many hours and served as an appetizer or light meal.

▶ **Chilies:** types of peppers that come in a variety of different shapes, sizes, colors, and flavors. There are over 100 different types of chilies native to Mexico. They vary in level of spiciness from mild to hot, hotter, and hottest. Chilies are available fresh and dried.

▶ **Chili con carne:** a thick soup, usually called "chili" in America, made with tomatoes, onions, peppers, beans, and, of course, chilies for kick. Con carne means "with meat." The meat can be ground, shredded, or in chunks. Vegetarian chili contains no meat. Chili is often served with chopped raw onions and shredded cheese.

▶ **Chimichanga:** a flour tortilla filled with beef, chicken, cheese, and/or beans, then deep-fried and served topped with tomato-based sauce.

▶ **Chorizo:** Mexican pork sausage that is highly seasoned.

▶ **Churros:** a fried dough pastry, often dipped in hot chocolate or café con leche (coffee with milk).

▶ **Cilantro:** a leafy green herb with a distinctive flavor frequently used in Mexican cooking; it is also called coriander.

▶ **Empanadas:** a pastry turnover filled with savory ingredients, then baked or fried.

▶ **Enchiladas:** corn tortillas dipped in enchilada sauce, warmed on a flat grill with a small amount of oil, filled with either chicken, beef, or cheese, and then served topped with light tomato-based enchilada sauce.

▶ **Fajitas:** sautéed chicken or beef served with sautéed onions and green peppers, shredded lettuce, tomatoes, guacamole, sour cream, and a side of flour or corn tortillas. Usually you make your own fajitas at the table, and there's often enough food for two.

▶ **Flan:** baked custard with a caramel topping. Flan contains mainly sugar, eggs, cream, and whole or condensed milk.

▶ **Flautas:** a rolled taco filled with beef, cheese, or chicken, then deep-fried. Sometimes called a taquito.

▶ **Gazpacho:** spicy, cold tomato-based soup containing puréed or chopped tomatoes, cucumbers, peppers, and onions.

▶ **Guacamole:** mashed avocado, onion, tomatoes, garlic, lemon juice, and spices. Guacamole is served as a topping, as a dip with chips, or on the side. Avocado is high in fat: approximately 80 calories per one-quarter of a small avocado. The fat is mainly monounsaturated. Avocados contain no cholesterol.

▶ **Jalapeño:** a very small, spicy, green chile used to spice or top certain menu items.

▶ **Mole:** a traditional sauce used on chicken or meats or to top enchiladas. There are many varieties of the sauce, and each variety typically contains more than 20 different ingredients and seasonings.

▶ **Nopalitos:** a dish made with diced nopales—the flat stems of the prickly pear cactus. The nopales are often pickled.

▶ **Pastel de tres leches:** a sponge cake soaked in three types of milk: evaporated milk, condensed milk, and heavy cream.

▶ **Quesadillas:** a tortilla that is filled with cheese and heated. Other ingredients may include meats, vegetables, or beans.

▶ **Queso fundido:** a dish of hot melted cheese with spicy chorizo.

▶ **Refried beans:** pinto beans or black beans that have been cooked and then refried in lard and seasoned with onions, garlic, and chilies.

▶ **Salsa:** a hot red sauce made from tomatoes, onions, and chilies. Salsa appears automatically on the table of most Mexican restaurants.

▶ **Salsa verde:** a hot green sauce made from tomatillos, the Mexican green tomato, and other spices.

▶ **Sopapillas:** a deep-fried pastry typically eaten with sugar or honey.

▶ **Taco:** a corn or flour tortilla filled with meat or chicken, shredded cheese, lettuce, and tomatoes. In the United States, the tortilla is sometimes fried in the shape of a "U."

▶ **Tamale:** a spicy filling of either meat or chicken surrounded by moist cornmeal dough, which is wrapped in corn husks or banana leaves and then steamed.

► **Tortilla:** the "bread" of Mexico, a very thin circle of dough made from either corn or flour. Corn tortillas are often fried into taco shells or chips and served with salsa.

► **Tostadas:** a crisp fried tortilla, which then may be covered with various toppings such as cheese, beans, lettuce, tomato, and/or onions.

ⓘ What's Your Solution? Answers

a) Good job identifying the high-fat items in your meal and requesting less of these. By asking for just half the cheese and sour cream, you'll probably save about 100 calories. That's a good start, but you'll want to do more to meet your healthy eating goals.

b) Choosing brown rice over white rice, if available, will add about 2 grams of fiber to your meal and add a serving of whole grains, which may help you feel a bit fuller on fewer calories. Skipping the chips and sour cream will save you a few hundred calories.

c) Even a healthy burrito can come close to 1,000 calories, depending on the size and fillings. Taking half home is a smart way to get the flavors you crave with only half the calories.

d) The flour tortilla used to make burritos is often quite large, containing approximately 300 calories and 45 grams of carbohydrate. Two taco-size flour tortillas provide about 175 calories and 25 grams of carbohydrate, which makes ordering soft tacos a great portion-control strategy. Choosing beans instead of rice will give you more fiber, while requesting just a sprinkle of cheese will provide flavor without all the fat. Sharing the chips and guacamole is a great way to indulge without overdoing it. Set a goal for how many you will eat and stick to it.

CHAPTER 19

Italian

T oday, Italian food is served in a wide array of settings, from inexpensive eateries in airports or food courts to elegant four-star sit-down restaurants. Italian food, besides pizza (which is covered in Chapter 20), is served in lots of independent restaurants, as well as in a growing list of national sit-down chains, such as Buca di Beppo, Carmines, Carrabba's Italian Grill, Maggiano's Little Italy, Olive Garden, and Romano's Macaroni Grill. Other national chains with locations in food courts or along city streets are California Pizza Kitchen and The Old Spaghetti Factory. Then there are the order-at-the-counter restaurants, such as Sbarro, Fazoli's, and Noodles & Company.

Italian cuisine is so richly integrated into menus across America that you can find traditional Italian dishes on many menus, including those at American family-style restaurants. Even a few of the big pizza chains, such as Domino's and Pizza Hut, have widened their menus to now include a few pasta dishes. Speaking of pizza, it is, without a doubt, one of the foods Americans—particularly children and young families—eat most frequently in and from restaurants. This statement is truer today than ever before as more people look for fast and easy meals that please the palates of all family members. Chapter 20 (page 390) will tell you everything you want to know (and more) about eating pizza healthfully. Yes, it can be done!

On the Menu

Italian cuisine ranks in the top three on Americans' hit parade of ethnic favorites. There is no doubt that you can eat healthfully in Italian restaurants; a cup of minestrone, linguine with white clam sauce, and a demitasse of espresso, for example, are great choices for a meal. At the opposite end of the spectrum, however, you can easily end up with a meal loaded with fat, cholesterol, and sodium. An unhealthy Italian meal might start with garlic bread slathered with butter and an antipasto of Italian cheeses, Genoa salami, marinated artichokes, and olives followed by an entrée of fettuccini Alfredo, and a cannoli for dessert.

A wide range of choices, from healthy to not so healthy, awaits you at Italian restaurants. And portion sizes are often large. Portion control, as usual, will be a key skill to help you avoid overeating in Italian restaurants.

Upscale Italian restaurants typically follow a traditional Italian meal structure, which includes several courses—appetizers, a pasta course, a meat course, and more. If you're tempted to follow the old adage of "when in Rome," think twice. Italians typically only eat each of these courses during celebratory meals. Plus they keep portions in check and walk a lot to burn off any large influx of calories. One Italian strategy you'll want to follow is sharing, which works wonderfully at family-style restaurants such as Buca di Beppo and Maggiano's Little Italy. Just remember, order several fewer dishes than there are people at the table.

Pasta, the quintessential Italian dish, can be a surprisingly healthy choice as long as you top it wisely and control the portion size. Yes, you read this correctly. Pasta has unfairly gotten a bad rap with criticism of its carbohydrate content and glycemic effect. The reality is that pasta can hold the line on fat and calories better than some burger-and-fry combinations. Pasta *can* fit with today's diabetes nutrition goals: it is low in fat and protein and moderate in carbohydrate. Enjoy pasta in reasonable quantities and top it wisely. Though healthier whole-grain pastas are very available on supermarket shelves, they're still a rarity on restaurant menus. Too bad, because that would make pasta an even healthier option. Today you can request whole-grain pasta at Olive Garden. Maybe in time it will be available in other restaurants as well.

Another benefit is that vegetables are plentiful in Italian dishes, from vegetable-based soups and tomato sauces to sautéed vegetables served on top of pasta or as a side. Take advantage of this and load up on low-calorie vegetables to feel full and keep pasta portions in check. Don't bury them in cream and cheese sauces.

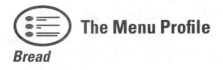 **The Menu Profile**

Bread

Ah, the bread. Italians have mastered the art of bread baking. As the menu is placed in front of you in an Italian restaurant, crusty Italian bread with butter or olive oil, garlic rolls, breadsticks, or focaccia (Italian flatbread) may well land on the table too. Unadulterated whole-grain bread is your best option, but it's a rarity in Italian restaurants. Before you reach out for the bread basket, make sure that the bread is really worth the carbohydrate grams. If your calorie and carbohydrate-gram goals allow for it, have one piece of bread and ask for a small dish of tomato (or marinara) sauce or balsamic vinegar to dip it in. If you have more calories and fat grams to spare, dip it in olive oil (rather than spreading on butter). With olive oil, you'll eat some good fats and limit unhealthy ones. After grabbing one piece, pass the bread as far away from you as possible. Keep in mind that a request to take it back to the kitchen is perfectly reasonable.

Antipasti (Appetizers)

Antipasti typically include starters like charcuterie (an assortment of Italian deli meats), cheeses, bruschetta, and vegetables. Sometimes you'll find shrimp, calamari (squid), mussels, or clams on the menu. At fast casual or more Americanized restaurants, the chefs love to fry, so you'll likely find deep-fried mozzarella and zucchini sticks as well as an assortment of flatbreads.

When you look at the menu, can you spot the all-star appetizers versus those that should get the boot? For a healthy starter try shrimp, squid, mussels, or clams in a tomato sauce or a sauce that uses any combination of lemon, garlic, herbs, and/or wine. Or select an antipasto of marinated vegetables—peppers, pickles, and olives—if you've got some wiggle room with your sodium count.

You may find fresh tomatoes featured as the star ingredient in crostini or bruschetta (tomatoes and garlic brushed on slices of Italian bread), but these options can be high in calories and carbohydrate depending on the thickness of the bread slices. Caprese salad, in which slices of fresh tomato, fresh mozzarella, and basil are layered, is a frequent appetizer option in Italian restaurants. Fresh mozzarella, like most cheese, has a significant amount of total and saturated fat; fat providing about 75% of the calories in a Caprese appetizer. If the Caprese is calling your name, go ahead and enjoy, but limit the cheese and other high-fat items you eat throughout the rest of your meal. You may also want to ask if they can add extra tomatoes to your dish.

Antipasti loaded with cheeses and Italian cold cuts, such as in charcuterie, are high in fat with a goodly dose of saturated fat. Avoid these options. Steer clear of deep-fried calamari, mozzarella, and zucchini sticks as well.

Soups and Salads

If you don't find any healthy antipasti on the menu, you're sure to have better luck with a soup or salad. Popular Italian soups are minestrone, stracciatella, pasta e fagioli, and Italian wedding. These are all tomato- or broth-based soups, making them a relatively low-calorie way to begin your meal. The beans in the minestrone and the pasta e fagioli can even add a bit of fiber to your meal.

Insalata, the innocent-sounding crunchy greens, can be filling and low in calories (depending on what's atop the greens). Look for salads made with radicchio (red leaves), arugula (a peppery-tasting green), endive, tomatoes, broccoli, mixed baby field greens, spinach, beets, peppers, onions, and/or other raw or marinated vegetables. A few olives or condiments like sun-dried tomatoes aren't a problem, but some Italian salads are loaded with high-fat items like cheese, pasta salad, proscuitto (Italian ham), bacon, pancetta (Italian cured bacon), or nuts. Avoid these high-fat items.

Order salad dressing on the side and try to choose a light option. Or, better yet, try a bit of olive oil with a vinegar of your choosing or a few squeezes of fresh lemon wedges. Some Italian restaurants use a variety of vinegars, from red wine and balsamic to flavored vinegars, such as tarragon or rosemary. If you spot one of these vinegars used on the menu, you know it's in the kitchen. Ask for vinegar on the side to use alone or to stretch the dressing you've ordered. (You can use it to dip your bread in as well.)

Caesar salad, with egg, grated cheese, anchovies, and thick and creamy dressing, is one salad option you need to limit. Just so you know, a traditional Caesar salad is dressed with an oil and lemon–based dressing, which is a healthier choice. Upscale restaurants often serve them dressed this way. If you've just got to have a Caesar salad ask them to go light on the cheese and serve dressing on the side with lemon wedges.

Panini

If you eat Italian for lunch, you may be tempted to order a panini, the Italian version of a toasted or grilled sandwich. The bread can often be hefty and the sandwich is usually oozing with high-fat cheese. Your best strategy is to order a half of a panini or split one with a dining companion. Pair it with a cup of healthy soup or a salad for a more balanced, lower-calorie lunch. If the kitchen won't accommodate a half-panini order and there's no one willing to share, then request a carry-out container and immediately put half of your sandwich in it to enjoy tomorrow.

Primo Piatto (First Course)

A featured item on most Italian menus is pasta, which is traditionally offered as the first course in a multi-course meal. Pasta is made by combining flour, water, and eggs (optional). Pasta takes many different shapes and forms, some large, some small, some stuffed, some not. Familiarize yourself with the variety of pastas at the end of this chapter (*Know Your Pasta*, page 388). Some healthier pasta choices include angel hair, linguini, fusilli, fettuccini, or ziti. Try flavored pastas: spinach, squid ink, or tomato.

Pasta on its own contains no fat; it's just carbohydrate with a bit of protein. One cup of cooked pasta (with no sauce) has about 220 calories and about 43 grams of carbohydrate. Though whole-grain pasta isn't typically available, it's beginning to make an appearance. Restaurants like Fazoli's, Olive Garden, and Noodles & Company have added it as an option on their menus. Perhaps the other large national chains will follow suit in the not too distant future. Order it if it's an option; you'll pick up a couple of grams of fiber and some other nutrients from the whole grain.

One of the challenges of eating pasta in restaurants is that it's served in huge portions. What's your portion-control weaponry? Split an order, take home half, or order an appetizer-size serving. Calories are another challenge when it comes to pasta. The calories in pasta dishes can add up fast depending on what your pasta is topped or stuffed with. Is the sauce tomato-based and loaded with onions and garlic, such as a marinara sauce? Or is it a sauce that's loaded with high-fat ingredients such as cheeses, sausage, cream, and/or bacon, such as a carbonara sauce? Your strategy is to keep an eye out for the *Green-Flag Words* for Italian cuisine and avoid menu items that use or contain the terms listed under *Red-Flag Words* (find both on page 377).

No need to sweat it. You can always find healthy pasta choices. Look for pasta marinara, pasta primavera (sautéed vegetables), or pasta with red or white clam sauce or Bolognese sauce. Limit stuffed items such as ravioli, cannelloni, and manicotti because they are usually stuffed with cheese or ingredients that are combined with cheese or butter. You can order one of these stuffed pastas if it's stuffed with vegetables, but ask for details before you order—it may be topped with a cream sauce.

If you are carefully watching your calories and fat grams, then leave pesto alone. Pesto is made with basil, which is a good start, but then three high-fat ingredients are usually blended in: pignoli (pine) nuts, olive oil, and Parmesan cheese. Just because it's green doesn't mean it's healthy. But, if you've got a few extra calories and fat grams to spare, go ahead. A small amount of flavorful pesto spreads around a small pile of pasta.

Two other primo piatto treats found more commonly in upscale Italian restaurants are risotto and polenta, which are grain-based dishes native to Italy. Risotto is made with Arborio rice, a short-grain rice with stubby kernels. It traces its ancestry to the Po Valley region of Italy, where it is grown in abundance. Unfortunately, chefs typically prepare risotto with lots of butter, cheese, sausage, and other high-fat ingredients. The taste might be great, but the calories count and fat and cholesterol content will be high. If you wish to try it, look for a risotto dish that blends spices, herbs, and vegetables. For example: risotto with spinach and mushrooms or risotto primavera. Polenta is like cornmeal pudding. Cornmeal, water, and salt are the three main ingredients. Polenta is a staple in the Veneto region of Italy. It is often served with sauces, many of which may load on the fat, so use caution if you order polenta. Sometimes you'll see triangles of polenta that have been grilled. These are low in fat grams.

Secondo Piatto (Main Course)

Moving on to the traditional secondo piatto, or main course, you might find *pollo, pesce,* or *carne*—that's poultry, seafood, or meat. If you're having pasta, don't feel compelled to order a main course, unless you split it or take half home. Most main courses are simply too much protein for one meal. When you do order a main course, try to choose grilled fish, scallops, or chicken breast. Again, as with pasta, the magic question is "how is it prepared?" Look for tomato-based sauces or sauces with vegetable, mushroom, or wine prepared without cream. It's common to see different proteins prepared with the same sauces on the menus. Limit the high-fat and high-sodium Prosciutto ham, pancetta, cheese, and cream sauces. Also, tread lightly with anything prepared parmigiana (or Parmesan) style, such as chicken or eggplant parmigiana. Anything prepared in this style has been deep-fried, then layered with cheese. Give these dishes the boot.

One popular Italian entrée is veal. Misconceptions about veal exist. Many people believe that veal is relatively low in calories, fat, and cholesterol. It's true that veal cutlet, the lean cut often used in Italian restaurants, is low in calories (about 40–50 per cooked ounce), but the cholesterol content is similar to that of lean beef (about 20–25 milligrams per ounce cooked). On the other side of the veal spectrum is veal breast, which is higher in fat at about 60–70 calories per cooked ounce. The main problem is that veal is most often prepared by being dredged in flour before being sautéed in butter or oil. If you have a few extra calories to spare, veal marsala, cacciatore, or piccata is a decent choice. If calories are tight, stick with grilled fish or chicken and enjoy veal cutlet at home, where you can prepare it healthfully.

Contorni (Side Dishes)

Traditional Italian side dishes are often served alongside the main course. They are usually vegetables served hot or cold, raw or cooked. Grilled asparagus, Brussels sprouts, sautéed broccolini or broccoli rabe, and roasted mushrooms are just a few options you may find on the menu. As always, be on the lookout for high-fat sauces that may be added to the vegetables. If there is a vegetable you like on the menu, but it has a red-flag word in the description, ask if it can be prepared differently. Most restaurants can easily accommodate this request.

Dolce (Dessert)

For dessert, Italian menus list items such as panna cotta, spumoni, cannoli, gelato, sorbetto, Italian ices, and fresh berries with liqueur and whipped cream to quench the sweet tooth. Think about splitting a dessert among several diners or choose a lower-fat Italian ice or sorbet. Better yet, go for the fresh berries. Another option: End the meal as they do in Italy—with a demitasse of espresso. Buon appetito!

The Lowdown on Olives and Olive Oil

In central and southern Italy, olive oil replaces butter as the fat of choice in recipes. Today, olives and olive oil wear a nutrition halo. That's because the fats in olive oil, mainly monounsaturated and (less so) polyunsaturated fats, are being touted for their health value. Olive oil contains minimal saturated fats. Monounsaturated fats help lower LDLs (bad cholesterol) without decreasing HDLs (good cholesterol). Fatty ingredients that contain mainly monounsaturated fats and don't come from animals, such as olive, canola, and peanut oils and nuts, and avocado, have the added benefit of being cholesterol-free. For these reasons, olive oil is one of the healthier fats you can consume both at home and away from home. However, do remember that any type of olive oil contains the same number of calories (50 calories per teaspoon) as every other fat, from butter to lard and hard shortening.

When it comes to olives themselves, try the many varieties available. Enjoy them on salads, in Italian sauces, or just as a tasty side item. Remember, however, that they fall into the high-sodium food category and, just like the oil that they are processed into, they contain mainly fat.

Nutrition Snapshot

Health Busters

Category	Restaurant Name	Dish Name	Serving Size	Cal.	Total Fat (g)	Carb. (g)	Sod. (mg)
Appetizers	Olive Garden	Calamari	1 portion	890	54	64	2340
Appetizers	The Old Spaghetti Factory	Bay Shrimp Crostini	1 portion	720	41	54	1510
Appetizers	The Old Spaghetti Factory	Portuguese Linguica	1 portion	1080	75	52	2830
Breads	Sbarro	Garlic Rolls	1 roll	170	5	28	370
Breads	The Old Spaghetti Factory	Sicilian Garlic Cheese	1 order	1310	76	110	2510
Caesar Salad Entrées	The Old Spaghetti Factory	Entrée Chicken Caesar	1 portion	1130	90	29	2240
Caesar Salad Entrées	The Old Spaghetti Factory	Chicken Caesar	1 portion	870	67	21	1780
Caesar Salad Entrées	Olive Garden	Grilled Chicken Caesar	1 portion	610	40	19	1230
Raviolis	Bertucci's	Four Cheese Ravioli	1 portion	950	29	118	2110
Raviolis	Romano's Macaroni Grill	Mushroom Ravioli	1 portion	900	31	52	1020

(table continues on next page)

Health Busters

Category	Restaurant Name	Dish Name	Serving Size	Cal.	Total Fat (g)	Carb. (g)	Sod. (mg)
Raviolis	Olive Garden	Cheese Ravioli w/Meat Sauce	1 portion	790	28	88	1510
Raviolis	Fazoli's	Ravioli w/ Alfredo Sauce	1 portion	710	40	55	2450
Lasagnas	Bertucci's	Rustica	1 portion	1310	65	119	2960
Lasagnas	Olive Garden	Rollata Al Forno	1 portion	1170	68	90	2510
Lasagnas	Fazoli's	Four Cheese	1 portion	1000	49	79	2560
Pasta Alfredos	Romano's Macaroni Grill	Fettuccine w/Chicken	1 portion	1470	43	94	2560
Pasta Alfredos	Olive Garden	Fettuccine	1 portion	1220	75	99	1350
Pasta Alfredos	Bertucci's	Fettuccine w/Shrimp & Asparagus	1 portion	1210	41	142	1660
Pasta Alfredos	Bertucci's	Rigatoni Broccoli & Shrimp w/Cream Sauce	1 portion	970	31	117	1290
Pasta Alfredos	Romano's Macaroni Grill	Fettucine w/Chicken	1 portion	1470	43	94	2560
Pasta Alfredos	Olive Garden	Seafood	1 portion	1020	52	88	2430
Pasta Entrées (Other)	Bertucci's	Spaghetti w/Meatballs and Bolognese Sauce	1 portion	1880	84	198	3740
Pasta Entrées (Other)	Romano's Macaroni Grill	Mom's Ricotta Meatballs & Spaghetti (Bolognese)	1 portion	1190	19	95	3310

(table continues on next page)

Health Busters

Category	Restaurant Name	Dish Name	Serving Size	Cal.	Total Fat (g)	Carb. (g)	Sod. (mg)
Pasta Entrées (Other)	Olive Garden	Spaghetti & Meatballs (dinner)	1 portion	920	36	98	1770
Eggplant Entrées	Bertucci's	Roasted Eggplant Panini	1 portion	1010	54	85	1550
Eggplant Entrées	Olive Garden	Eggplant Parmigiana	1 portion	850	35	98	1900
Chicken Entrées	Fazoli's	Chicken Parmigano	1 portion	920	32	106	2420
Chicken Entrées	Olive Garden	Chicken Parmigiana	1 portion	1090	49	79	3380
Veal Entrées	Romano's Macaroni Grill	Veal Saltimbocca	1 portion	1320	73	81	1770
Salmon Entrées	Bertucci's	Grilled Salmon	1 portion	520	35	1	70
Salmon Entrées	Romano's Macaroni Grill	Grilled King Salmon	1 portion	1110	68	71	1220
Desserts	Bertucci's	Cheesecake	1 slice	940	68	67	660
Desserts	Romano's Macaroni Grill	New York Style Cheesecake	1 slice	760	52	61	520
Desserts	Romano's Macaroni Grill	Tiramisu	1 portion	690	48	54	160
Desserts	Fazoli's	New York Style Cheesecake w/ Strawberry Topping	1 slice	630	45	49	630
Desserts	Olive Garden	Tiramisu	1 portion	510	32	48	75

Healthier Bets

Category	Restaurant Name	Dish Name	Serving Size	Cal.	Total Fat (g)	Sat. Fat (g)	Carb. (g)	Pro. (g)	Fiber (g)	Chol. (mg)	Sodium (mg)	Exchanges/ Choices
Appetizers	Tony Roma's	Kids' Appetizer Celery & Carrots w/ Buttermilk Dressing	1 portion	190	19	4	3	1	1	24	407	1 Vegetable, 4 Fat
Soups	Pizzeria Uno Chicago Grill	Veggie	1 bowl	90	1	0	18	4	3	0	620	3 1/2 Vegetable
Soups	Pizzeria Uno Chicago Grill	Italian Wedding	1 bowl	120	3.5	1	16	6	2	15	730	1/2 Starch, 2 Vegetable, 1/2 Lean Protein, 1/2 Fat
Soups	Bertucci's	Tuscan Minestrone	1 cup	100	2.5	1.5	14	6	2	n/a	640	1/2 Starch, 2 Vegetable, 1/2 Fat
Salads	Sbarro	Caesar Salad	1 portion	80	5	1	6	2	1	5	200	1 Vegetable, 1 Fat
Salads	Olive Garden	Garden-Fresh Salad (without dressing)	1 portion	130	4	0.5	19	4	4	n/a	530	1/2 Starch, 2 Vegetable, 1 Fat

(table continues on next page)

Healthier Bets

Category	Restaurant Name	Dish Name	Serving Size	Cal.	Total Fat (g)	Sat. Fat (g)	Carb. (g)	Pro. (g)	Fiber (g)	Chol. (mg)	Sodium (mg)	Exchanges/Choices
Salads	Tony Roma's	Dinner Caesar Side Salad	1 portion	215	18	4	10	6	2	21	578	2 Vegetable, 1/2 Medium-Fat Protein, 3 Fat
Salads	Olive Garden	Garden-Fresh Salad (without dressing)	1 portion	130	4	0.5	19	4	4	50	700	1/2 Starch, 2 Vegetable, 1 Fat
Salads	Pizzeria Uno Chicago Grill	Power Salad	1 portion	270	6	2	34	21	5	n/a	867	1 1/2 Fruit, 2 Vegetable, 2 1/2 Lean Protein, 1/2 Fat
Salads	Bertucci's	Insalata, w/out Dressing	1 portion	150	6	2.5	21	7	5	n/a	710	1/2 Starch, 2 Vegetable, 1 Fat
Kids' Meals	Bertucci's	Kids' 4 Cheese Ravioli w/ Pasta Sauce (chicken added)	1 portion	440	13	4.5	47	33	3	n/a	n/a	2 1/2 Starch, 2 Vegetable, 3 Medium-Fat Protein

(table continues on next page)

Healthier Bets

Category	Restaurant Name	Dish Name	Serving Size	Cal.	Total Fat (g)	Sat. Fat (g)	Carb. (g)	Pro. (g)	Fiber (g)	Chol. (mg)	Sodium (mg)	Exchanges/ Choices
Kids' Meals	Bertucci's	Kids' 4 Cheese Ravioli w/ Pasta Sauce	1 portion	290	8	4	38	16	3	n/a	n/a	2 Starch, 1 1/2 Vegetable, 1 High-Fat Protein
Kids' Meals	Olive Garden	Cheese Ravioli	1 portion	290	8	3.5	43	12	3	n/a	760	2 1/2 Starch, 1 Vegetable, 1 1/2 Fat
Kids' Meals	Fazoli's	Three Cheese Baked Ravioli	1 portion	340	19	11	26	17	2	80	940	1 1/2 Starch, 1 Vegetable, 1 1/2 High-Fat Protein, 1 Fat
Pasta Entrées	Romano's Macaroni Grill	Lasagna Bolognese	1 portion	510	18	0.5	46	41	4	n/a	1860	3 Starch, 5 Lean Protein, 1 Fat
Pasta Entrées	Fazoli's	Spaghetti w/ Meatballs	1 portion	300	7	2.5	45	12	3	n/a	n/a	2 1/2 Starch, 1 Vegetable, 1 Medium-Fat Protein

(table continues on next page)

Healthier Bets

Category	Restaurant Name	Dish Name	Serving Size	Cal.	Total Fat (g)	Sat. Fat (g)	Carb. (g)	Pro. (g)	Fiber (g)	Chol. (mg)	Sodium (mg)	Exchanges/ Choices
Pasta Entrées	Bertucci's	Spaghetti w/ Meatballs (kids)	1 portion	530	13	4.5	82	23	5	n/a	900	4 Starch, 3 Vegetable, 2 Medium-Fat Protein
Pasta Entrées	The Old Spaghetti Factory	Kids' Spaghetti w/ Meat Sauce	1 portion	410	6	1.5	70	18	4	15	650	4 Starch, 2 Vegetable, 1 Medium-Fat Protein
Pasta Entrées	Romano's Macaroni Grill	Capellini Pomodoro	1 portion	340	11	1	55	7	6	n/a	n/a	2 1/2 Starch, 2 Vegetable, 2 Fat
Pasta Entrées	Olive Garden	Linguine Alla Marinara (lunch)	1 portion	310	4	1	55	12	5	n/a	n/a	3 Starch, 2 Vegetable, 1 Fat
Pasta Entrées	The Old Spaghetti Factory	Spaghetti Marinara	1 portion	370	3.5	0	72	13	5	0	580	4 Starch, 2 Vegetable
Pasta Entrées	Fazoli's	Spaghetti w/ Marinara Sauce	1 portion	220	1	0	43	7	3	0	330	2 1/2 Starch, 1 Vegetable

(table continues on next page)

Healthier Bets

Category	Restaurant Name	Dish Name	Serving Size	Cal.	Total Fat (g)	Sat. Fat (g)	Carb. (g)	Pro. (g)	Fiber (g)	Chol. (mg)	Sodium (mg)	Exchanges/ Choices
Salmon Entrée	Tony Roma's	Salmon, Pan Seared w/ Sesame Crusted and Fish Grill Toppings— Mojo Glace	1 portion	397	12	1	13	54	3	207	1198	1 Starch, 7 Lean Protein
Salmon Entrée	Tony Roma's	Asian Salad w/ Grilled Salmon (lunch)	1 portion	407	16	3	33	32	3	84	783	1 1/2 Starch, 2 Vegetable, 4 Lean Protein, 1 Fat
Vegetables	Pizzeria Uno Chicago Grill	Roasted Seasonal Vegetables	1 portion	80	4.5	0	10	2	3	0	160	2 Vegetable, 1 Fat
Vegetables	Sbarro	Mixed Vegetables	1 portion	190	15	3	14	3	4	0	330	1/2 Starch, 1 Vegetable, 3 Fat

Green-Flag Words

Ingredients:

▶ Artichoke hearts—not marinated in oil
▶ Broccoli, broccolini, broccoli rabe
▶ Capers (high in sodium)
▶ Grilled chicken, fish, seafood
▶ Herbs (basil and oregano)
▶ Marinated vegetables—not in oil
▶ Olives, olive oil
▶ Pasta (all types other than those stuffed with cheese)
▶ Spinach, kale, and other greens
▶ Sun-dried tomatoes
▶ Tomatoes—raw or cooked
▶ Tomatoes, onions, peppers, mushrooms

Cooking Methods/Menu Descriptions:

▶ Light mushroom and wine sauce
▶ Light red- or white-wine sauce
▶ Lightly sautéed with onions and shallots
▶ Piccata
▶ Primavera (without cream)
▶ Tomato sauce and meatballs
▶ Tomato-based sauces—marinara, Bolognese, cacciatore, pomodoro, puttanesca
▶ White or red clam sauce

Red-Flag Words

Ingredients:

▶ Butter
▶ Cheese—mozzarella, Gorgonzola, Parmesan, provolone
▶ Eggplant or zucchini (if fried)
▶ Italian cold cuts
▶ Pancetta, prosciutto, or bacon
▶ Sausage, veal, or pork

Cooking Methods/Menu Descriptions:

- ► Alfredo
- ► Cannelloni
- ► Carbonara
- ► Charcuterie
- ► Creamy sauces (wine, mushroom, cheese)
- ► Fried or deep-fried
- ► Lasagna
- ► Manicotti
- ► Parmigiana (veal, chicken, eggplant)
- ► Saltimbocca
- ► Stuffed shells
- ► Stuffed with cheese

At the Table:

- ► Butter
- ► Grated cheese
- ► Salad dressing

Healthy Eating Tips and Tactics

- ► Share multiple courses with your dining companions. This lets you sample a lot of different dishes without overdoing it.
- ► Make marinara sauce (or light tomato sauce) your go-to sauce. Use it as a topping for your pasta or as a dip for your bread.
- ► Ask for a take-home container. Even when you share a dish, in some restaurants you'll still have plenty left over to enjoy for a meal on another day.
- ► Along with pasta, munch on a healthy garden salad to fill yourself up but not out.
- ► The red pepper flakes you'll probably find sitting right on your table (or in your spice cabinet for takeout) will add zip to your pizza, pasta, or salad without adding calories.
- ► Decline the bread basket before it even hits your table.

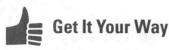 **Get It Your Way**

► Manage your portions. Request a half-order (possibly called "appetizer size") of pasta if you don't have someone to split it with. Or take home half of a regular order.

► Swap sauces. Instead of a cream- or oil-based sauce, ask that your pasta be tossed with a tomato-based sauce, such as marinara or Bolognese sauce.

► Add in extra vegetables. See a favorite pasta dish on the menu? Ask that broccoli or another favorite vegetable be added to it. This will help you fill up on fewer calories.

► Request that the chef hold or use less cheese, bacon, olives, or pine nuts in your dish.

 Tips and Tactics for Gluten-Free Eating

► Avoid all meats, poultry, and seafood that has been dredged in flour, breaded, battered, or fried. Meatballs typically contain breadcrumbs, so they probably contain gluten. Order a protein that has been roasted, baked, broiled, or grilled on clean surfaces. Check all sauces, marinades, and seasonings for gluten.

► All breads and pasta, unless otherwise stated as gluten-free, are made from wheat. Beware of restaurants that make their own pasta from scratch as there may be residual flour in the air.

► Order risotto or polenta prepared in a gluten-free broth.

► Fresh vegetables or salad with balsamic or red wine vinegar and olive oil on the side are good choices. Try a Caprese salad with sliced tomatoes, mozzarella, and basil.

► Olive Garden stocks gluten-free rotini to serve on request and will give you additional nutrition or food allergy information and gluten-free menu items upon request. Make sure that gluten-free pasta is cooked in fresh, clean water and that a clean strainer, tongs, etc., are used to serve it.

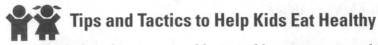 **Tips and Tactics to Help Kids Eat Healthy**

▶ Think about how you can add a vegetable serving to your child's meal. At many Italian restaurants, pasta or chicken strips (grilled or deep-fried) are the default kids' meal options and vegetables are nowhere to be found. Can you order a side of broccoli to share with your child? Or a cup of minestrone soup?

▶ Choose marinara over cream-based sauces. Sure, it's messy, but, like you, your child will benefit from this tomato-based topping that's low in fat. Now is a good time to use that old napkin-as-a-bib trick.

▶ Take advantage of family-style ordering to give your child the grown-up responsibility of picking a dish that the whole family will share. Want to increase the odds that your child will eat his or her veggies? Ask your child to pick the vegetable dish for the table.

▶ Share, share, share! Most portions at Italian restaurants are big enough for two or three to share. Rather than order a special kids' meal for your child, bring him or her in on the sharing of regular menu items, just like the Italians do.

? **What's Your Solution?**

Your family is at a festive Italian restaurant where the food is served family style. You recently set a family wellness goal together to eat more healthfully, which involves watching portions and eating more vegetables. Yet most of the choices that your family members are requesting are large portions of foods topped with layers of cheese.

What can you say and do to help your family stick to the wellness goal everyone agreed to?

    a) Establish a plan for the meal in advance. Agree to order at least one to two servings of vegetables. Then, depending on the number of people and the individual preferences of each person, decide how many pasta and entrée dishes you will order.

b) Start with a big family-style salad. Nosh on that while you peruse the rest of the menu.

c) Request that take-home containers hit your table at the same time as your entrées.

d) Make special requests. Challenge every family member to think of a way to make each dish a little bit healthier. For example, request that no extra cheese top your meal before it leaves the kitchen. Decline the bread basket. Substitute marinara or a light wine sauce for a heavy cream-based sauce.

See page 389 for answers.

Menu Samplers

Light 'N' Healthy

Menu Samplers Section	Menu Item	Amount	Calories	Fat (g)	% Calories from Fat	Saturated Fat (g)	Chol. (mg)	Sodium (mg)	Carb. (g)	Fiber (g)	Protein (g)	Exchanges/ Choices
Light 'N' Healthy (Women)	Pasta e fagioli soup	1 cup	130	3		1	10	600	17	6	9	1 Starch, 1 1/2 Lean Protein
	Seafood cannelloni	1/2 entrée	255	12		7	95	800	20	2	15	1 Starch, 2 Lean Protein, 2 Fat
	House salad (greens, tomatoes, cucumber, and red pepper) without croutons and cheese	2 cups	16	0		0	0	0	3	1	1	1 Vegetable
	Oil and vinegar dressing	2 teaspoons olive oil	80	7		1	0	0	0	0	0	1 Fat
	Whole-wheat roll	1 roll (1 oz)	74	1		0	0	147	14	2	3	1 Starch
Totals			535	23	38	9	105	1547	54	11	28	3 Starch, 1 Vegetable, 3 1/2 Lean Protein, 3 Fat

(table continues on next page)

Light 'N' Healthy

Menu Samplers Section	Menu Item	Amount	Calories	Fat (g)	% Calories from Fat	Saturated Fat (g)	Chol. (mg)	Sodium (mg)	Carb. (g)	Fiber (g)	Protein (g)	Exchanges/ Choices
Light 'N' Healthy (Men)	Veal piccata	1/2 entrée	246	15		9	80	320	4	0	23	3 Medium-Fat Protein
	Pasta	1 cup	200	2		1	10	450	40	2	7	2 1/2 Starch
	Italian green beans	1 side order	55	3		1	0	190	6	5	2	1 Vegetable
	Breadstick	1 breadstick (4 inches long)	140	5		1	0	260	19	1	5	1 Starch, 1 Fat
	House salad (greens, tomatoes, cucumber, and red pepper) without croutons and cheese	2 cups	16	0		0	0	0	3	1	1	1 Vegetable
	Oil and vinegar dressing	2 teaspoons olive oil	80	7		1	0	0	0	0	0	1 Fat
Totals			**717**	**32**	**40**	**13**	**90**	**1220**	**72**	**9**	**38**	**3 1/2 Starch, 2 Vegetable, 3 Medium-Fat Protein, 2 Fat**

(table continues on next page)

Hearty 'N' Healthy

Menu Samplers Section	Menu Item	Amount	Calories	Fat (g)	% Calories from Fat	Saturated Fat (g)	Chol. (mg)	Sodium (mg)	Carb. (g)	Fiber (g)	Protein (g)	Exchanges/ Choices
Hearty 'N' Healthy (Women)	Bruschetta	3/4 appetizer	310	17		3	0	500	35	1.5	4	2 Starch, 3 Fat
	Chicken marsala with mushrooms	1/2 dinner entrée	185	17		5	45	800	5	1	30	4 Lean Protein, 1 Fat
	Pasta	1 1/2 cups	318	2		0	0	30	60	3	12	4 Starch
	Broccoli sautéed with olive oil and garlic	1 cup	110	7		1	0	65	11	5	3	2 Vegetable, 1 Fat
Totals			**923**	**43**	**42**	**9**	**45**	**1395**	**111**	**11**	**49**	**6 Starch, 2 Vegetable, 4 Lean Protein, 5 Fat**

(table continues on next page)

Hearty 'N' Healthy

Menu Samplers Section	Menu Item	Amount	Calories	Fat (g)	% Calories from Fat	Saturated Fat (g)	Chol. (mg)	Sodium (mg)	Carb. (g)	Fiber (g)	Protein (g)	Exchanges/Choices
Hearty 'N' Healthy (Men)	Eggplant parmesan	1/2 entrée	475	17		4.5	25	800	45	7	16	3 Starch, 1 Vegetable, 3 1/2 Fat
	Seafood portofino	1/2 entrée	400	17		7	90	900	43	8	21	3 Starch, 3 Lean Protein, 2 Fat
	House salad (spinach, shredded carrots, tomato, cucumber) without croutons and cheese	2 cups	16	0		0	0	0	3	1	1	1 Vegetable
	Oil and vinegar dressing	1/2 Tbsp olive oil	60	7		1	0	0	0	0	0	1 Fat
Totals			891	41	41	12.5	115	1700	91	16	38	6 Starch, 2 Vegetable, 3 Lean Protein, 6 1/2 Fat

(table continues on next page)

Lower Carb 'N' Healthy

Menu Samplers Section	Menu Item	Amount	Calories	Fat (g)	% Calories from Fat	Saturated Fat (g)	Chol. (mg)	Sodium (mg)	Carb. (g)	Fiber (g)	Protein (g)	Exchanges/ Choices
Lower Carb 'N' Healthy (Women)	Minestrone soup	1 cup	125	2		0	20	900	24	3	4	1 1/2 Starch, 1/2 Lean Protein
	Breadstick	1/2 breadstick (4 inches long)	70	2.5		0.5	0	130	9	1	2.5	1/2 Starch
	Oil and vinegar dressing	2 teaspoons olive oil	80	7		1	0	0	0	0	0	1 Fat
	Beef and pork ravioli	1 appetizer	360	16		2.5	70	780	39	2	20	2 Starch, 3 Medium-Fat Protein
	House salad (spinach, shredded carrot, cherry tomatoes, and cucumber) without croutons and cheese	2 cups	16	0		0	0	0	3	1	1	1 Vegetable
Totals			631	28	40	4	90	1810	75	7	28	4 Starch, 1 Vegetable, 3 1/2 Medium-Fat Protein, 1 Fat

(table continues on next page)

Lower Carb 'N' Healthy

Menu Samplers Section	Menu Item	Amount	Calories	Fat (g)	% Calories from Fat	Saturated Fat (g)	Chol. (mg)	Sodium (mg)	Carb. (g)	Fiber (g)	Protein (g)	Exchanges/Choices
Lower Carb 'N' Healthy (Men)*	Lasagna primavera with grilled chicken	1 entrée	420	15		6	120	1125	36	5	35	2 Starch, 5 1/2 Lean Protein
	Wild mushroom goat cheese flatbread	1/3 appetizer	303	15		6	10	520	28	2	13	2 Starch, 1 Medium-Fat Protein, 2 Fat
	Steamed broccoli	1 cup	15	0		0	0	10	2	2	1	1 Vegetable
Totals			738	30	37	12	130	1655	66	9	49	4 Starch, 1 Vegetable, 6 1/2 Medium-Fat Protein, 2 Fat

*Cholesterol is higher than recommended due to the chicken entrée.

Know Your Pasta

Pasta, meaning "paste" or "dough," is found on the menu of every Italian restaurant. Pasta is created from flour (durum or all-purpose flour), water, and sometimes eggs. These ingredients are used to create a wide variety of different shapes of pasta, from angel hair to ziti. Unlike in Italy of yesteryear, you see many different-colored pastas available in America today: whole-wheat and whole-grain pastas (though not served in most restaurants) and flavored pastas, such as tomato, spinach, artichoke, and more. This pasta primer will help you "know your pasta" and have an easier time distinguishing the healthy from the not-so-healthy choices.

- ▶ **Agnolotti:** pieces of pasta, often shaped like crescents, that are stuffed with one ingredient or a combination of cheese, meat, and spinach.
- ▶ **Angel hair:** the thinnest and finest of the "long" pasta family. It is quite light in consistency and is often served topped with light, vegetable-based sauces.
- ▶ **Cannelloni:** large, tubular pasta, similar to manicotti. It is stuffed with one ingredient or a combination of cheese, meat, and spinach.
- ▶ **Capelletti:** (meaning "little hats") these are small, stuffed pastas that look like little tortellini. They're often stuffed with cheese or meats.
- ▶ **Fettuccini:** flat, long noodles about 1 inch wide (wider than linguine).
- ▶ **Fusilli:** spiral-shaped long pasta.
- ▶ **Gnocchi:** little dumplings in 1/2-inch pieces made from either flour or potatoes, or a combination of the two.
- ▶ **Lasagna:** the widest noodle among the long, flat pastas. It has either smooth or scalloped edges. Typically, lasagna is used in making a multi-layered casserole dish that is served in squares.
- ▶ **Linguine:** flat, long noodles about 1/8 inch wide (thinner than fettuccini).
- ▶ **Manicotti:** long, tubular noodles about 2 inches in diameter. Manicotti is most often stuffed with cheese and/or meat and served with tomato sauce.
- ▶ **Mostaccioli:** short, tubular noodles about 1 1/2 inches long.
- ▶ **Penne:** short, tubular noodle quite similar to mostaccioli and rigatoni.
- ▶ **Ravioli:** two pieces of pasta with a pocket in the middle. Traditionally, they come in 2-inch squares, but today they are often found smaller and are either square or round. Ravioli are traditionally stuffed with

cheese, spinach, and/or meats, but today you can find most anything stuffed in ravioli from butternut squash to duck confit.

► **Rigatoni:** short, tubular noodles quite similar to penne and mostaccioli.

► **Shells:** noodles in the shape of conch shells. These are called conchiglie in Italian, and can be found in a variety of sizes. Sometimes the larger ones are stuffed, and most are served topped with tomato sauce.

► **Spaghetti:** a round pasta, which is the most commonly known and eaten pasta in America. Spaghetti is available in a variety of widths.

► **Tortellini:** small pasta that is stuffed and joined at the ends to form a ring; a larger version of capellitti.

► **Ziti:** a short, tubular pasta similar to mostaccioli.

(i) What's Your Solution? Answers

a) Developing a plan in advance is a key strategy to eating out. Agree on your priorities and choices before you're tempted by the sights and smells of the restaurant.

b) Starting with a healthy salad is a great way to get in an extra serving or two of vegetables. It will also help satiate you from the start, making it less likely that everyone will over-eat. Just be sure to order the salad wisely: limit meats and cheeses and get the dressing on the side.

c) When dining family style, sometimes everyone wants a special dish. Rather than deprive someone of his or her order, go ahead and order all requests (within reason), but plan to box up extra portions. Leaving uneaten food in the center of the table can be tempting, even when everyone feels full. You'll hopefully have dinner for the next night ready to just heat and eat.

d) Little changes can add up to big nutrition differences. Making special requests can help ensure that you get all your family's favorites while still meeting your wellness goals. It's a wonderful idea to involve your whole family in implementing healthy eating strategies!

CHAPTER 20

Pizza

Pizza is ubiquitous in America today and is served for many a meal. You find it sold almost everywhere, in airports and food courts, at sporting events and kid- and family-focused events, as well as at the obvious places: pizzerias, moderately priced Italian restaurants, and many American and family-style restaurants.

Believe it or not, according to the *Dietary Guidelines for Americans* 2010 report, pizza was the fifth leading source of calories for Americans! That's not because it's so high in calories, but because we eat it so often!

Pizza ranks number one among the foods delivered most frequently to homes, offices, and more. In other words, Americans have grown a bit dependent on pizza. Pizza is Italian in origin, but because it's now such a central food item in American cuisine, it gets its own chapter in this book. For information on other Italian fare, see Chapter 19 (page 361).

Many national chains are dedicated to serving pizza both in their sit-down restaurant and as carryout orders, so you can whisk the pizza home (or elsewhere) and enjoy it at your dining room table. Among the big pizza chains of this type are Pizza Hut, Godfather's Pizza, Cici's Pizza, Uno Pizzeria & Grill, and Round Table Pizza. Some of the largest pizza chains, like Domino's, Papa John's Pizza, Little Caesars, and Papa Murphy's Take 'N' Bake offer pizza for takeout or delivery only. Sbarro's specialty is lining food courts or airport terminals, and Chuck E. Cheese's caters to the younger crowd by integrating food and free-for-all playtime into one kid-friendly experience. Then there are the more upscale, sit-down pizza establishments, which boast pizza made in wood-fired or brick ovens and sport a wide array of less-common toppings, such as goat cheese, spinach, pesto, and roasted red peppers. Bertucci's and California Pizza Kitchen are two national sit-down restaurant chains in this category. A plethora of independent pizzerias line America's highways, byways, and city streets as well.

On the Menu

Pizza is a favorite with every age group. Eat it hot or cold. You can have it for lunch, dinner, a late-night snack, or even eat a leftover slice for breakfast.

Pizza can be healthy—in fact, it can be healthier than many a burger-and-fries meal—if you put *The 10 Skills and Strategies for Healthier Restaurant Eating* (Chapter 4, page 29) into action. One of the best things about pizza is it's most often made to order, making it easy to customize your pizza and make it as healthy as you can.

But you've got decisions to make along the way if you're going to enjoy a healthy piece or two of pizza. You'll need to choose the thickness of the crust, the amount of cheese you want, the toppings, and most importantly, how many pieces you're going to eat. Not overeating is the biggest challenge with pizza. One or two slices seem to always be left on the tray, begging you to chow them down.

Put these portion-control strategies to work when ordering pizza: Practice portion control from the start by ordering fewer slices or a smaller-size pie and stop eating when you're full. Then pack up the extra pieces to go.

Thin, thick, stuffed crust, deep dish—yes, the thickness of the crust is the next decision to tackle. Most pizza restaurants offer a variety from thin to thick. If calories and your carbohydrate count are your biggest concern, then thin crust is the way to go. Generally, the thicker the crust, the higher the calorie and carbohydrate counts. If you enjoy a thicker crust and you've got the calories and carbohydrate grams to spare, then order a thicker-crust pizza but eat only a few slices.

Another bit of advice: enjoy a salad alongside your pizza. Not only will a salad allow you to check off one or two more vegetable servings that day, but it will also fill you up and won't leave as much room for that extra piece of pizza that you shouldn't really have. Most restaurants that serve pizza sit-down style also offer salads. Even most corner pizza parlors offer a garden or Greek salad. Don't forget the salad mantras: watch higher-fat add-ons and order dressing on the side. Munch on the salad first, prior to eating the pizza. Chapter 15 (page 250) provides all the information you need to keep your salads healthy and dress them for success.

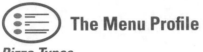 **The Menu Profile**

Pizza Types

Styles of pizza have been influenced by regions around the country and globe. You may even have a unique style in your own hometown. Some pizzerias offer several types of pizza, while others serve just one type. While any type of pizza can be made more or less healthy depending on which topping you order, some pizza styles are inherently lower in calories, thanks largely to their thin crust. Thinner crusts generally have fewer calories than thicker crusts, plus they physically can't hold the weight of lots of cheese and other high-fat toppings. This helps them win a few extra points toward healthfulness.

Here's a brief overview of a few of the pizza styles served across the United States.

▶ **Chicago-Style Deep Dish Pizza:** This is a knife-and-fork pizza that is almost akin to a casserole, since it's baked in a deep pan. It has a buttery crust and is layered from the bottom up with sliced (yes, sliced) mozzarella, meats, and veggies, then topped with sauce and more cheese (this time grated). An "individual size" deep dish pizza topped with cheese and tomato at Uno Pizzeria & Grill weighs in at 1750 calories, more than half of which come from fat! If the occasion calls for deep dish, limit yourself to just one piece and opt for low-calorie vegetables as your toppings.

▶ **Gourmet Pizza:** Pizzas are considered "gourmet" when high-quality and/or unique toppings are emphasized. You may find gourmet pizzas at upscale Italian restaurants, at the new crop of "bake at home" pizzerias, or at California Pizza Kitchen, the restaurant chain that originally made gourmet pizzas with inventive toppings go mainstream. Peanut sauce and Thai veggies on your pizza? When it comes to gourmet pizzas, take advantage of the wide array of vegetables available, the whole-grain crust options, and the leaner protein topping choices such as grilled chicken, turkey sausage, or shrimp.

- **Neapolitan Pizza:** These thin-crust pizzas are usually about 10 inches in diameter and are made in a traditional wood-burning oven. The crust is moist and chewy toward the center of the pizza and slightly puffy and charred toward the crust. Perhaps the most popular Neapolitan pizza is the Margherita, which is topped with fresh tomato sauce, fresh buffalo mozzarella, and basil (the colors of the Italian flag). As far as pizzas go, Neapolitan pizzas are generally lower in calories and fat than other versions, thanks to the thinner crust and lighter hand used when sprinkling on the cheese. However, most restaurants that serve Neapolitan pizzas will suggest that the pizza is the perfect size for one person. Think again. You're better off getting your own salad and sharing the pizza.

- **New York–Style Pizza:** A true New York–style pizza is big, thin, and has a crust that somehow manages to be both crisp and chewy. It generally has just one or two toppings, so the crust remains crisp, but anything goes with this type of pizza. Because the slices are large and thin, people often fold the slice while eating it. One or two slices will be enough.

- **Pan Pizza:** Pan pizza is cooked in a pan with a rim, although not as deep as the Chicago-style deep dish pizza, and has a buttery, uniform crust. At Pizza Hut, one slice from a 12-inch pan pizza has 50 calories more than a slice from a 12-inch thin-and-crispy pizza. So you can see how calories can add up just from the crust or style of pizza you choose.

- **Stuffed-Crust Pizza:** The crust is literally stuffed with cheese and sometimes other toppings, such as pepperoni. This is a quick way to add even more saturated fat to an already high-fat pizza. Is it worth it?

- **Stuffed Pizza:** Often confused with deep dish, this pizza, which also hails from Chicago, is cooked in a deep pan and has a top layer of crust. It's usually densely packed with toppings. These are generally high in fat, high in calories, and high in carbohydrate. Giordano's, the famous Chicago pizzeria, brags that their stuffed pizzas are 40% bigger than their competitors' deep dish pizza. In implementing your healthy eating strategy, this is one bragging right to stay away from.

- **Thin-Crust Pizza:** Generally, the thinner the crust, the lower the calorie and carbohydrate count. If the crust is extra thin and crispy, that means extra oil may have been used to achieve the cracker-like crunch.

While thin-crust pizza is generally a better choice than, say, a deep dish or stuffed pizza, you'll still need to engage your willpower to stop at just one or two slices.

▶ **Calzones and Strombolis:** These are not exactly pizza, but more like pizza's first cousins. A calzone has all the same ingredients as pizza (dough, tomato sauce, and toppings), but it is folded in half before baking to form a half-crescent with the toppings nestled inside. Strombolis have the same dough and toppings as a pizza, but are rolled into a long cylinder shape. The sauce is often served on the side, but sometimes you'll find it within the stromboli. As with a pizza, the healthfulness of these options depends on the serving size and the type and amount of toppings (or, in this case, fillings) you order.

Dough

In addition to the amount of dough used for your pizza crust, what the dough is made from also matters. The dough used for most restaurant-made pizzas is basically flour, yeast, salt, and water, which means it has no fat, no cholesterol, and few calories. Unfortunately, at this point, none of the large pizza chains have introduced a whole-wheat crust. Pizzas made with whole-wheat crusts could markedly increase the dietary fiber intake of Americans just because we eat so much pizza!

You may find an independent or small chain pizza establishment that offers the option of a whole-grain crust. If it's available, order it. If not, ask for it; if restaurants hear the plea enough, they may eventually add whole-wheat or whole-grain crusts to the menu. Papa John's Pizza introduced a whole-grain crust in 2008, but discontinued it shortly after. In 2013, Pizza Hut began testing whole-grain crust in various cities. The bottom line is that if restaurants notice a demand for whole-grain crust, they will add it to and keep it on their menus.

Sauces

Tomato sauce, the most popular pizza sauce, is a low-calorie item. Sauces may contain some sugar and salt, so use your taste buds and your glucose results after eating to help you determine the sauce ingredients. Does the sauce taste sweet to you? If so, look at the nutrition information and check the number of carbohydrate grams. Read the ingredient list (large restaurants provide ingredients on their web site) or simply ask if there's sugar in their sauce. If you eat pizza regularly around your neighborhood or other areas you frequent, consider scouting out a pizza restaurant that uses a relatively low-sugar and low-salt sauce.

White pizzas are another story entirely, and they require you to read the description on the menu more closely. A white pizza is defined by the color of the pizza, not the sauce. Sometimes this means no sauce is added at all, while other times it means that a high-fat cream-based sauce, like a béchamel, is used. You will get your fill of fat with the cheese that tops a pizza, so there is no need to add insult to injury with a high-fat sauce. Avoid white pizzas that have a cream-based sauce.

Cheeses

The amount and type of cheese used on pizzas can vary drastically. Cheese is high in both saturated fat and sodium. (No wonder saturated fat and sodium intakes are higher than desirable in Americans.) Your best strategy is to request that less, not more, cheese be added to your pizza. Since most pizzas are made to order, this is an easy request to make. You likely won't even miss it. Or you can go all out and request that no cheese be used at all (yes, it's possible and can be quite tasty with enough healthy toppings).

Toppings

The final step in preparing a pizza before baking is to add toppings. Will you choose low-calorie mushrooms, onions, spinach, and tomato slices, or will you order high-fat toppings such as extra cheese, pepperoni, and sausage? Consider choosing more inventive toppings. There seems to be a move afoot, particularly in upscale pizza chains and restaurants, to be more creative with the ingredient combinations used on pizza. That is great for the nutrition-conscious diner, because some of these ingredients are vegetables and other lower-calorie foods (see *Green-Flag Toppings* below). Choose toppings wisely, and remember, the more vegetables and lower-calorie items, the healthier your pizza will be.

Nutrition Snapshot

Health Busters

Category	Restaurant Name	Dish Name	Serving Size	Cal.	Total Fat (g)	Carb. (g)	Sod. (mg)
Appetizers	Papa Gino's Pizzeria	Fried Chicken Wings—Buffalo (large)	1 portion	1800	140	36	7200
Appetizers	Old Chicago Pizza & Pasta	Original Buffalo Wings	1 portion	1423	111	7	1997
Breads	Papa Romano's	Papa's Cheezy Bread (16 pieces)	1 portion	1835	50	254	3072
Breads	Mellow Mushroom	Garlic	1 portion	615	23	87	1167
Breads	Mellow Mushroom	Cheese	1 portion	875	42	90	1792
Breads	Papa Gino's Pizzeria	Breadsticks	1 breadstick	250	9	31	650
Pizza	Pizza Hut	14" Large Hand-Tossed Style—Meat Lover's	1 slice	440	23	38	1250

(table continues on next page)

Health Busters

Category	Restaurant Name	Dish Name	Serving Size	Cal.	Total Fat (g)	Carb. (g)	Sod. (mg)
Pizza	Pizza Hut	14" Large Pan—Ultimate Cheese Lover's	1 slice	400	21	36	800
Pizza	Pizza Hut	14" Large Pan—Veggie Lover's	1 slice	330	15	38	690
Pizza	Pizza Hut	14" Large Pan—Triple Meat Italiano	1 slice	420	23	37	1000
Pizza	Pizza Hut	14" Large Hand-Tossed Style—Ultimate Cheese Lover's Garlic Parmesan	1 slice	360	15	38	880
Pizza	Pizza Hut	14" Large Pan—Ultimate Cheese Lover's	1 slice	400	21	36	800
Pizza	Pizza Hut	14" Large Pan—Veggie Lover's	1 slice	330	15	38	690
Pizza	Pizza Hut	14" Large Stuffed Crust—Pepperoni Lover's	1 slice	430	21	40	1230
Pizza	Pizza Hut	14" Large Stuffed Crust—Meat Lover's	1 slice	480	26	39	1380

(table continues on next page)

Health Busters

Category	Restaurant Name	Dish Name	Serving Size	Cal.	Total Fat (g)	Carb. (g)	Sod. (mg)
Calzones	Godfather's Pizza	Cheese	1 calzone	1660	51	200	2920
Calzones	Godfather's Pizza	Combo	1 calzone	1450	40	199	2900
Calzones	Old Chicago Pizza & Pasta	Monterey Chicken (includes dipping sauces)	1 calzone	1283	59	118	2306
Sandwiches	Papa Gino's Pizzeria	Mushroom Swiss Double Burger	1 burger	1300	93	39	1090
Sandwiches	California Pizza Kitchen	Italian Deli with Herb Cheese	1 sandwich	1260	n/a	88	2862
Sandwiches	Papa Gino's Pizzeria	Steak & Cheese	1 large sub	1240	62	102	2540
Sandwiches	California Pizza Kitchen	Italian Deli with Herb Onion	1 sandwich	1206	n/a	89	2715
Sandwiches	Donatos Pizza	Meatball on Wheat	1 sub	1119	63	78	3108

Healthier Bets

Category	Restaurant Name	Dish Name	Serving Size	Cal.	Total Fat (g)	Sat. Fat (g)	Carb. (g)	Pro. (g)	Fiber (g)	Chol. (mg)	Sodium (mg)	Exchanges/ Choices
Appetizers	Pizza Hut	Bone Out Wings— Honey BBQ	2 pieces	220	8	1.5	27	10	1	20	720	2 Starch, 1 Medium-Fat Protein
Appetizers	Pizza Hut	Bone Out Wings— Spicy Asian	2 pieces	210	8	1.5	24	10	1	20	690	1 1/2 Starch, 1 Medium-Fat Protein, 1/2 Fat
Appetizers	Domino's Pizza	Boneless Chicken	3 pieces	150	6	1	14	12	1	20	440	1 Starch, 1 Lean Protein
Salads	Papa Gino's Pizzeria	Greek	1 salad	180	11	6	12	11	4	30	710	1/2 Starch, 1 Vegetable, 1 High-Fat Protein, 1 Fat
Salads	Papa Gino's Pizzeria	Caesar	1 salad	190	10	3.5	18	9	5	40	380	1/2 Starch, 2 Vegetable, 1/2 High-Fat Protein, 1 Fat

(table continues on next page)

Healthier Bets

Category	Restaurant Name	Dish Name	Serving Size	Cal.	Total Fat (g)	Sat. Fat (g)	Carb. (g)	Pro. (g)	Fiber (g)	Chol. (mg)	Sodium (mg)	Exchanges/ Choices
Salads	Papa Murphy's Pizza	Italian (no dressing)	1 salad	263	19	9	13	14	6	40	738	1/2 Starch, 1 Vegetable, 1 1/2 High-Fat Protein, 1 Fat
Salads	Papa Murphy's Pizza	Garden (no dressing)	1 salad	192	11	6	15	11	6	23	463	1/2 Starch, 1 Vegetable, 1 High-Fat Protein, 1 Fat
Pizza	CiCi's Pizza	Cheese, 12"	1 slice	150	3.5	2	20	6	1	10	330	1 1/2 Starch, 1 Lean Protein
Pizza	Pizza Hut	12" Medium Thin 'N Crispy— Ultimate Cheese Lover's	1 slice	220	11	5	21	10	1	25	600	1 1/2 Starch, 1 High-Fat Protein, 1/2 Fat

(table continues on next page)

Healthier Bets

Category	Restaurant Name	Dish Name	Serving Size	Cal.	Total Fat (g)	Sat. Fat (g)	Carb. (g)	Pro. (g)	Fiber (g)	Chol. (mg)	Sodium (mg)	Exchanges/ Choices
Pizza	Pizza Hut	12" Medium Thin 'N Crispy— Cheese Only	1 slice	190	8	4	22	9	1	25	550	1 1/2 Starch, 1 High-Fat Protein
Pizza	Pizza Hut	14" Large Thin 'N Crispy— Cheese Only	1 slice	260	11	6	29	12	1	35	740	2 Starch, 1 High-Fat Protein, 1/2 Fat
Pizza	CiCi's Pizza	Veggie, 12"	1 slice	130	2	0.5	20	4	1	5	280	1 Starch, 1 Vegetable, 1/2 Fat
Pizza	Pizza Hut	14" Large Thin 'N Crispy— Veggie Lover's	1 slice	240	9	4	30	10	2	20	710	1 1/2 Starch, 1 1/2 Vege-table, 1/2 High-Fat Protein, 1 Fat

(table continues on next page)

Healthier Bets

Category	Restaurant Name	Dish Name	Serving Size	Cal.	Total Fat (g)	Sat. Fat (g)	Carb. (g)	Pro. (g)	Fiber (g)	Chol. (mg)	Sodium (mg)	Exchanges/ Choices
Pizza	East of Chicago Pizza	14" Thin Small Garden Vegetable	1 slice	210	7	3	29	9	1	15	520	1 1/2 Starch, 1 1/2 Vegetable, 1/2 High-Fat Protein, 1/2 Fat
Pizza	Little Caesar's Pizza	Just Cheese 14"	1 slice	250	9	4	32	12	1	20	440	2 Starch, 1 High-Fat Protein
Pizza	Pizza Hut	12" Fit 'N Delicious— Green Pepper, Red Onion & Diced Red Tomato	1 slice	150	4	1.5	24	6	2	10	400	1 1/2 Starch, 1 Fat
Pizza	CiCi's Pizza	Zesty Veggie, 12"	1 slice	120	3	1	20	4	1	5	320	1 Starch, 1 Vegetable, 1/2 Fat

(table continues on next page)

Healthier Bets

Category	Restaurant Name	Dish Name	Serving Size	Cal.	Total Fat (g)	Sat. Fat (g)	Carb. (g)	Pro. (g)	Fiber (g)	Chol. (mg)	Sodium (mg)	Exchanges/ Choices
Pizza	CiCi's Pizza	Veggie, 12"	1 slice	130	2	0.5	20	4	1	5	280	1 Starch, 1 Vegetable, 1/2 Fat
Pizza	Pizza Hut	12" Medium Pan—Veggie Lover's	1 slice	230	9	3.5	28	9	2	15	500	2 Starch, 1/2 High-Fat Protein, 1 Fat
Pizza	CiCi's Pizza	Cheese, 12"	1 slice	150	4	2	20	6	1	10	330	1 1/2 Starch, 1/2 Medium-Fat Protein
Pizza	Pizza Hut	12" Medium Pan— Cheese Only	1 slice	240	10	4.5	27	11	1	25	530	2 Starch, 1 High-Fat Protein
Pizza	CiCi's Pizza	Pepperoni & Jalapeño, 12"	1 slice	150	5	2	20	6	1	10	390	1 1/2 Starch, 1/2 Medium-Fat Protein

(table continues on next page)

Healthier Bets

Category	Restaurant Name	Dish Name	Serving Size	Cal.	Total Fat (g)	Sat. Fat (g)	Carb. (g)	Pro. (g)	Fiber (g)	Chol. (mg)	Sodium (mg)	Exchanges/ Choices
Pizza	Pizza Hut	12" Medium Hand-Tossed Style—Ham & Pineapple Garlic Parmesan	1 slice	210	6	3	28	9	1	20	570	2 Starch, 1/2 Medium-Fat Protein, 1/2 Fat
Pizza	Pizza Hut	12" Medium Hand-Tossed Style— Pepperoni & Mushroom Garlic Parmesan	1 slice	210	8	3.5	26	10	1	20	570	2 Starch, 1/2 High-Fat Protein, 1/2 Fat

(table continues on next page)

Healthier Bets

Category	Restaurant Name	Dish Name	Serving Size	Cal.	Total Fat (g)	Sat. Fat (g)	Carb. (g)	Pro. (g)	Fiber (g)	Chol. (mg)	Sodium (mg)	Exchanges/ Choices
Pizza	Pizza Hut	14" Large Hand-Tossed Style—Ham & Pineapple	1 slice	290	9	4.5	40	13	2	25	810	2 1/2 Starch, 1 Medium-Fat Protein, 1 Fat
Pizza	Pizza Hut	14" Large Hand-Tossed Style—Ham & Pineapple Garlic Parmesan	1 slice	300	9	4.5	41	14	2	25	840	2 1/2 Starch, 1 Medium-Fat Protein, 1 Fat

(table continues on next page)

Healthier Bets

Category	Restaurant Name	Dish Name	Serving Size	Cal.	Total Fat (g)	Sat. Fat (g)	Carb. (g)	Pro. (g)	Fiber (g)	Chol. (mg)	Sodium (mg)	Exchanges/ Choices
Pizza	Pizza Hut	14" Large Hand-Tossed Style— Pepperoni & Mushroom Garlic Parmesan	1 slice	320	11	5	39	14	2	30	840	2 1/2 Starch, 1 High-Fat Protein, 1/2 Fat
Calzones	Old Chicago Pizza & Pasta	Lunch Cheese Only (includes dipping sauces)	1 calzone	352	10	4	56	12	3	5	624	3 Starch, 1 Vegetable, 2 Fat

(table continues on next page)

Healthier Bets

Category	Restaurant Name	Dish Name	Serving Size	Cal.	Total Fat (g)	Sat. Fat (g)	Carb. (g)	Pro. (g)	Fiber (g)	Chol. (mg)	Sodium (mg)	Exchanges/ Choices
Calzones	Papa Murphy's Pizza	Chicken Florentine (large)	1 calzone	447	13	5	46	20	1	40	987	3 Starch, 2 Lean Protein, 2 Fat
Sandwiches	Old Chicago Pizza & Pasta	Chicken Wrap (half)	1 sand-wich	299	11	3	31	18	3	34	961	2 Starch, 2 Lean Protein, 1 Fat
Sandwiches	Old Chicago Pizza & Pasta	Burger, Old Chicago Plain Chicken Breast	1 sand-wich	466	11	2	41	46	2	102	831	2 1/2 Starch, 5 1/2 Lean Protein

✅ Green-Flag Toppings

- Anchovies (high in omega-3s, but also high in sodium)
- Artichoke hearts
- Black olives
- Broccoli
- Chicken
- Eggplant
- Feta cheese, part-skim cheese (high in sodium)
- Fresh herbs
- Garlic
- Green and red peppers
- Ham, Canadian bacon
- Jalapeño or other chilies
- Mushrooms
- Onions
- Pineapple
- Roasted peppers
- Shrimp or crabmeat
- Sliced tomatoes
- Spinach

❌ Red-Flag Toppings

- Alfredo sauce
- Bacon
- Extra cheese, four cheese, six cheese
- Feta cheese
- Meatballs, hamburger meat
- Mozzarella cheese
- Pepperoni
- Prosciutto
- Sausage, Italian sausage

🍎 Healthy Eating Tips and Tactics

- Stick with the thin crust and load up on the veggies.
- If your favorite chain does not publish nutrition information, check the nutrition information for similar items from two

other pizza chains. This gives you ballpark figures to base your choice on.

► If your dining partner requests less-healthy pizza toppings, order healthier toppings on one half of the pizza and let your partner handle the other.

► If you count grams of carbohydrate, make sure the slices you eat are average in size. If they are bigger or smaller, change your carbohydrate estimate based on the carbohydrate information/nutrition information available. Let your eyes guide you.

► Start with a healthy garden salad to help squelch your appetite before the pizza even arrives.

► If you know a few extra pieces of pizza will be left over, package them up before you take your first bite.

Get It Your Way

► Ask for your pizza to be made with less cheese, or better yet, no cheese at all.

► Substitute spicy chicken for the pepperoni or sausage on a pizza.

► Instead of extra cheese, request extra vegetables.

► Order just enough pizza for everyone at the table, to avoid that just-one-more-piece syndrome.

Tips and Tactics for Gluten-Free Eating

► Unless the pizza restaurant has a completely separate preparation area for gluten-free pizzas, there is a very high risk for cross-contamination with gluten. Always question the staff carefully about their preparation areas and methods.

► Make sure any toppings are in the dedicated gluten-free area of the restaurant and any utensils used to handle gluten-free ingredients are dedicated as well.

Tips and Tactics to Help Kids Eat Healthy

► When kids are hungry, they can easily devour more calories from pizza than their growing bodies need, especially if slices are placed in front of them with the expectation that they finish them. Try to limit the number of slices put in front of your child, and make sure they don't feel pressure to eat beyond the point of fullness.

▶ Order a healthy appetizer—a garden salad or cup of soup—to help satiate your child's appetite before the pizza arrives. Or order a garden salad to accompany the pizza.

▶ Introduce a new vegetable as a topping. Since kids are so familiar with pizza, and typically love it so much, it is a great vehicle to help kids feel comfortable with the idea of a new vegetable.

▶ There is no need for kids to get their own personal pizza. Order a pizza that can feed your whole family so that your child gets used to following the same healthy eating strategies that you follow.

? What's Your Solution?

You are watching a sporting event with a group of friends. Your friend, who is hosting the get-together, plans to order pizza for everyone to eat while you watch the game. You don't want to be a high-maintenance guest, but you know your friend won't order healthy pizzas if left to his own devices.

How can you maintain your healthy eating plan even in this peer-pressured situation?

a) Text your friend before the game starts to let him know you will bring a vegetable tray for everyone to share.

b) Offer to phone-in the order. On the sly, request that all the pizzas be made with less cheese. Your buddies probably won't even notice.

c) Speak up at the start of the get-together to place your order: a thin crust pizza with grilled chicken, red onions, and tomatoes, easy on the cheese.

d) Keep your mouth shut and enjoy two large slices of pepperoni pizza, but stop at that and enjoy the vegetables you brought along.

See page 417 for answers.

▦ Menu Samplers

(table continues on next page)

Light 'N' Healthy

Menu Samplers Section	Menu Item	Amount	Calories	Fat (g)	% Calories from Fat	Saturated Fat (g)	Chol. (mg)	Sodium (mg)	Carb. (g)	Fiber (g)	Protein (g)	Exchanges/ Choices
Light 'N' Healthy (Women)	Sausage and pepper pizza	1 1/2 Slices (pf 14" pizza)	506	27		9	50	1020	50	3	18	3 Starch, 3 Medium-Fat Protein, 1 Fat
	House salad (spinach, cucumber, and red onion) without croutons and cheese	2 cups	16	0		0	0	0	3	1	1	1 Vegetable
	Oil and vinegar dressing	2 teaspoons olive oil	30	7		1	0	0	0	0	0	1 Fat
Totals			**532**	**34**	**53**	**10**	**50**	**1020**	**53**	**4**	**19**	**3 Starch, 1 Vegetable, 3 Medium-Fat Protein, 2 Fat**

Light 'N' Healthy

Menu Samplers Section	Menu Item	Amount	Calories	Fat (g)	% Calories from Fat	Saturated Fat (g)	Chol. (mg)	Sodium (mg)	Carb.(g)	Fiber (g)	Protein (g)	Exchanges/ Choices
Light 'N' Healthy (Men)	Artisan spinach feta chicken pizza	3 square pieces (from 13 × 9" pizza)	368	16		7	47	837	36	2	22	2 1/2 Starch, 1 Vegetable, 2 Medium-Fat Protein, 1 Fat
	Garden fresh salad	2 cups	280	4		10	40	320	20	8	16	4 Vegetable, 1 1/2 Lean Protein
	Oil and vinegar dressing	2 teaspoons olive oil	80	7		1	0	0	0	0	0	1 Fat
Totals			**708**	**27**	**34**	**18**	**87**	**1157**	**56**	**10**	**38**	**2 1/2 Starch, 5 Vegetable, 3 1/2 Medium-Fat Protein, 2 Fat**

(table continues on next page)

Hearty 'N' Healthy

Menu Samplers Section	Menu Item	Amount	Calories	Fat (g)	% Calories from Fat	Saturated Fat (g)	Chol. (mg)	Sodium (mg)	Carb. (g)	Fiber (g)	Protein (g)	Exchanges/Choices
Hearty 'N' Healthy (Women)	Hawaiian BBQ chicken pizza (with bacon, ham, pineapple, and red peppers)	2 slices (of 14" pizza)	700	24		10	70	1630	92	4	30	5 Starch, 1 Fruit, 2 Medium-Fat Protein, 3 Fat
	House salad (spinach, cucumber, and red onion) without croutons and cheese	2 cups	15	0		0	0	0	3	1	1	1 Vegetable
	Oil and vinegar dressing	2 teaspoons olive oil	80	7		1	0	0	0	0	0	1 Fat
Totals			**776**	**31**	**36**	**11**	**70**	**1630**	**95**	**5**	**31**	**5 Starch, 1 Fruit, 1 Vegetable, 2 Medium-Fat Protein, 4 Fat**

(table continues on next page)

Hearty 'N' Healthy

Menu Samplers Section	Menu Item	Amount	Calories	Fat (g)	% Calories from Fat	Saturated Fat (g)	Chol. (mg)	Sodium (mg)	Carb. (g)	Fiber (g)	Protein (g)	Exchanges/ Choices
Hearty 'N' Healthy (Men)	Philly cheese steak pizza (steak, onion, peppers, and mushrooms)	3 slices (of 10" pizza)	750	36		15	90	1520	72	3	33	4 1/2 Starch, 1 Vegetable, 2 1/2 Medium-Fat Protein, 4 Fat
	House salad (greens, tomatoes, cucumber, and red pepper) without croutons and cheese	2 cups	16	0		0	0	0	3	1	1	1 Vegetable
	Oil and vinegar dressing	2 teaspoons olive oil	80	7		1	0	0	0	0	0	1 Fat
Totals			**826**	**43**	**47**	**16**	**90**	**1520**	**75**	**4**	**34**	**4 1/2 Starch, 2 Vegetable, 2 1/2 Medium-Fat Protein, 5 Fat**

(table continues on next page)

Lower Carb 'N' Healthy

Menu Samplers Section	Menu Item	Amount	Calories	Fat (g)	% Calories from Fat	Saturated Fat (g)	Chol. (mg)	Sodium (mg)	Carb. (g)	Fiber (g)	Protein (g)	Exchanges/ Choices
Lower Carb 'N' Healthy (Women)	Sausage and veggie pizza	2 slices (of 14" pizza)	400	20		2	10	980	50	2	17	3 Starch, 1 Vegetable, 3 Medium-Fat Protein, 1 Fat
	House salad (romaine, tomatoes, cucumber, and red pepper) without croutons and cheese	2 cups	16	0		0	0	0	3	1	1	1 Vegetable
	Oil and vinegar dressing	2 teaspoons olive oil	80	7		1	0	0	0	0	0	1 Fat
Totals			**476**	**27**	**51**	**3**	**10**	**980**	**53**	**3**	**18**	**3 Starch, 2 Vegetable, 3 Medium-Fat Protein, 2 Fat**

(table continues on next page)

Lower Carb 'N' Healthy

Menu Samplers Section	Menu Item	Amount	Calories	Fat (g)	% Calories from Fat	Saturated Fat (g)	Chol. (mg)	Sodium (mg)	Carb. (g)	Fiber (g)	Protein (g)	Exchanges/ Choices
Lower Carb 'N' Healthy (Men)	Cheese pizza with spinach	2 slices (of 14" pizza)	580	22		9	40	890	71	2	24	4 1/2 Starch, 1 Vegetable, 2 Medium-Fat Protein, 2 Fat
	House salad (spinach, tomatoes, red onion, and red pepper) without croutons and cheese	2 cups	16	0		0	0	0	3	1	1	1 Vegetable
	Oil and vinegar dressing	2 teaspoons olive oil	80	7		1	0	0	0	0	0	1 Fat
Totals			**656**	**29**	**40**	**10**	**40**	**890**	**74**	**3**	**25**	**4 1/2 Starch, 2 Vegetable, 2 Medium-Fat Protein, 3 Fat**

(i) What's Your Solution? Answers

a) Nice job being proactive! A vegetable tray will give everyone something healthy to chew on before the pizza arrives, making it easier to limit your pizza to just one or two slices.

b) Good job taking charge and looking after everyone's health! Requesting less cheese is a great way to slash calories and fat. But you're better off being upfront about it.

c) This is a smart order. The thin crust helps you keep your carbohydrate count in check, while the lean protein and vegetable toppings keep the pizza low in fat. Going easy on the cheese is always a key strategy. Just be sure you don't overdo it on the number of slices you eat, especially if you'll be the only one eating this pizza.

d) You know your friends best. If you don't feel comfortable speaking up or don't want to, then your best strategy is to limit your portion size. You may want to bring a stick of sugar-free chewing gum with you to chew on after those two slices. This will help prevent you from reaching for a third slice.

CHAPTER 21

Chinese

C hinese food ranks in the top three of Americans' favorite ethnic cuisines. While Chinatowns in major cities are one place to find Chinese food, today it's common to see Chinese restaurants in shopping malls and urban, suburban, and rural neighborhoods. Some of these restaurants have tables for eating in, as well as plenty of containers for takeout. Others offer only takeout. Many Chinese restaurants are single, family-owned establishments and reflect the foods typical in a specific region of China.

There are currently only a handful of national Chinese food chains. Typically, these chains offer a more Americanized version of Chinese food than independent restaurants. Panda Express, the largest national chain serving Chinese food, can be found in food courts, airports, casinos, and even in the food courts in the Pentagon, just outside of Washington, D.C.

Today, due to the increasing popularity of other Asian cuisines, Panda Express has integrated a few Thai, Japanese, and Vietnamese dishes into their menu, so it's no longer purely Chinese cuisine. Two other fast casual Chinese chains on the rise are Pei Wei Asian Diner, which offers dishes from a variety of Asian cuisines, and a relatively small Minneapolis-based chain called Leeann Chin. If you're looking for upscale Chinese restaurants, P.F. Chang's China Bistro (locations nationwide) and Big Bowl (locations in Chicago, Minneapolis, and Washington, D.C.) offer sit-down service and an array of Chinese and Thai dishes.

There's also a crop of Mongolian barbeque restaurant chains, in which a waiter serves you but you make a trip (or unlimited trips) to a food bar to pick out your own ingredients, which are then stir-fried on a large grill by a chef. Despite the Mongolian name, this type of cooking is believed to have originated in Taiwan, China. Great Khan's, Genghis Grill, BD's Mongolian Grill, and Flat Top Grill are four of the chains that offer this type of cuisine.

Chinese dishes, such as stir-fry chicken, vegetables, and chop suey, also show up on many family and American-style restaurant menus, but you'll find these dishes discussed in this chapter. Chapter 22 (page 448) will give you a more in-depth look at Thai cuisine and Chapter 23 (page 475) covers Japanese cuisine.

On the Menu

Chinese foods, markets, and cooking styles were virtually unknown in America prior to the mid-1800s. Initially, when people from China came to the United States, it was common for them to settle in enclaves that became known as Chinatowns. Well-known Chinatowns were located bi-coastally—in Boston and New York and in Los Angeles and San Francisco. The streets of Chinatowns were (and still are) dotted with restaurants and bakeries where you can enjoy a sit-down meal or grab a quick order of pork buns.

Though Americans initially became accustomed to eating only Cantonese-style Chinese food, today Chinese restaurants serve cuisines from various regions of China, such as Szechuan, Hunan, and Peking (Beijing). Many times, dishes on a Chinese menu will be named for the particular region from which the cooking method originated. Examples are Peking duck, Szechuan spicy chicken, and Hunan crispy beef. Opinions vary as to whether China actually has three, four, or five regional cuisines, but in reality, if you consider all the subtle regional differences the food can reflect, there are many types of Chinese cuisine.

Interestingly, Chinese cuisine wears a halo of health because people think of Chinese food as heavy on vegetables and light on fat. This perception may be true when foods are prepared traditionally or in China, but it's not true when most Chinese foods are prepared in America. The Americanized preparation methods often mean added fat, fried noodles with soup, fried appetizers, and battered and fried meats (shrimp, pork, chicken, beef) in dishes coated with sweet sauces. Keep this in mind when you order and try to eat more vegetable-dense and traditional dishes.

The fat content of many Chinese dishes is one of the main roadblocks to eating healthfully at Chinese restaurants. However, it's easier to limit the amount of fat in dishes at Chinese restaurants than at family-style American restaurants. Special requests—which are easy to make because the food, at least in sit-down Chinese restaurants, is generally prepared to order—will help you limit the fatty ingredients, added oils, and high-sodium and thick, sugary sauces in your meal.

What types of fat are used in Chinese cooking? Traditionally, lard (pork fat) was used. Thank goodness healthier liquid oil is generally used today. Peanut oil is commonly used because of its high smoking point, not its health quotient, but it's reasonably healthy too. Peanut oil gives a slightly nutty flavor to dishes. It is mainly a monounsaturated fat, which is thought to help lower bad blood cholesterol (LDL). Sesame oil is also used, but in smaller quantities. Sesame oil is a polyunsaturated fat, which also assists in lowering blood cholesterol. The oils used in Chinese cooking are generally healthy, but the problem is excess use.

The most common Chinese cooking method is stir-frying in a wok (a common bowl-shaped cooking vessel). A wok can also be used for other cooking methods, such as braising and steaming. Wok cooking can be quite healthy. A minimal amount of oil can be used, and foods are cooked only briefly, so they retain their much of their vitamins and minerals.

One other health villain is the high sodium content of Chinese food. Many dishes contain high-sodium soy sauces, light and dark, and monosodium glutamate (MSG). MSG is the sodium salt of the amino acid glutamic acid. It's approved for use by the FDA and is used in foods as a flavor enhancer. It contains about one-third of the sodium in salt. Other sauces such as oyster, black bean, and hoisin (or plum sauce) also contain large amounts of sodium. For a frame of reference, 1 tablespoon of soy sauce has about 1,000 milligrams of sodium.

A few special requests can quickly decrease the sodium content of your meal. You can request that the kitchen use less soy sauce and no MSG in your dish. Many Chinese restaurants today note on their menu that no MSG is used. Do not try to eliminate soy sauce or sauces altogether because the end product simply will not be tasty. You don't want that. There is a happy medium! Think about using hot oil, chile sauce, or hot mustard as low-sodium flavorings to add some zip to your food. All things considered, however, Chinese food might not be the optimal choice, at least on a frequent basis, if you need to keep your sodium intake in check.

Another important note: people with diabetes often find that Chinese food can wreak havoc on their blood glucose levels. That's not a surprise. There are hidden grams of carbohydrate in Chinese foods, from the sugar in marinades for meats to the cornstarch that's used to thicken dishes in the wok. Then there are high-sugar sauces, such as the sauce used in sweet-and-sour dishes, hoisin sauce, and the duck sauce on the table. Limit your use of heavy, potentially sugar-dense sauces. Request that the chef leave sugar and corn-starch out of your dishes if possible. (However, you may be told that these ingredients are already premixed into marinades or sauces.)

One of the biggest perks of eating Chinese food is that the common way of ordering and eating is family style, and sharing is ideal for people practicing portion control. Don't feel compelled to order one dish per person. Order fewer dishes than the number of people at the table and get ready to share. Order protein-focused dishes and complement them with vegetable-focused dishes. This balance can help you meet your healthy eating goals.

Another plus is that vegetables are abundant in Chinese cooking. Be sure to look at the descriptions of menu items and cast your eyes on the vegetarian listings. You are familiar with many of the vegetables used in Chinese cuisine: broccoli, cabbage, carrots, mushrooms, snow peas, water chestnuts, bamboo shoots, and onions. Others vegetables on the menu may be less familiar, such as bok choy, napa cabbage, wood ears, and lily buds. For descriptions of these ingredients, see *Menu Lingo* (page 446) at the end of this chapter. Load up on vegetables at Chinese restaurants, and try some unfamiliar veggies if you're feeling adventurous.

Chopsticks are the eating utensils of choice in Chinese restaurants, though forks and spoons are available if you are not adept with chopsticks. However, lack of aptitude with chopsticks might be a blessing in disguise. A lack of dexterity can slow your pace of eating. So go ahead, be daring and use chopsticks, but put your napkin squarely on your lap to catch the misfires.

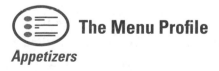 **The Menu Profile**

Appetizers

Decisions, decisions—it's appetizer time. Many Chinese appetizers are simply off-limits to those who follow a healthy eating plan because they are fried or high in fat. The appetizers to avoid include fried noodles, fried shrimp, wontons, chicken wings, spareribs, and egg rolls, to name just a few. Some healthier appetizer options are spring rolls (fresh, not fried), steamed Peking raviolis (preferably vegetable or shrimp rather than pork), roasted pork strips, and barbecued or teriyaki beef or chicken (if sodium is not a big concern).

Soups

Think about skipping high-fat appetizers and filling up, instead, on a bowl of low-calorie broth-based soup, especially if your dining partners are indulging in high-fat appetizers. Notice that no creamy soups are served in Chinese restaurants. Hot-and-sour, sizzling rice, egg drop, or wonton soup are all healthy soups unless you're watching your sodium intake. Like most soups, the soups you'll find in Chinese restaurants are loaded with sodium. Hot-and-sour soup is likely the highest in sodium, and egg drop or wonton soup the lowest. Soup can take the edge off your appetite, fill you up, and help you decrease the total amount of food you eat over the course of the meal.

Entrées

You'll likely have a wide array of choices when it comes to the source of protein in your entrée, including beef, pork, chicken, duck, seafood, and tofu (bean curd). Beef, pork, and duck are typically higher in fat and calories than chicken, seafood, and tofu. But of course, preparation method matters. Just because an entrée contains a lean source of protein—or at least one that was lean before it was surrounded by batter and hit the deep-fryer—doesn't mean the final dish will be healthy. Three popular chicken dishes, Kung Pao chicken, honey chicken, and General Tso's chicken are often high in calories and fat, as the chicken is usually deep-fried. But don't be shy about asking to have your protein sautéed instead of fried.

Likewise, shrimp, prawns, scallops, calamari (squid), and whole or pieces of finfish are common on Chinese menus. But read the menu descriptions with care. Much seafood is also battered and fried before it reaches your table.

At Pei Wei Asian Diner, most entrées can be prepared in two ways: the traditional way (cooked in oil) or what they call "stock velveted," a method in which the source of protein in the dish is cooked (steamed) in seasoned water. This restaurant provides nutrition information for both the traditionally prepared and stock velveted (steamed) versions of each entrée, when applicable. To give you an idea of the difference that this small change in preparation method makes, it usually reduces the dish's fat grams by half or more. If possible, try to get your dishes stock velveted in the Chinese restaurants you frequent to reduce fat grams and calories. Thanks, Pei Wei Asian Diner! Maybe other restaurants will follow suit.

In addition to the cooking method, you'll want to pay close attention to the sauces used in or on the dishes you order. Sauces like sweet-and-sour, duck, and plum are thick, sugar-dense sauces that contain extra carbohydrate and should be used minimally. The same goes for menu items that are honey battered; they offer a double whammy of sugar and fat.

Always peruse the menu and look for dishes with lots of vegetables. You might find the words "assorted vegetables" or "broccoli and water chestnuts." If it's not obvious, ask if the dish has vegetables and what types of vegetables are used. You can always request that extra vegetables be added to your dish. Another strategy is to complement a protein-focused dish with a vegetarian one. Try spicy green beans, spinach and garlic, or the vegetarian delight. However, make sure none of the items in the dish, such as the tofu, are deep-fried prior to being served. If an item is usually fried, ask for the item to be prepared in a different way. Skip Szechuan eggplant, which is loaded with fat.

At Mongolian barbeque–style restaurants, the biggest perk is that you have full control over your meal. As you assemble your dish, fill your bowl with plenty of vegetables. You'll be surprised at how much they shrink down when cooked. Use your discretion when you ladle on the sauces. Flavored waters and spices are often available and are a healthful way to add flavor to your meal without adding sugar or lots of sodium. Your biggest red flag at this type of restaurant is the promise of unlimited trips to the food bar. Fill up on vegetables and lean sources of protein to help curb the temptation to keep returning. Then just fold your hands in your lap when you know you've had all you should eat.

Rice and Noodles

On to the starches: rice and noodles. Both are always available in Chinese restaurants in different forms. Some are healthy, some are not. Obviously, steamed brown rice is ideal, but it's not available in many Chinese restaurants. Steamed white rice is more common. It's steamed with no added salt or fats. Fried rice is white rice stir-fried (which adds oil) with soy sauce that turns it brown and adds sodium. If you order fried rice, stick with the vegetable variety and avoid the fat and protein added by pork or other meats. Similar advice holds true for lo mein and pan-fried noodles. Order these dishes with vegetables rather than high-fat proteins. The basic noodle is healthy, though it has very little fiber or whole grains, but the health quotient goes downhill as chefs add oils and high-sodium sauces. It's easy to eat a lot of carbohydrate from rice and noodles, so eat only a small amount of these dishes.

Dessert

Dessert in Chinese restaurants is usually low key. Often, you don't even order it. Pineapple, orange sections, or lychee nuts simply appear at the table with one fortune cookie for each diner. Desserts on the menu sometimes include ice cream or fried bananas. You are best off skipping menu desserts. And you'll leave the table a bit healthier, and maybe wiser, if you read your fortune but leave the cookie.

Nutrition Snapshot

Health Busters

Category	Restaurant Name	Dish Name	Serving Size	Cal.	Total Fat (g)	Carb. (g)	Sod. (mg)
Appetizers	Kona Grill	Grilled Chicken Wrap	1 portion	1120	58	83	2390
Appetizers	Kona Grill	Pot Stickers	1 portion	860	52	59	2250
Appetizers	T.G.I. Friday's	Pan-Seared Pot Stickers	1 portion	780	42	80	2150
Appetizers	Elephant Bar	Wok-Fired Chicken & Lettuce Wrap	1 portion	570	37	26	2030
Appetizers	Yang Kee Noodle	Imperial Spring Rolls	4 pieces	650	26	53	1676
Noodles	Kona Grill	Pan-Asian	1 portion	1060	35	166	5250
Noodles	Noodles & Company	Buttered Noodles (regular)	1 portion	930	39	114	970
Rice, Fried	Yang Kee Noodle	Fried Rice w/Chicken	1 portion	1069	32	116	2303
Rice, Fried	Panda Express	Fried Rice	1 portion	530	16	82	820

(table continues on next page)

Health Busters

Category	Restaurant Name	Dish Name	Serving Size	Cal.	Total Fat (g)	Carb. (g)	Sod. (mg)
Vegetable Entrées	Pei Wei Asian Diner	Vegetables & Tofu	1 portion	530	20	74	1400
Vegetable Entrées	Pei Wei Asian Diner	Vegetables & Tofu—Kung Pao	1 portion	430	20	44	3260
Vegetable Entrées	Pei Wei Asian Diner	Vegetables & Tofu—Mandarin Kung Pao	1 portion	380	22	31	1980
Vegetable Entrées	Pei Wei Asian Diner	Vegetables & Tofu—Orange Peel	1 portion	350	15	41	1730
Chicken Entrées	Pei Wei Asian Diner	Chicken—Kung Pao	1 portion	510	25	40	3180
Chicken Entrées	Pei Wei Asian Diner	Chicken Sweet & Sour, Gluten-Free	1 portion	380	12	43	1150
Chicken Entrées	P.F. Chang's	Moo Goo Gai Pan on Brown Rice	1/2 portion	380	13	43	1000
Chicken Entrées	P.F. Chang's	Moo Goo Gai Pan	1/3 portion	247	13	13	823
Beef Entrées	Elephant Bar	Wok-Fired Mongolian Beef	1 portion	1330	92	64	3030

(table continues on next page)

Health Busters

Category	Restaurant Name	Dish Name	Serving Size	Cal.	Total Fat (g)	Carb. (g)	Sod. (mg)
Beef Entrées	Pei Wei Asian Diner	Beef—Ginger Broccoli	1 portion	290	13	24	2130
Beef Entrées	Pei Wei Asian Diner	Beef—Caramel	1 portion	540	29	49	1580
Pork Entrées	Elephant Bar	Kona BBQ Pork Ribs—Half Rack	1 portion	1480	97	84	2460
Pork Entrées	Panda Express	BBQ Pork	1 portion	360	19	13	1310
Seafood Entrées	Pei Wei Asian Diner	Shrimp—Mandarin Kung Pao	1 portion	320	18	26	1950
Seafood Entrées	Pei Wei Asian Diner	Shrimp—Caramel	1 portion	320	16	35	1510
Seafood Entrées	Panda Express	Honey Walnut Shrimp	1 portion	370	23	27	470
Seafood Entrées	Elephant Bar	Quick-Seared Ahi Tuna with Ponzu	1 portion	390	17	28	2390
Seafood Entrées	Elephant Bar	Blackened Ahi Tuna with Tropical Fruit Salsa (no rice)	1 portion	640	38	24	1951
Combination Entrées	Yoshinoya	BBQ Style Beef & Chicken Plate w/ Fried Rice & Noodle	1 portion	950	38	101	1530

Healthier Bets

Category	Restaurant Name	Dish Name	Serving Size	Cal.	Total Fat (g)	Sat. Fat (g)	Carb. (g)	Pro. (g)	Fiber (g)	Chol. (mg)	Sodium (mg)	Exchanges/ Choices
Appetizers	Hissho Sushi	Garden Spring Roll	1 roll	130	3	1	23	4	3	2	173	1 Starch, 1 Vegetable, 1/2 Fat
Appetizers	Hissho Sushi	Grilled Chicken Spring Roll	1 roll	140	4	1	19	8	3	20	164	1 Starch, 1 Vegetable, 1 Lean Protein
Appetizers	Tokyo Joe's	Spring Rolls Chicken	1 roll	219	8	1.4	21	16	4	n/a	150	1 Starch, 1 Vegetable, 2 Lean Protein, 1/2 Fat
Soups	Rice King	Egg Drop Soup	1 bowl	62	2	0	8	4	n/a	25	398	1/2 Starch, 1/2 Lean Protein
Soups	Rice King	Hot & Sour Soup	1 bowl	55	2	0	7	3	n/a	38	445	1/2 Starch, 1/2 Fat
Noodles	Rice King	Chicken Chow Mein Noodles	1 portion	218	8	1	26	11	n/a	13	418	1 1/2 Starch, 1 Lean Protein, 1 Fat

(table continues on next page)

Healthier Bets

Category	Restaurant Name	Dish Name	Serving Size	Cal.	Total Fat (g)	Sat. Fat (g)	Carb. (g)	Pro. (g)	Fiber (g)	Chol. (mg)	Sodium (mg)	Exchanges/ Choices
Noodles	P.F. Chang's	Gluten-Free Singapore Street Noodles	1/3 portion	300	7	1	41	11	3	n/a	980	2 1/2 Starch, 1 Vegetable, 1 Lean Protein, 1 Fat
Noodles	Sansai Japanese Grill	Linguine Noodle Salad (with dressing)	1 portion	189	3	0	36	3.5	6	0	251	2 Starch, 1/2 Fat
Rice	Rice Garden	Fried Rice	1 portion	196	5	1	33	4	1	31	331	2 Starch, 1 Fat
Rice	Rice King	Chicken Fried Rice	1 portion	249	9	2	31	11	1	56	380	2 Starch, 1 Lean Protein, 1 Fat
Rice	Panda Express	Fried Rice	1 portion	530	16	3	82	12	1	150	820	5 1/2 Starch. 2 1/2 Fat
Rice	Teriyaki Experience	Brown Rice	1 portion	207	1.2	0	45	5	2	1	9	3 Starch

(table continues on next page)

Healthier Bets

Category	Restaurant Name	Dish Name	Serving Size	Cal.	Total Fat (g)	Sat. Fat (g)	Carb. (g)	Pro. (g)	Fiber (g)	Chol. (mg)	Sodium (mg)	Exchanges/ Choices
Rice	Teriyaki Experience	White Rice	1 portion	285	0.6	0	62	6	1	0	2	4 Starch
Vegetable Entrées	Pei Wei Asian Diner	Vegetables & Tofu—Thai Dynamite	1 portion	250	13	2	22	12	6	5	930	1 Starch, 2 Vegetable, 1 1/2 Medium-Fat Protein, 1 Fat
Vegetable Entrées	Pei Wei Asian Diner	Vegetables & Tofu—Sweet & Sour	1 portion	310	10	1.5	44	11	6	5	620	2 Starch, 2 Vegetable, 1 Medium-Fat Protein, 1 Fat
Vegetable Entrées	Manchu Wok	Mixed Vegetables	1 portion	130	10	1.5	11	2	3	0	510	2 Vegetable, 2 Fat
Chicken Entrées	Pei Wei Asian Diner	Chicken—Honey Seared	1 portion	430	15	2.5	49	22	4	50	640	3 Starch, 1 Vegetable, 2 Lean Protein, 1 1/2 Fat

(table continues on next page)

Healthier Bets

Category	Restaurant Name	Dish Name	Serving Size	Cal.	Total Fat (g)	Sat. Fat (g)	Carb. (g)	Pro. (g)	Fiber (g)	Chol. (mg)	Sodium (mg)	Exchanges/ Choices
Chicken Entrées	Pei Wei Asian Diner	Chicken—Sweet & Sour	1 portion	350	10	2	48	22	5	50	690	3 Starch, 1 Vegetable, 2 Lean Protein, 1/2 Fat
Chicken Entrées	Pei Wei Asian Diner	Chicken—Thai Dynamite	1 portion	310	12	2	26	22	6	50	1000	1 1/2 Starch, 1 Vegetable, 2 1/2 Lean Protein, 1 Fat
Chicken Entrées	Yang Kee Noodle	Chicken Satays	1 portion	466	18	7	22	38	1	78	366	1 1/2 Starch, 1 Vegetable, 5 Lean Protein, 1 Fat
Chicken Entrées	Manchu Wok	Pineapple Chicken	1 portion	170	9	1.5	19	6	1	20	260	1/2 Starch, 1 Fruit, 1 Lean Protein, 1 Fat
Chicken Entrées	Manchu Wok	Chicken with Snow Peas	1 portion	140	9	1.5	11	7	2	20	710	2 Vegetable, 1 Lean Protein, 1 Fat

(table continues on next page)

Healthier Bets

Category	Restaurant Name	Dish Name	Serving Size	Cal.	Total Fat (g)	Sat. Fat (g)	Carb. (g)	Pro. (g)	Fiber (g)	Chol. (mg)	Sodium (mg)	Exchanges/ Choices
Chicken Entrées	Pei Wei Asian Diner	Chicken Honey Seared (kid's, without rice or noodles)	1 portion	180	5	1	21	11	2	20	300	1 Starch, 1 Vegetable, 1 Lean Protein, 1/2 Fat
Beef Entrées	Yoshinoya	Kids' Meal Beef	1 portion	350	11	5	48	13	3	30	700	3 Starch, 1 Vegetable, 1 Medium-Fat Protein, 1 Fat
Beef Entrées	Teriyaki Experience	Beef Pan Asian	1 portion	464	14	3	41	44	3	98	259	2 1/2 Starch, 1 Vegetable, 5 Lean Protein
Beef Entrées	Panda Express	Broccoli Beef	1 portion	120	4	0.5	13	9	3	10	660	1/2 Starch, 1 Vegetable, 1 Medium-Fat Protein

(table continues on next page)

Healthier Bets

Category	Restaurant Name	Dish Name	Serving Size	Cal.	Total Fat (g)	Sat. Fat (g)	Carb. (g)	Pro. (g)	Fiber (g)	Chol. (mg)	Sodium (mg)	Exchanges/ Choices
Combination Entrées	Teriyaki Experience	Chicken & Beef Yakisoba	1 portion	552	9	3	65	50	4	103	769	4 Starch, 1 Vegetable, 5 Lean Protein
Shrimp Entrées	Pei Wei Asian Diner	Shrimp Sweet & Sour, Gluten-Free	1 portion	240	7	1	39	8	4	20	590	2 Starch, 1 Vegetable, 1/2 Lean Protein, 1 Fat
Shrimp Entrées	Pei Wei Asian Diner	Shrimp Lo Mein (kid's, without rice or noodles)	1 portion	110	8	1.5	5	4	0	25	520	1/2 Starch, 1/2 Lean Protein, 1 Fat
Shrimp Entrées	Pei Wei Asian Diner	Shrimp Teriyaki (kid's, without rice or noodles)	1 portion	180	8	1	19	4	0	20	950	1 Starch, 1 Vegetable, 1/2 Lean Protein, 1 Fat

(table continues on next page)

Healthier Bets

Category	Restaurant Name	Dish Name	Serving Size	Cal.	Total Fat (g)	Sat. Fat (g)	Carb. (g)	Pro. (g)	Fiber (g)	Chol. (mg)	Sodium (mg)	Exchanges/ Choices
Shrimp Entrées	Pei Wei Asian Diner	Shrimp— Thai Coconut Curry	1 portion	240	14	10	20	12	4	55	730	1 Starch, 1 Vegetable, 1 Lean Protein, 2 Fat
Desserts	P.F. Chang's	Mini Tres Leche Lemon Dream	1 portion	180	8	4	31	1	1	n/a	125	2 Other Carbohydrate, 1 1/2 Fat
Desserts	P.F. Chang's	Mini Apple Pie	1 portion	190	7	2	29	2	1	n/a	170	2 Other Carbohydrate, 1 1/2 Fat

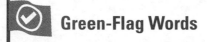 **Green-Flag Words**

Ingredients:

- ▶ Assorted vegetables (broccoli, mushrooms, onions, carrots, cabbage, bok choy, water chestnuts, bamboo shoots, lily buds, wood ears, bean sprouts)
- ▶ Bean curd (tofu)—sautéed, not fried
- ▶ Broth (for both-based soups)
- ▶ Chicken, roast pork
- ▶ Chile sauce
- ▶ Chinese hot mustard
- ▶ Chinese spices
- ▶ Fish, shrimp, scallops, squid
- ▶ Garlic
- ▶ Ginger
- ▶ Hot oil
- ▶ Pineapple
- ▶ Soy sauce (high in sodium)
- ▶ Tomatoes

Cooking Methods/Menu Descriptions:

- ▶ Brown sauce, oyster sauce, black bean sauce (these can be high in hidden sugars and sodium)
- ▶ Chop suey
- ▶ Chow mein
- ▶ Hot and spicy tomato sauce
- ▶ Light wine sauce
- ▶ Lobster sauce
- ▶ Moo shi (or moo shu)
- ▶ Served on sizzling platter
- ▶ Simmered or braised
- ▶ Slippery white sauce or velvet sauce
- ▶ Steamed
- ▶ Stir-fried with vegetables

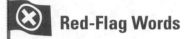

Red-Flag Words

Ingredients:

- ► Cashews or peanuts
- ► Chinese noodles
- ► Duck with skin (typically served with skin)
- ► Hoisin sauce, plum sauce, sweet (duck) sauce (these can be high in hidden sugars and sodium)
- ► Water chestnut flour

Cooking Methods/Menu Descriptions:

- ► Battered or breaded and fried
- ► Crispy
- ► Fried, deep-fried, deep-fried until crispy
- ► General Tso's
- ► Honey sauce, honey battered
- ► Kung Pao
- ► Orange peel or orange flavored (chicken, beef, etc.; all are deep-fried)
- ► Served in bird's nest (which is fried)
- ► Spare ribs
- ► Sweet-and-sour
- ► Whole fish (usually fried)

At the Table:

- ► Chinese noodles

Healthy Eating Tips and Tactics

- ► To keep sodium low, don't dip appetizers in sweet (carbohydrate-containing) or soy-based (sodium-containing) sauces or limit their use. Hot Chinese mustard might be a flavorful option.
- ► Choose steamed white or brown rice rather than fried rice. Brown rice is healthiest when available.
- ► You'll be better able to control your order if you choose a sit-down Chinese restaurant, where you can easily custom order, rather than one in a food court or an all-you-can-eat Chinese buffet.

▶ Rely on hot mustard sauce or hot chile sauce to add zing to your meal with minimal additional sodium, sugar, and fat.

▶ If you eat family style, order fewer dishes than the number of people at the table. This controls portions from the start. And make at least one of the dishes you order vegetables only.

▶ Use chopsticks. They will slow down your eating, particularly if you haven't mastered using them yet.

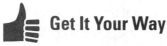 ## Get It Your Way

▶ Ask to have extra vegetables added to a dish to make it more healthful and filling. You might have to pay a bit more.

▶ Dishes are made to order in sit-down Chinese restaurants, so feel free to ask that one item be left out or others be added in.

▶ You may want to order a sauce on the side and use the dipping technique to limit the amount of sauce you eat. This may help decrease both your sodium and sugar intake. However, make sure that you don't sacrifice flavor and taste so much that you'll feel deprived.

▶ Request that no MSG or cornstarch be used in your dish, to limit sodium and carbohydrate, respectively.

▶ Ask what type of oil is used for stir-frying. If lard or another type of saturated fat is used, request that peanut oil or some type of vegetable oil be used instead.

▶ Request that the protein source in your dish be sautéed rather than breaded and deep-fried.

Tips and Tactics for Gluten-Free Eating

▶ Most soy sauce is made from wheat, which means that gluten-free diners should avoid it, and it is included in many typical sauces served in Chinese restaurants. Ask about thickeners, marinades, and seasoning ingredients, as they typically will contain soy sauce.

▶ Noodles, crispy chow mein noodles, lo mein, egg roll and wonton wrappers, and other deep-fried foods typically contain wheat unless otherwise noted. Fortune cookies are made from wheat.

▶ Try plain steamed or stir-fried meats, poultry, fish, or seafood dishes with vegetables that are prepared without soy sauce in a clean wok.

▶ Order plain rice or rice noodles (make sure they are labeled gluten-free) or brown rice if they have it. Bring your own gluten-free soy sauce to the restaurant.

▶ Ingredients such as rice wine, rice vinegar (wheat may be added to some Asian black rice vinegars), dried mushrooms, cornstarch, garlic, ginger root, spring onions, oyster sauce (if it contains soy, it's most likely not gluten-free), rice, sesame oil, chile paste, and tofu (plain is gluten-free, but fried may not be) are gluten-free.

Tips and Tactics to Help Kids Eat Healthy

▶ Avoid ordering off the kids' menu if there is one. The kids' menu often has items that are high in fat, such as fried rice or deep-fried honey chicken. Instead, go family style and share one or two dishes that have been steamed or lightly stir-fried in a wok, rather than deep-fried. Remember, you're having a healthier meal and serving up lifelong healthier restaurant eating skills at the same time.

▶ Order brown rice rather than white rice. If your child is new to brown rice, consider ordering a side of white rice and a side of brown rice. Combine them to gradually introduce your child to the taste of brown rice.

▶ Rather than fried rice, consider a side of steamed vegetables, which you can dice at the table and add to steamed rice if you'd like.

What's Your Solution?

You and your friends decide to visit Chinatown to celebrate a friend's recent promotion at work. Your friend chooses a traditional Chinese restaurant, which has a menu that is written in both in English and Chinese. Yet, language is still a barrier between you and your server.

What can you do to ensure the healthfulness of your meal, determine your insulin dose, and maintain your blood glucose control, even though the language barrier will make it difficult for you to inquire about the details of dishes or make substitutions?

   a)   Request hot and sour soup as your appetizer if your friends are splitting high-fat appetizers.

   b)   If the group is ordering family style, be the one to suggest at least one vegetarian selection.

   c)   Convince your friends to order family style, then use your eyes and taste buds to help guide you on which dishes will fit within your strategy.

   d)   Ask your server to bring a few takeout containers along with your entrées.

See page 447 for answers.

Menu Samplers

Light 'N' Healthy

Menu Samplers Section	Menu Item	Amount	Calories	Fat (g)	% Calories from Fat	Saturated Fat (g)	Chol. (mg)	Sodium (mg)	Carb. (g)	Fiber (g)	Protein (g)	Exchanges/ Choices
Light 'N' Healthy (Women)*	Grilled teriyaki chicken	1/2 entrée (5 oz)	250	11		3	150	440	7	0	30	1/2 Other Carbohydrate, 4 Lean Protein
	Stir-fried vegetables	1 cup	70	5		0	0	530	13	5	4	2 Vegetable, 1 Fat
	Brown rice	3/4 cup	190	2		0	0	3	40	3	4	2 1/2 Starch
Totals			**510**	**18**	**32**	**3**	**150**	**973**	**60**	**8**	**38**	**2 1/2 Starch, 1/2 Other Carbohydrate, 2 Vegetable, 4 Lean Protein, 1 Fat**

*Cholesterol levels are above recommended due to chicken dish.

(table continues on next page)

Light 'N' Healthy

Menu Samplers Section	Menu Item	Amount	Calories	Fat (g)	% Calories from Fat	Saturated Fat (g)	Chol. (mg)	Sodium (mg)	Carb. (g)	Fiber (g)	Protein (g)	Exchanges/Choices
Light 'N' Healthy (Men)	Chicken pot stickers	4 pot stickers (4 oz total)	330	16		3	30	320	34	2	10	2 Starch, 1 Lean Protein, 3 Fat
	Beef and broccoli	1/2 entrée (6 oz)	290	12		3	40	1500	21	2	24	1 Other Carbohydrate, 1 Vegetable, 3 Medium-Fat Protein
	Brown rice	3/4 cup	190	2		0	0	3	40	3	4	2 1/2 Starch
Totals			**810**	**30**	**33**	**6**	**70**	**1823**	**95**	**7**	**38**	**4 1/2 Starch, 1 Other Carbohydrate, 1 Vegetable, 4 Medium-Fat Protein, 3 Fat**

(table continues on next page)

Hearty 'N' Healthy

Menu Samplers Section	Menu Item	Amount	Calories	Fat (g)	% Calories from Fat	Saturated Fat (g)	Chol. (mg)	Sodium (mg)	Carb.(g)	Fiber (g)	Protein (g)	Exchanges/ Choices
Hearty 'N' Healthy (Women)	Veggie spring rolls	3 rolls	160	9		2	0	750	33	6	6	2 Starch, 1/2 Vegetable, 2 Fat
	Hot and sour soup	1 cup	76	2		1	10	100	10	1	4	1 Other Carbohydrate
	Pepper steak (beef with onions and peppers)	1/2 entrée (8 oz)	261	13		3	60	1000	14	1	21	1/2 Other Carbohydrate, 1 Vegetable, 2 1/2 Medium-Fat Protein
	Brown rice	1 cup	218	2		0	0	20	46	4	5	3 Starch
Totals			**715**	**26**	**32**	**6**	**70**	**1870**	**103**	**12**	**36**	**5 Starch, 1 1/2 Other Carbohydrate, 1 1/2 Vegetable, 2 1/2 Medium-Fat Protein, 2 Fat**

(table continues on next page)

Hearty 'N' Healthy

Menu Samplers Section	Menu Item	Amount	Calories	Fat (g)	% Calories from Fat	Saturated Fat (g)	Chol. (mg)	Sodium (mg)	Carb. (g)	Fiber (g)	Protein (g)	Exchanges/ Choices
Hearty 'N' Healthy (Men)*	Asian noodles (served with braised cabbage, green peppers, and Chinese black mushrooms)	1 cup	490	22		4	0	1060	65	4	13	3 Starch, 1 Other Carbohydrate, 1 Vegetable, 4 Fat
	Asian glazed salmon	4 oz, cooked	295	18		3	140	710	7	3	28	1/2 Other Carbohydrate, 4 Lean Protein, 1 Fat
	Brown rice	1/2 cup	109	1		0	0	10	23	2	2	1 1/2 Starch
Totals			**894**	**41**	**41**	**7**	**140**	**1780**	**95**	**9**	**43**	**4 1/2 Starch, 1 1/2 Other Carbohydrate, 1 Vegetable, 4 Lean Protein, 5 Fat**

*Higher than recommended cholesterol levels are due to the salmon dish.

(table continues on next page)

Lower Carb 'N' Healthy

Menu Samplers Section	Menu Item	Amount	Calories	Fat (g)	% Calories from Fat	Saturated Fat (g)	Chol. (mg)	Sodium (mg)	Carb. (g)	Fiber (g)	Protein (g)	Exchanges/ Choices
Lower Carb 'N' Healthy (Women)	Wonton soup	6 oz	85	3		1	10	570	9	0	6	1/2 Starch, 1 Fat
	Veggie spring rolls	3 oz	160	7		1	0	540	22	4	4	1 Starch, 1 Vegetable, 1 Fat
	Tofu lettuce wraps with mushrooms and water chestnuts	3 lettuce cups with filling	147	7		1	0	600	13	2	8	3 Vegetable, 1/2 Lean Protein, 1 Fat
	Seared ahi tuna (without glaze)	1/2 of 4 oz (cooked) entrée	100	5		1	45	100	5	1	11	1 1/2 Lean Protein
	Brown rice	1/3 cup	72	1		0	0	5	15	1	2	1 Starch
Totals			**564**	**23**	**37**	**4**	**55**	**1815**	**64**	**8**	**31**	**2 1/2 Starch, 4 Vegetable, 2 Lean Protein, 3 fat**

(table continues on next page)

Lower Carb 'N' Healthy

Menu Samplers Section	Menu Item	Amount	Calories	Fat (g)	% Calories from Fat	Saturated Fat (g)	Chol. (mg)	Sodium (mg)	Carb. (g)	Fiber (g)	Protein (g)	Exchanges/ Choices
Lower Carb 'N' Healthy (Men)	Hot and sour soup	1 cup	76	2		1	10	100	10	1	4	1 Vegetable, 1 Fat
	Spicy tofu eggplant	6 oz	310	24		3	0	570	20	3	7	1 Other Carbohydrate, 1 Lean Protein, 4 Fat
	Chicken with Chinese mushrooms	3 oz	102	4		1	25	400	5	1	10	1 Vegetable, 1 Lean Protein
	Brown rice	1 cup	218	2		0	0	20	46	4	5	3 Starch
Totals			**706**	**32**	**41**	**5**	**35**	**1090**	**81**	**9**	**26**	**3 Starch, 1 Other Carbohydrate, 2 Vegetable, 2 Lean Protein, 5 Fat**

Menu Lingo

- **Bean curd:** is made from soybeans and formed into cubes. It is known as "tofu" to Americans. You'll see it used in soups and other dishes. Be careful to request that it not be fried because it is often fried in entrées.
- **Black bean sauce:** a thick, brown sauce made of fermented soybeans, salt, and wheat flour. It is frequently used in Cantonese cooking.
- **Bok choy:** looks like a cross between celery and cabbage. It is also known as Chinese chard.
- **Five-spice powder:** a reddish-brown powder that combines star anise, fennel, cinnamon, cloves, and Szechuan pepper. It is often used in Szechuan dishes.
- **Hoisin sauce:** a thick, sweet-and-spicy sauce, also called plum sauce, made from soybeans, sugar, garlic, chilies, and vinegar. Served with moo shu dishes.
- **Lily buds:** dried, golden-colored buds with a light, flowery flavor. They are also called lotus buds and tiger lily buds and are often used in entrées and soups.
- **Lychees, or lychee nuts:** a crimson-colored fruit with translucent flesh around a brown seed. They closely resemble white grapes.
- **Monosodium glutamate (MSG):** a white powder used in small amounts to bring out and enhance the flavors of ingredients. (Note: MSG doesn't contain gluten.) It contains sodium, but not as much as salt.
- **Napa cabbage:** also referred to as Chinese cabbage, it has thick-ribbed stalks and crinkled leaves.
- **Oyster sauce:** a rich, thick sauce made of oysters, their cooking liquid, and soy sauce (which may contain gluten). It is frequently used in Cantonese dishes.
- **Plum sauce:** an amber-colored, thick sauce made from plums, apricots, hot peppers, vinegar, and sugar; it has a spicy sweet-and-sour flavor.
- **Sesame oil:** oil extracted from sesame seeds. It has a strong sesame flavor and is used as seasoning for soups, seafood, and other dishes.
- **Soy sauce:** either light or dark, is used in lieu of salt in virtually all Chinese dishes.

▶ **Sweet-and-sour sauce:** a thick sauce made from sugar, vinegar, and soy sauce (which may contain gluten). Meat, chicken, or shrimp served in this sauce usually have been dipped in batter and fried.

▶ **Wood ear:** a variety of tree lichen, which is brown and resembles a wrinkled ear; it is soaked before use. Found in soups and some vegetable dishes.

(i) **What's Your Solution? Answers**

a) Ordering soup at a Chinese restaurant is always a smart choice. The soups are generally low in calories and can help take the edge off your appetite.

b) Requesting a vegetarian entrée, or even a vegetable-based side dish, can help balance out all the sources of protein in the dishes on the table.

c) Sharing dishes family style is one of the best strategies you can take. Not only will this help with portion control, but, given the language barrier, it will give you the opportunity to gauge the healthfulness of the dishes based on appearance and a small taste. Then you can decide what you want to put on your plate.

d) Smart move! It's easy to overeat when there is a lot of food on the table, especially when you're enjoying leisurely conversation with friends. Boxing up some of the food from the start will help keep you (and your friends) from overeating.

CHAPTER 22

Thai

Thai restaurants are a relatively new addition to America's restaurant landscape. While they don't have the stateside longevity of other ethnic cuisines, Thai restaurants have quickly gained popularity in the last decade or so. Today, you'll find Thai restaurants in cities of all sizes and even in suburban strip malls. Most of them are independently run with a few locations (or just one) in the same geographic area.

While there are no Thai chain restaurants to date, restaurateurs have noticed the mass appeal of Thai flavors. So it's no surprise that Thai dishes and flavors are being added to the menu in a variety of restaurants, including P.F. Chang's, Pei Wei Asian Diner, Noodles & Company, and even California Pizza Kitchen, which offers a Thai-style pizza. From pad thai, the favorite noodles dish on nearly every Thai menu, to Thai-inspired salads and pizzas at family restaurants, Thai food has developed a strong following in America.

On the Menu

Thai cuisine is often compared to Chinese cuisine, though the similarities don't go much beyond the preparation method of stir-frying, the central role of rice and noodles, and a cadre of similar vegetables. As for end results, Thai food differs substantially due to the use of many different herbs and spices. In fact, in terms of taste, Thai food more closely resembles Indian fare with its use of aromatic flavors and spices, such as coriander, cumin, cardamom, and cinnamon, to name a few. The similarities among these three types of cuisine make sense because India and China are both Thailand's neighbors.

Thai cooking is generally light and healthy, but fat does creep in from various sources, though not nearly as much fat as you'll find in Chinese food. Most Thai appetizers are deep-fried and many entrées are stir-fried. If you frequent a particular Thai restaurant, ask what type(s) of oil they cook with. Make sure they say "no" to animal-based fats (such as lard) in favor of vegetable oils.

Another source of fat is coconut milk, which is used frequently in Thai cuisine to create dishes with curry sauces. Coconut milk, similar to coconut oil, contains saturated fat, as well as a hefty dose of calories. One-quarter cup of coconut milk—the amount you might have in a Thai curry dish that you split in half—contains 110 calories, most of which are from saturated fat. To limit your intake of this unhealthy ingredient, limit the amount of dishes with coconut milk you eat, such as curry entrées and some soups.

The sodium content of Thai food can run high. The spicing and flavor profiles of Thai food are not as dependent on soy sauces as Chinese cuisine. However, it is not uncommon to see soy sauce and/or salt added to main dishes, soups, rice (other than steamed), and noodle dishes. Some Thai sauces, such as yellow bean paste, shrimp paste, and fish sauce, also add sodium to dishes.

People with diabetes should be on the alert and realize that, in similar fashion to many Southeast Asian cuisines, a small amount of sugar is used in many Thai dishes. On average, 1 teaspoon to 2 tablespoons of sugar might be added to a dish. Some sauces, like the sweet soy sauce used in the noodle dish pad see ew, have a bit more sugar than others. Sometimes, Thai people use palm sugar in their cuisine. If you feel that your blood glucose generally rises after eating Thai meals, adjust your insulin (if you are able), limit certain items that add sugars and starches to your Thai meal, and/or use your favorite portion-control techniques to eat less of the higher-carbohydrate foods.

Thai dishes in sit-down restaurants are generally made to order. This makes special requests easy to grant; don't hesitate to make them. Family-style eating is commonplace in Thai cuisine. So, don't feel compelled to order an entrée just for yourself. Practice the key portion-control strategy of splitting or sharing a few menu items among your entire dining party.

≣ The Menu Profile

Appetizers

Thai food features its fair share of deep-fried appetizers, but there are also a handful of healthy options available. Try fresh basil or vegetable rolls (the ones that aren't fried), or meat or chicken satay. Just be on guard when you dip your appetizers into the tasty sauces. Peanut sauce, served with satay, is loaded with fat from the nuts, whereas tamarind sweet-and-sour sauce is high in sugar. Dip lightly or use the chile sauce that is often on the table at Thai restaurants to add a flavor kick to your appetizer.

As is often the case with appetizers, many Thai appetizers are deep-fried and dense in fat, including Thai rolls, tod mun, crab Rangoon, and stuffed chicken wings. However, portions are small and it's common to split appetizers. If you've got a few calories to spare and dining partners to share with, enjoy a few tastes. If not, just dive into a bowl of clear soup and a healthy entrée.

Soups and Salads

Soup is filling and can take the edge off your appetite. Thai soups can be divided into two groups: those that are healthy and those you should avoid. Clear-broth soups like tom yum koong and poh taek have a bit of protein (from poultry or seafood) and great flavor thanks to Thai spices such as lemon grass, chile paste, and lime juice. The calorie count of these soups is low, but they are high in sodium. The soups to avoid (unless you've got calories and fat grams to spare) are tom ka gai, which is a chicken coconut soup, and any other soups with coconut milk. When in doubt, read the soup's description to determine whether its base is clear or made cloudy with coconut milk. Stick with soups you can see through.

Salads are unusual in some Southeast Asian cuisines, like Chinese, but these items are regulars on Thai menus. Thai salads range from simple garden salads to salads that combine less common ingredients such as green papaya and dried shrimp. Salads often combine vegetables and/or fruit with beef, chicken, seafood, or a combination of proteins—yam yai, for example, is a combo of shrimp, chicken, and pork. Nam tok, a steak salad, is devoid of the types of vegetables we often associate with salads. It really consists of mostly steak with herbs and a lime-based marinade.

Thai salad dressings are light and made with spices such as lemon grass, chilies, lime juice, and sometimes peanut sauce. Remember to ask for dressing on the side when you order a salad. Or request a few slices of fresh lime to use instead. Try eating a salad while others are digging into fried appetizers. Or you can order a seafood or beef salad as your main course with a bowl of steamed rice on the side; split it with your dining partner(s) as one of the group's entrée choices.

Entrées

You'll find many healthy entrées in Thai restaurants. Some load on the vegetables and are cooked in light sauces. Think about which source(s) of protein you want—chicken, shrimp, scallops, fish, beef, or pork. Try to choose a lean protein to reduce your fat intake. Complement a protein-dense dish with a vegetable-rich side dish. Or choose a vegetable or tofu (bean curd) dish for a meal that is light on animal protein and saturated fat. However, if you order tofu, ask them not to fry it.

You may find peanuts, cashews, or peanut sauce added into or on top of many Thai dishes. If you want to skim fat grams from your meal, tell the waitperson to leave these ingredients in the kitchen. But you can leave them on if you want a few grams of healthier fats. If calories are a prime concern for you, lighter basil, chile, and lime juice sauces are lower-calories options.

Curry dishes in Thai restaurants often contain coconut milk, which adds saturated fat—the artery-clogging variety of fat. It's best not to overload on curry sauces, whether yellow, green, red, or mussaman, which is the thickest type of curry. Order one curry dish to share among a group and make an effort to minimize the amount of sauce you spoon onto your plate. On the plus side, curry dishes can be packed with veggies. Make sure the curry dish you choose is full of vegetables by reading the menu descriptors or asking your waitperson. You can always ask to add more of one vegetable or another to your dish. Thai kitchens usually have plenty of broccoli, green beans, eggplant, and carrots, because these are frequently used in other Thai dishes.

Rice and Noodles

Several rice and noodle offerings are up for grabs in Thai restaurants. Hands down, the best choice, which arrives with your meal without even a request, is steamed brown rice (or white if you can't get brown). It's long grain, often with a sprinkling of jasmine grains. Fried rice is also usually available. Thai fried rice is a bit lighter in fat and color than most Chinese versions of fried rice. Like Chinese fried rice, Thai fried rice comes in varieties such as vegetable, pork, seafood, or combination. Stick with the vegetable if you must and eat only a small amount. There's no doubt about it, you up the fat and sodium content of your meal when you switch from steamed brown or white rice to fried rice.

Pad thai is the omnipresent Thai noodle dish. It consists of noodles, stir-fried with finely chopped peanuts, bean sprouts, egg, tofu, scallions, and often a slice of lime on the side. It's served either with tofu or with chicken or shrimp. Like fried rice, pad thai gains fat and sodium in the cooking process. A whole serving of pad thai at P.F. Chang's has more than 3,500 milligrams of sodium. Wow! If you order pad thai, ask that the restaurant limit the use of soy sauce and plan to enjoy a smaller portion of the dish, supplementing it with steamed vegetables. Several other noodle dishes, such as drunken noodles, are often on the menu. They all spend time in a wok being tossed with oil and sodium-containing sauces, so use the same strategies suggested for eating pad thai. Be on the lookout for hidden sugars in Thai noodle dishes, such as the sweet soy sauce used in the noodle dish pad see ew.

Desserts

The dessert listings in most Thai restaurants are minimal and easy to pass by. You might find rambutan or lychee nuts, which are common Southeast Asian fruits, and puddings or custards. The rambutan and lychee nuts are fine, but a nice, relaxing cup of coffee or tea might just make a satisfying end to your meal with fewer calories.

Drinks

Most Thai restaurants offer Thai iced coffee or iced tea. Don't be fooled into thinking that these items are just like regular coffee or tea. They contain plenty of sugar and milk or cream, so you are better off resisting these beverages. For tips on choosing healthy beverages in restaurants, see Chapter 9 (page 87).

Nutrition Snapshot

Health Busters

Category	Restaurant Name	Dish Name	Serving Size	Cal.	Total Fat (g)	Carb. (g)	Sod. (mg)
Appetizers	Yang Kee Noodle	Imperial Spring Rolls	4 eggrolls	650	26	53	1676
Appetizers	California Pizza Kitchen	Sesame Ginger Chicken Dumplings	1 portion	465	13	63	1801
Appetizers	Yang Kee Noodle	Chicken Satay	1 portion	466	18	22	366
Soups	Noodles & Company	Thai Curry (regular)	1 portion	470	18	70	1900
Soups	Yang Kee Noodle	Saigon Noodle w/Beef	1 portion	529	25	44	2560
Soups	Yang Kee Noodle	Saigon Noodle w/Chicken	1 portion	623	21	44	2584
Salads	California Pizza Kitchen	Thai Crunch w/Avocado (full)	1 salad	1212	77	80	1081
Salads	Yang Kee Noodle	Sesame Spinach w/Chicken	1 salad	674	25	60	436
Noodles, Pad Thai	Elephant Bar	Bangkok w/Vegetables & Chicken	1 portion	1190	50	120	2520
Noodles, Pad Thai	Noodles & Company	Regular Pad Thai	1 portion	830	18	151	2050
Noodles, Pad Thai	Pei Wei Asian Diner	Vegetables & Tofu Pad Thai	1 portion	750	23	111	2680

(table continues on next page)

Health Busters

Category	Restaurant Name	Dish Name	Serving Size	Cal.	Total Fat (g)	Carb. (g)	Sod. (mg)
Noodles, Pad Thai	Pei Wei Asian Diner	Chicken Pad Thai	1 portion	720	20	105	2570
Noodles, Pad Thai	Yang Kee Noodle	Classic Pad Thai	1 portion	940	35	77	2471
Rice, Fried	Yang Kee Noodle	Fried Rice w/Pork	1 portion	1036	41	116	2300
Rice, Fried	Panda Express	Regular Fried Rice	1 portion	530	16	82	820
Rice, Fried	Pei Wei Asian Diner	Vegetables & Tofu Fried Rice	1 portion	530	20	74	1400
Rice, Fried	Pei Wei Asian Diner	Fried Rice w/Steak	1 portion	520	16	68	1380
Entrées	Yang Kee Noodle	Island Green Curry	1 portion	1088	55	77	3464
Entrées	Kokoro Restaurant	Chicken Curry Bowl (regular)	1 portion	520	11	75	670
Entrées	Yang Kee Noodle	Firecracker Chicken	1 portion	1201	36	142	2214
Entrées	Elephant Bar	Wok-Fired Sesame Ginger Chicken	1 portion	1180	46	132	5170
Entrées	P.F. Chang's	Sweet & Sour Pork	1/2 portion	460	14	72	950
Entrées	Yang Kee Noodle	Crispy White Sea Bass	1 portion	859	19	128	1916
Entrées	Kona Grill	Sweet Chili Glazed Salmon	1 portion	910	39	85	2440
Entrées	Teriyaki Stix	Curry Bowl	1 bowl	704	15	110	n/a

Healthier Bets

Category	Restaurant Name	Dish Name	Serving Size	Cal.	Total Fat (g)	Sat. Fat (g)	Carb. (g)	Pro. (g)	Fiber (g)	Chol. (mg)	Sodium (mg)	Exchanges/ Choices
Appetizers	California Pizza Kitchen	Tortilla Spring Roll Thai Chicken w/ Thai Peanut Sauce	1 roll	320	15	4	33	13	3	n/a	747	2 Starch, 1 Lean Protein, 2 1/2 Fat
Appetizers	Yang Kee Noodle	Imperial Spring Rolls	1 eggroll	163	6	2	13	3	1	17	419	1 Starch, 1 1/2 Fat
Appetizers	P.F. Chang's	Pork Dumplings (steamed)	1 dumpling	60	2	1	6	4	0	n/a	125	1/2 Starch, 1/2 Lean Protein
Soups	Au Bon Pain	Thai Coconut Curry (large)	1 bowl	230	10	3	29	6	3	5	1490	2 Starch, 2 Fat
Soups	Au Bon Pain	Thai Coconut Curry (small)	1 bowl	110	5	1	14	3	1	5	740	1 Starch, 1 Fat

(table continues on next page)

Healthier Bets

Category	Restaurant Name	Dish Name	Serving Size	Cal.	Total Fat (g)	Sat. Fat (g)	Carb. (g)	Pro. (g)	Fiber (g)	Chol. (mg)	Sodium (mg)	Exchanges/ Choices
Soups	Souplantation	Thai Peanut & Red Pepper (vegan)	1 cup	220	11	2	23	7	5	0	430	1 Starch, 1 Vegetable, 1/2 High-Fat Protein, 1/2 Fat
Soups	Souplantation	Curried Pineapple & Ginger (low-fat, non-vegetarian)	1 cup	200	2	0	40	6	2	0	560	1 1/2 Starch, 1 Fruit, 1 Vegetable
Soups	Noodles & Company	Thai Curry (small)	1 portion	230	9	6	35	3	2	0	950	1 1/2 Starch, 2 Vegetable, 2 Fat
Soups	Pei Wei Asian Diner	Thai Wonton (cup—6 oz)	1 cup	110	6	2	5	10	1	30	1030	1 Vegetable, 1 Lean Protein, 1 Fat

(table continues on next page)

Healthier Bets

Category	Restaurant Name	Dish Name	Serving Size	Cal.	Total Fat (g)	Sat. Fat (g)	Carb. (g)	Pro. (g)	Fiber (g)	Chol. (mg)	Sodium (mg)	Exchanges/ Choices
Noodles	Noodles & Company	Bangkok Curry (small)	1 portion	240	7	4.5	40	4	4	0	430	2 Starch, 2 Vegetable, 1 Fat
Rice, Fried	Rice King	Fried Rice	1 portion	197	9	2	25	5	4	55	380	1 1/2 Starch, 2 Fat
Rice, Fried	Rice Garden	Fried Rice	1 portion	196	5	1	33	4	1	31	331	2 Starch, 1 Fat
Rice, Fried	Panda Express	Fried Rice	1 portion	530	16	3	82	12	1	150	820	5 Starch, 1 Vegetable, 3 Fat
Rice	Teriyaki Experience	Brown Rice	1 portion	207	1	0	45	5	2	1	9	3 Starch
Rice	Teriyaki Experience	White Rice	1 portion	285	1	0	62	6	1	0	2	4 Starch
Entrées	P.F. Chang's	Buddha's Feast— Steamed on White Rice	1/2 portion	235	1	0	45	10	3	n/a	575	3 Starch

(table continues on next page)

Healthier Bets

Category	Restaurant Name	Dish Name	Serving Size	Cal.	Total Fat (g)	Sat. Fat (g)	Carb. (g)	Pro. (g)	Fiber (g)	Chol. (mg)	Sodium (mg)	Exchanges/ Choices
Entrées	Pei Wei Asian Diner	Vegetables & Tofu— Thai Coconut Curry	1 portion	340	20	11	27	15	8	5	820	1 Starch, 2 Vegetable, 1 Medium-Fat Protein, 3 Fat
Entrées	Pei Wei Asian Diner	Vegetables & Tofu— Sweet & Sour	1 portion	310	10	1.5	44	11	6	5	620	2 Starch, 2 Vegetable, 1 Medium-Fat Protein, 1 Fat
Entrées	Pei Wei Asian Diner	Chicken— Thai Dynamite	1 portion	310	12	2	26	22	6	50	1000	1 1/2 Starch, 1 Vegetable, 2 1/2 Lean Protein, 1 Fat
Entrées	Pei Wei Asian Diner	Chicken— Thai Coconut Curry	1 portion	320	16	10	21	26	4	55	710	1 Starch, 1 Vegetable, 3 Lean Protein, 2 Fat

(table continues on next page)

Healthier Bets

Category	Restaurant Name	Dish Name	Serving Size	Cal.	Total Fat (g)	Sat. Fat (g)	Carb. (g)	Pro. (g)	Fiber (g)	Chol. (mg)	Sodium (mg)	Exchanges/ Choices
Entrées	Pei Wei Asian Diner	Chicken— Sweet & Sour	1 portion	360	10	2	48	22	5	50	590	3 Starch, 2 Lean Protein, 1 Fat
Entrées	P.F. Chang's	Sweet & Sour Chicken	1/3 portion	370	19	3	38	12	0	n/a	367	2 1/2 Starch, 1 Lean Protein, 3 Fat
Entrées	P.F. Chang's	Ginger Chicken w/ Broccoli	1/3 portion	273	11	2	18	28	2	n/a	1457	1/2 Starch, 2 Vegetable, 3 Lean Protein, 1 Fat
Entrées	Pei Wei Asian Diner	Beef—Thai Coconut Curry	1 portion	350	21	12	24	20	5	20	890	1 1/2 Starch, 2 1/2 Medium-Fat Protein, 1 Fat
Entrées	Kokoro Restaurant	Beef Curry Bowl (regular)	280	5	1.5	40	18	0	30	820	2 1/2 Starch, 2 Lean Protein

(table continues on next page)

Healthier Bets

Category	Restaurant Name	Dish Name	Serving Size	Cal.	Total Fat (g)	Sat. Fat (g)	Carb. (g)	Pro. (g)	Fiber (g)	Chol. (mg)	Sodium (mg)	Exchanges/ Choices
Entrées	Pei Wei Asian Diner	Beef—Thai Dynamite	1 portion	230	10	3	17	18	2	20	970	1/2 Starch, 2 Vegetable, 3 Medium-Fat Protein
Entrées	Pei Wei Asian Diner	Shrimp— Thai Coconut Curry	1 portion	240	14	10	20	12	4	55	730	1 Starch, 1 Vegetable, 1 Lean Protein, 2 Fat
Entrées	Pei Wei Asian Diner	Shrimp— Ginger Broccoli	1 portion	190	6	1	20	15	2	75	2000	1 Starch, 1 Vegetable, 1 Lean Protein, 1 Fat
Entrées	P.F. Chang's	Asian Grilled Norwegian Salmon on White Rice	1/2 portion	345	5	1	50	22	1	n/a	570	3 1/2 Starch, 2 Lean Protein
Entrées	P.F. Chang's	Norwegian Salmon Steamed w/ Ginger	1/2 portion	330	19	3	12	31	3	n/a	605	1 Starch, 4 Lean Protein, 1 1/2 Fat

Green-Flag Words

Ingredients:

- ► Chile, chile paste, crushed or dried chilies, chile sauce
- ► Basil or basil leaves
- ► Bean curd (tofu)—sautéed, but not fried
- ► Chicken
- ► Fish sauce (high in sodium)
- ► Fish, shrimp, scallops, squid
- ► Green beans, broccoli, carrots, tomatoes
- ► Green papaya
- ► Lemon grass
- ► Lime juice, Kaffir limes
- ► Mint or mint leaves
- ► Napa cabbage, bamboo shoots, black mushrooms
- ► Pineapple
- ► Soy sauce (high in sodium)

Cooking Methods/Menu Descriptions:

- ► Barbecued
- ► Basil sauce
- ► Braised
- ► Fresh
- ► Lime sauce
- ► Marinated
- ► Sautéed
- ► Sizzling
- ► Soup made with clear broth
- ► Stir-fried
- ► Thai salad

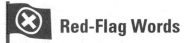

Red-Flag Words

Ingredients:

- ► Cashews
- ► Coconut milk

- ▶ Fried tofu
- ▶ Peanuts, ground peanuts
- ▶ Roasted duck (skin and fat are usually left on)

Cooking Methods/Menu Descriptions:

- ▶ Crispy
- ▶ Curry sauce
- ▶ Deep-fried
- ▶ Fried
- ▶ Golden brown
- ▶ Mee-krob (crispy noodles)
- ▶ Curry sauce (red, green, yellow, massaman)
- ▶ Served with peanut sauce
- ▶ Soup made with coconut milk
- ▶ Tamarind sauce

Healthy Eating Tips and Tactics

- ▶ If you order an appetizer, choose nonfried options or clear-broth soups.
- ▶ Don't overload on curry sauces. Order one curry dish to share among a group and make an effort to minimize the amount of sauce you spoon on your rice or noodles.
- ▶ Ask for extra plates to make sharing easy.
- ▶ Use chopsticks to slow down your eating, particularly if you haven't mastered using them.
- ▶ Takeout boxes are aplenty. Request one (or more) to wrap up half your meal before you dig in. Enjoy the leftovers for dinner the next night.

Get It Your Way

- ▶ Use a bit of chile sauce on your appetizer in place of tamarind or peanut sauce. Chile sauce contains very few calories.
- ▶ Ask what kind of oil is used to prepare your foods. If coconut oil or lard is the answer, request that vegetable oil be used instead.

- Request that salt and soy sauce be used sparingly in your dishes.
- Replace beef or pork with leaner sources of protein, such as tofu, chicken, scallops, or shrimp. And ask that your protein be sautéed rather than deep-fried. Remember deletions, substitutions, and additions are easy to make.
- Double up. Ask that double the amount of your favorite vegetables be added to your dish.
- Give your dish a kick. Ask that your dish be made with the heat (spiciness) equivalent of two or three chilies. This is a great way to add lots of flavor to a dish, especially after you cut back on the oil or other sauces. Added bonus: the strong flavor may keep you from overeating.

Tips and Tactics for Gluten-Free Eating

- Most authentic Thai cuisine is naturally gluten-free. Most dishes are made with rice or rice noodles and rice spring roll wrappers, but ask someone to make sure.
- Check to see if the dish you want contains soy sauce. Traditional Thai soy sauce is gluten-free, but some restaurants may use Chinese wheat-based soy sauce. Ask about the fish and oyster sauces as well to be sure they do not contain wheat.
- Coconut milk is gluten free.

Tips and Tactics to Help Kids Eat Healthy

- Order à la carte for or with your child (depending on age). Chicken satay, steamed noodles or rice, and steamed vegetables make for a kid-friendly meal.
- Try tofu as the source of protein. While it's not often thought of as "kid food," its mild flavor and texture and mouth feel lend it some serious kid-appeal.
- Order clear-broth soups. Thai soups, like other Asian soups, are often served with a ladle-like spoon that kids get a kick out of. Plus, Thai soups are a great low-calorie way to start a meal and take the edge off a child's hunger.

(?) What's Your Solution?

You often order Thai food and have it delivered to your home, especially when you are having dinner alone and don't have the time or energy to prepare a meal. The crab Rangoon and pad thai have been your go-to favorites and you usually eat the full serving while unwinding in front of the TV.

What tweaks can you make to this routine to help it better fit with your new healthier-eating strategies?

    a) Order the fresh spring rolls (not fried) instead of the crab Rangoon.

    b) Request that the pad thai be made with less oil and soy sauce and ask that they leave the peanuts off.

    c) Ask for the same changes to the pad thai as above (option b), plus request that they add an extra veggie of your choice to the dish.

    d) When you place your order, ask them to split the pad thai into two containers.

See page 474 for answers.

Menu Samplers

Light 'N' Healthy

Menu Samplers Section	Menu Item	Amount	Calories	Fat (g)	% Calories from Fat	Saturated Fat (g)	Chol. (mg)	Sodium (mg)	Carb. (g)	Fiber (g)	Protein (g)	Exchanges/ Choices
Light 'N' Healthy (Women)	Vegetable tom yum soup	2 cups	140	4		1	10	500	25	2	8	1 Other Carbo-hydrate, 2 Veg-etable, 1/2 Lean Protein
	Pork larb with green onion in lettuce cups	6 oz	298	9		2	100	630	8	1	34	1 1/2 Vege-table, 4 Medium-Fat Protein
	Green papaya salad	1 cup	80	0		0	0	20	20	4	0	1 1/2 Fruit
	Brown rice	1/2 cup	109	0		0	0	0	23	2	2	1 1/2 Starch

(table continues on next page)

Light 'N' Healthy

Menu Samplers Section	Menu Item	Amount	Calories	Fat (g)	% Calories from Fat	Saturated Fat (g)	Chol. (mg)	Sodium (mg)	Carb.(g)	Fiber (g)	Protein (g)	Exchanges/ Choices
Totals			**627**	**13**	**19**	**3**	**110**	**1150**	**76**	**9**	**44**	**1 1/2 Starch, 1 1/2 Fruit, 1 Other Carbohydrate, 3 1/2 Vegetable, 4 1/2 Medium-Fat Protein**
Light 'N' Healthy (Men)	Chicken satay	3 skewers	286	18		2	63	350	6	1	25	1/2 Other Carbohydrate, 3 Lean Protein, 2 Fat
	Peanut sauce	1 1/2 Tbsp	59	4		1	0	96	4	0	2	1 Fat

(table continues on next page)

Light 'N' Healthy

Menu Samplers Section	Menu Item	Amount	Calories	Fat (g)	% Calories from Fat	Saturated Fat (g)	Chol. (mg)	Sodium (mg)	Carb. (g)	Fiber (g)	Protein (g)	Exchanges/ Choices
	Vegetable pad thai	1 cup	287	7		0	0	700	50	6	7	2 1/2 Starch, 1 Vegetable, 1 1/2 Fat
	Savory Thai stir-fried vegetables	1/2 cup	193	5		1	1	439	24	2	4	1 Other Carbohydrate, 1 Vegetable, 1 Fat
Totals			825	34	37	4	64	1585	84	9	38	2 1/2 Starch, 1 1/2 Other Carbohydrate, 2 Vegetable, 3 Lean Protein, 5 1/2 Fat

(table continues on next page)

Hearty 'N' Healthy

Menu Samplers Section	Menu Item	Amount	Calories	Fat (g)	% Calories from Fat	Saturated Fat (g)	Chol. (mg)	Sodium (mg)	Carb. (g)	Fiber (g)	Protein (g)	Exchanges/ Choices
Hearty 'N' Healthy (Women)	Thai chili chicken	4 oz	250	13		2	96	800	14	1	36	1 Other Carbohydrate, 5 Lean Protein
	Savory Thai stir-fried vegetables	3/4 cup	288	15		2	2	655	36	3	5	1 Other Carbohydrate, 2 Vegetable, 3 Fat
	Brown rice	1/2 cup	109	0		0	0	0	23	2	2	1 1/2 Starch
Totals			**647**	**28**	**39**	**4**	**98**	**1455**	**73**	**6**	**43**	**1 1/2 Starch, 2 Other Carbohydrate, 2 Vegetable, 5 Lean Protein, 3 Fat**

(table continues on next page)

Hearty 'N' Healthy

Menu Samplers Section	Menu Item	Amount	Calories	Fat (g)	% Calories from Fat	Saturated Fat (g)	Chol. (mg)	Sodium (mg)	Carb. (g)	Fiber (g)	Protein (g)	Exchanges/ Choices
Hearty 'N' Healthy (Men)	Green papaya salad	1 cup	80	0		0	0	20	20	4	0	1 1/2 Fruit
	Lemon grass beef with side of vegetable pad thai (broccoli and shredded carrots)	1/2 cup noodles, 3 oz beef	710	30		4	70	740	71	3	45	3 Starch, 1 Other Carbohydrate, 2 Vegetable, 4 Medium-Fat Protein
	Coconut rice with mango slices	1/2 cup	150	5		2.5	0	520	27	2	2	1 Starch, 1 Fruit, 1 Fat
Totals			**940**	**35**	**34**	**6.5**	**70**	**1280**	**118**	**9**	**47**	**4 Starch, 2 1/2 Fruit, 1 Other Carbohydrate, 2 Vegetable, 4 Medium-Fat Protein, 1 Fat**

(table continues on next page)

Lower Carb 'N' Healthy

Menu Samplers Section	Menu Item	Amount	Calories	Fat (g)	% Calories from Fat	Saturated Fat (g)	Chol. (mg)	Sodium (mg)	Carb. (g)	Fiber (g)	Protein (g)	Exchanges/ Choices
Lower Carb 'N' Healthy (Women)	Panang chicken curry with assorted vegetables	3 oz chicken, 1 cup of entrée	205	5		1	72	770	10	0	28	1/2 Other Carbohydrate, 1 Vegetable, 4 Lean Protein
	Brown rice	2/3 cup	146	0		0	0	0	31	2	3	2 Starch
	Green papaya salad	1 1/2 cups	120	0		0	0	30	30	6	0	2 Fruit
Totals			**471**	**5**	**10**	**1**	**72**	**800**	**71**	**8**	**31**	**2 Starch, 2 Fruit, 1/2 Other Carbohydrate, 1 Vegetable, 4 Lean Protein**

(table continues on next page)

Lower Carb 'N' Healthy

Menu Samplers Section	Menu Item	Amount	Calories	Fat (g)	% Calories from Fat	Saturated Fat (g)	Chol. (mg)	Sodium (mg)	Carb. (g)	Fiber (g)	Protein (g)	Exchanges/ Choices
Lower Carb 'N' Healthy (Men)	Vegetable tom yum soup	1 1/2 cups	105	3		1	7	375	20	2	6	1 Starch, 1 Vegetable, 1/2 Fat
	Soy plum glazed duck with scallions, cucumbers, and rice	1 1/2 cups	690	29		8	95	1300	65	1	52	3 Starch, 1 Other Carbohydrate, 1 Vegetable, 7 Medium-Fat Protein
Totals			**795**	**32**	**36**	**9**	**102**	**1675**	**85**	**3**	**58**	**4 Starch, 1 Other Carbohydrate, 2 Vegetable, 7 Medium-Fat Protein, 1/2 Fat**

Menu Lingo

- ▶ **Bamboo shoots:** an oriental vegetable commonly found in Thai entrées. They are light in color, crunchy, stringy in texture, and very low in calories.
- ▶ **Basil:** known as horapa in Thailand, this herb is used mainly in leaf form in Thai dishes. Several types of basil are common in Thai cooking.
- ▶ **Cardamom:** a member of the ginger family. Cardamom seeds are often used in curry mixtures and other dishes, either whole or ground.
- ▶ **Chilies:** various types of chilies are used in Thai dishes, depending on heat level of the dish. Red and green chilies are common and are used whole, chopped, or ground into paste for sauces. Chilies add zip with almost no calories. Chile icons on Thai menus often denote the level of heat in dishes or how much chile is used.
- ▶ **Cilantro:** a member of the carrot family. It is also called Chinese parsley or coriander (it's the coriander plant leaves). Cilantro is widely used in Mexican, Caribbean, and Asian cooking. Cilantro looks flat like Italian parsley but the leaves are more delicate.
- ▶ **Coconut milk:** a liquid extracted by grating fresh coconut (not the liquid from inside the coconut). Coconut milk is used for marinating foods (such as satay) and for making sauces, such as curry sauces. It is high in saturated fat and calories.
- ▶ **Coriander:** dried coriander seed is the main ingredient in curry mixtures. The seeds and leaves (cilantro; see above) are both essential flavors in Thai cooking.
- ▶ **Cumin:** another fragrant spice important to curry mixtures. It is used either as whole seeds or ground.
- ▶ **Curry:** a combination of spices—not a single spice as is often thought—used to flavor dishes and sauces. Different spice and food combinations create the green, red, and mussaman curry mixtures common in Thai cuisine.
- ▶ **Kapi:** a dried shrimp paste made from prawns or shrimp that is commonly used to flavor many Thai dishes.
- ▶ **Lemon grass:** also known as takrai in Thailand, this is an Asian plant whose bulbous base is used to add a lemony flavor to many soups

and entrées. It is usually cut into strips when used in dishes, and it is fibrous in nature.

- **Lime:** known as makrut in Thai. Lime leaves or the juice of Kaffir limes are commonly used in soups, salads, and entrées.
- **Nam pla:** a fish sauce used like soy sauce in Thai cooking. This thin, salty, brown sauce brings out the flavor of other foods. It's high in sodium.
- **Nam prik:** also called Thai shrimp sauce, it is used to flavor many Thai foods. Nam prik is made from shrimp paste, chilies, lime juice, soy sauce, and sugar.
- **Napa cabbage:** also referred to as Chinese cabbage, it has thick-ribbed stalks and crinkled leaves.
- **Palm sugar:** a strong-flavored, dark sugar obtained from the sap of coconut palms. It is boiled down until it crystallizes.
- **Scallions:** also called spring onions, these are white, slender, and have long green stems. Usually, they are chopped into short or long pieces and stir-fried into dishes.
- **Soy sauce:** is used in many Thai dishes to add a salty flavor and is made from soybeans.
- **Tamarind:** an acidy-tasting fruit from a large tropical tree that is used for its tart flavor.
- **Turmeric:** the spice that lends the yellow-orange color to commercial curry. It is a member of the ginger family.

(i) What's Your Solution? Answers

a) Good choice. While preparation methods vary, the fresh spring rolls generally have half the calories and fat of the crab Rangoon, which is deep-fried and stuffed with cream cheese.

b) The kitchen will prepare your dish as ordered, so requesting less oil and soy sauce is a reasonable way to improve the nutritional quality of your dish. If you're watching your calories, skipping the peanuts can help a bit.

c) Yes, please! While a heavy dose of vegetables isn't common in pad thai, bok choy, broccoli, or any vegetable you like makes a nice addition.

d) When you are eating alone at home, it can be tough to find the willpower needed to keep from devouring the whole serving. Asking the restaurant to divide the meal for you makes it easier to just pop one container directly into the fridge to eat for dinner the next day. Postponing your TV watching until after your dinner, so you can focus on savoring the flavor of your food, can also help.

CHAPTER 23

Japanese

Years ago, Japanese restaurants were mainly located in communities heavily populated by people of Japanese descent. Not so today! Now there are more Japanese restaurants in America than ever before, particularly sushi-focused restaurants. You'll spot them in metropolitan areas, suburbs, airports, and food courts. Generally speaking, these are one- or maybe two-location restaurants. A few Japanese restaurant chains exist, but they're mainly Japanese steak houses, which are part food and part theatre.

Menu offerings in Japanese restaurants vary. Many traditional Japanese restaurants serve the whole gamut of Japanese favorites, from tempura, sukiyaki, and teriyaki to lesser-known cooking preparations or dishes, such as agemono (fried protein or vegetables without a batter), yosenabe (a hearty soup with noodles, a type of protein, and/or vegetables), and donburi (a rice bowl with a source of protein and/or vegetables). These restaurants may also pride themselves on a busy sushi bar that keeps the hands of multiple sushi chefs busy rolling up both familiar and exotic rolls.

With the increasing popularity of sushi, many Japanese restaurants stick solely to just that, serving sushi. And as sushi and sashimi become more popular—for health and nutrition reasons and because it can be eaten on the run—a few local chain sushi restaurants are cropping up in locations where you'd expect them to be. Sugarfish, for example, has a handful of locations in the Los Angeles area, whereas Haru Sushi can be found in several locations in Manhattan and Boston.

Another category of Japanese restaurants popular with younger diners (kids) and families are Japanese steak houses. These restaurants shine the spotlight on chefs who turn meal preparation into a tableside acrobatic performance and turn out tempting chicken, shrimp, or beef teriyaki complemented with rice and vegetables. Most of these restaurants are independently owned, although Benihana is a national chain that you may see in your area.

Because Japanese foods and cuisine have become popular, you now often find Japanese foods and preparations integrated into the menus of Asian fusion restaurants and some family restaurants. You may find an increasing number of upscale restaurants incorporating traditional Japanese flavors into their modern fusion cuisine.

On the Menu

With Japanese restaurants of all types springing up, more Americans are eating Japanese food today. This is good news because Japanese food is both healthy and low in fat. This type of cuisine falls right in line with the *Dietary Guidelines for Americans;* it's heavy on vegetables, moderate on the starches, and light on proteins, and fats. The biggest thorns in the side of Japanese cuisine are its high sodium count and its deep-fried items—the best known being tempura, but there are others, like the less familiar agemono.

Japanese cuisine accentuates carbohydrate, in the form of rice, noodles, and vegetables, and minimizes added fats by using food preparation methods that require little or no oil or fat, such as steaming, braising, or simply serving food raw (sushi). Another big plus, especially in our world of big portions, is that small portion sizes are standard with Japanese fare.

The higher-than-desired sodium count in Japanese cuisine comes mainly from soy-based items. Marinades and sauces, whether for teriyaki, sukiyaki, or shabu-shabu, are generally made up of a combination of some or all of the following: shoyu, dashi, mirin, sugar, sake, and a bit of kombu. See *Menu Lingo* at the end of this chapter for more on these ingredients.

It's easy to control your fat gram count by selecting foods that are low in fat. For example, ordering fish, shellfish, or poultry rather than selecting beef or pork helps keep the fat down. When you see fats used in Japanese cooking, they're mainly the no-cholesterol varieties: cottonseed, olive, peanut, or sesame oil. Sesame oil is used in small quantity for its wonderful nutty flavor.

You'll also eat less fat if you order smaller portions. As with other Asian cuisines, it's easy to limit portions in Japanese restaurants by ordering and eating family style. Remember, when eating family style, order fewer dishes than there are mouths at the table.

As with Southeast Asian cuisines, it's typical to see sugar incorporated into many food preparations. Sugar is used in almost all the sauces and marinades. Sugar is also found in su (vinegared rice) used in sushi. Using sugar in the sushi rice gives it that sticky quality. In the end, most sauces and dishes will not provide you with more than a couple of teaspoons to a tablespoon of sugar. From a calorie standpoint that's minimal. But from a glucose-raising standpoint, it's worth noting due to the additional carbohydrate. If your glucose levels rise after eating your usual Japanese choices, you have one or two options. One is to carefully review what you order and make some changes that can reduce the sugar content. For starters, simply try eating less. Another tip: start your meal with a bowl of miso soup to fill up. Then up your vegetable count and lighten up on rice or noodles by making sure your sushi contains items like avocado and cucumber or by ordering noodle dishes that contain vegetables like broccoli, napa cabbage, and onions. If you take rapid-acting insulin based on your carbohydrate intake, you may have the option of taking a bit more insulin to cover the additional carbohydrate of your Japanese meal and/or changing the timing of your insulin. Refer to Chapter 8 (page 78) to learn more.

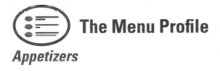 ## The Menu Profile

Appetizers

You'll find a number of healthy appetizers on Japanese menus. You can eat sushi and sashimi as an appetizer or make these items your entire meal. See page 479 to learn more about sushi. Beyond sushi there are many healthy appetizers. This is a rare delight since so many restaurants serve appetizers that are fried and high in fat. You'll find calorie and fat-wise appetizers that are barbecued, steamed, pickled, or served raw. Common hot appetizers are edamame (steamed soybeans in their shells that are lightly salted or glazed with a soy-based sauce), gyoza (small, crimped dumplings with protein-based or vegetarian fillings that are steamed or lightly fried), and shumai (small dumplings open at the top and filled with protein-based or vegetarian ingredients that are steamed or lightly fried) and the list of cold appetizers usually includes wakame (seaweed salad) and agedashi (fried tofu in a soy-based sauce).

Some appetizers are partnered with a dipping sauce. Often dipping sauces are high in sodium. Avoid the few fried items on the menu—tempura, agedashi, or agetofu (fried bean curd). The healthiest appetizers on the list are edamame, wakame, and steamed spinach.

Soups and Salads

Light and delicate broth-based soups are the mainstay soups in Japanese cuisine. You'll find miso soup on nearly every Japanese menu. It's mainly broth and bits of tofu and scallion (green onion). Or you'll see a simple, clear broth called sui-mono, which has a base of dashi and bits of vegetables or meat. Udon- or dashi-based noodle soups have a few more calories due to the noodles. Other varieties of udon have stir-fried beef, vegetables, or tempura items added. Stick with the broth-based noodle dishes su udon (thinner noodles) or yaki udon (thick noodles). Soup is a healthy and filling starter that allows you to put a dent in your appetite. Or you can order soup for a filling entrée, but slurp sparingly if sodium is a concern. Also, be aware of the portion size and carbohydrate load of the soup you choose. Order a small bowl if you can or be sure to split a large bowl.

You'll find salads in Japanese restaurants: either tossed greens, tofu, seaweed, or seafood salad. In Japan, salads are called sunomono or aemono. They consist of vinegared or otherwise dressed vegetables and seafood served in small quantities in elegant little bowls. The dressing is often a light miso dressing, which use a combination of the regular Japanese seasonings. This means the dressing is usually light in calories but contains sodium. The good news is that small salads equals minimal dressing.

Entrées

The majority of Japanese entrées are generally low in fat (and potentially low in saturated fat and cholesterol, if you choose wisely). Several styles of food preparation are usually stated on Japanese menus. You can have different proteins prepared in different fashions. For example, teriyaki is listed as a preparation method. You can order chicken, beef, or salmon prepared teriyaki style. The same goes for nabemonos: one-pot meals that are akin to a stew. Sukiyaki, yosenabi, and shabu-shabu all fall under the nabemonos category.

Donburi is a rice dish topped with broiled or fried protein, such as pork, fish, or poultry, with an egg on top and a soy-based sauce. Obviously, donburi is best topped with broiled items rather than the breaded and fried ones. Donburi, due to the whole eggs, might need to be avoided if you're watching your cholesterol count carefully. If you need to limit your cholesterol, simply request that the egg be left in the kitchen.

At teppanyaki-style restaurants (Japanese steak houses), like Benihana, the food is often plentiful. Stick with leaner sources of protein, like chicken or shrimp, and opt for steamed rice rather than fried rice. While portion sizes will be a challenge, the benefit of these restaurants is that you can see your meal being made, making it easy to voice any special requests directly to your acrobatic chef.

Sushi and Sashimi

Sushi and sashimi have a long heritage in Japanese dining. Many different fish, shellfish, eggs, and/or vegetables are used in their preparation. Interestingly, the preparation of sushi began centuries ago as a method of preserving fish. At that time, sushi was simply rice that had been vinegared (mixed with sugar and vinegar, likely for the purpose of preserving it) and served with a piece of dried fish. Later the thin piece of nori—the black seaweed that is used in sushi rolls today—was added to avoid getting one's fingers sticky from the rice.

You'll find sushi most commonly served in rolls, with pieces of fish served atop a bed of sushi rice (called nigiri), or in hand rolls, which contain fish or vegetables wrapped in su rice and nori. People who are unfamiliar with sushi often think that all sushi contains raw fish. A lot of sushi does, but this is not always the case. Raw tuna, salmon, yellowtail (tuna), and other fish are certainly popular choices. However, cooked fish, such as crab, shrimp, surimi (imitation crab), soft shell crab, eel, and others are commonly used. Sushi can also be enjoyed by vegetarians because it can be made without fish. Commonly used vegetables in vegetable sushi are cucumber and avocado. You can also hold the rice by opting for sashimi, which consists of bite-size pieces of raw fish served with soy sauce and wasabi paste but no rice.

The su rice used in sushi is flavored with vinegar, salt, and a bit of sugar, which lends to the sticky quality of the rice. The volume of rice used in sushi varies. A general observation is that the more expensive the sushi, the less rice is used. Expect to see more rice and less fish or other ingredients in all-you-can-eat sushi restaurants. To study this in restaurants you may frequent, use your eyes. You'll nearly always see sushi accompanied by wasabi and pickled ginger, which each provide a lot of flavor with almost no calories, fat, or sodium. Enjoy!

You can't go wrong, healthwise, with sushi and sashimi. But do watch out for some of the newfangled Americanized types of sushi, such as the Philadelphia roll, which uses cream cheese, and tempura rolls that use tempura-fried seafood or vegetables. A few bites if sharing is fine, but avoid ordering and eating whole orders of these items. Also, be on the lookout for sushi preparers who use a lot of mayonnaise-based spicy and/or seasoned sauces. All in all, the small amount of fat from these preparations doesn't hold a candle to the amount of fat you can down from a hamburger and french fries meal. If you frequent certain sushi bars and notice a heavy hand with mayonnaise-based sauces, simply request they use them sparingly or leave them off entirely.

A final note about sushi: great importance is placed on the creativity with which it's prepared, as well as freshness of the fish. To help ensure that you have a safe food experience, choose a reputable restaurant that serves a lot of sushi. This means there will be a lot of fish sold and fresh fish coming in regularly. Keep an eye on the sushi chefs. Make sure they are working with clean hands. Also take a look at the fresh fish on display even before you order. If the raw fish doesn't smell or look fresh to you, don't eat it. See Chapter 17 (page 298) for more guidance about the safety of seafood.

Drinks

A drink unique to Japanese restaurants is sake. Sake is a fermented rice wine. It is typically served in very small decanters and then poured into very small cups. It is served hot or cold and is sipped. Sake's calories come mainly from alcohol and a few are contributed by carbohydrate. An ounce contains about 40 calories. If it's a drink you enjoy, go ahead and sip a cup. Beer, either Japanese beer or common American varieties, is also commonly poured in Japanese restaurants. Explore Chapter 9 (page 87) to learn more about non-alcoholic and alcoholic beverages.

Desserts

Dessert in Japan is typically very minimal and doesn't receive much attention. You'll see a short list of desserts in full-menu Japanese restaurants: fresh fruit, ice cream, and maybe yo kan (a sweet bean cake). Obviously, fresh fruit is the way to go from a health standpoint.

Nutrition Snapshot

Health Busters

Category	Restaurant Name	Dish Name	Serving Size	Cal.	Total Fat (g)	Carb. (g)	Sod. (mg)
Appetizers	T.G.I. Friday's	Tapa-Tizer Skewers—Grilled Chicken	1 portion	750	20	105	3110
Appetizers	Tokyo Joe's	Yakitori Bowl	1 portion	678	17	88	1167
Appetizers	T.G.I. Friday's	Tapa-Tizer Skewers—Black Angus Sirloin	1 portion	620	18	73	1700
Appetizers	Sansai Japanese Grill	Tempura Plate	1 portion	972	97	8.5	85
Salads	Yard House	Ahi Crunchy w/ Soy Vinagrette	1 salad	693	39	47	1472
Salads	Pei Wei Asian Diner	Spicy Chicken (without dressing)	1 salad	520	22	58	1210
Salads	Pei Wei Asian Diner	Spicy Shrimp	1 salad	510	26	61	1120
Tempura	Elephant Bar	Salmon Roll	1 roll	710	27	100	1410
Tempura	Sansai Japanese Grill	Shrimp and Veggie	1 portion	686	71	6	52
Tempura	Sansai Japanese Grill	Kid's Plate	1 portion	682	68	6	52

(table continues on next page)

Health Busters

Category	Restaurant Name	Dish Name	Serving Size	Cal.	Total Fat (g)	Carb. (g)	Sod. (mg)
Tempura	Sansai Japanese Grill	Plate	1 portion	972	97	9	85
Sushi	Kona Grill	Sushi Sampler	1 portion	720	32	79	2010
Sushi	Kona Grill	Volcano Roll	1 roll	660	50	35	1720
Sushi	Yard House	Spicy Tuna Roll	1 roll	577	34	25	1433
Sushi	Kona Grill	Dragon Roll	1 roll	520	13	78	1760
Sashimi	Yard House	Seared Ahi	1 portion	436	28	16	912
Sashimi	Kona Grill	Freshwater Eel	1 portion	390	19	23	580
Entrées	Pei Wei Asian Diner	Chicken—Teriyaki (dinner portion, no side)	1 portion	490	13	67	1980
Entrées	Pei Wei Asian Diner	Vegetables & Tofu Japanese Teriyaki Bowl w/ White Rice	1 portion	560	13	95	1620
Entrées	Elephant Bar	Grilled Teriyaki Chicken Rice Bowl (brown rice)	1 portion	830	25	99	1570
Entrées	T.G.I. Friday's	Japanese Hibachi Entrée— Black Angus Sirloin	1 portion	1390	53	186	3840
Desserts	Nothing but Noodles	New York Cheesecake	1 piece	770	53	59	0

Healthier Bets

Category	Restaurant Name	Dish Name	Serving Size	Cal.	Total Fat (g)	Sat. Fat (g)	Carb. (g)	Pro. (g)	Fiber (g)	Chol. (mg)	Sodium (mg)	Exchanges/ Choices
Appetizers	Pei Wei Asian Diner	Edamame	1 portion	160	7	1.5	9	15	9	0	490	1/2 Starch, 2 Lean Protein, 1/2 Fat
Appetizers	Tokyo Joe's	Edamame	1 portion	147	5	0	16	12	12	n/a	400	1 Starch, 1 1/2 Lean Protein
Appetizers	Tokyo Joe's	Tataki-Seared Ahi Tuna	1 portion	73	0	0	9	7	1	n/a	28	1/2 Starch, 1 Lean Protein
Soups	Yoshinoya	Miso	1 bowl	60	1.5	0	8	3	0	0	380	1/2 Starch, 1/2 Fat
Soups	Kona Grill	Miso (bowl)	1 bowl	60	2	n/a	6	4	1	0	760	1/2 Starch, 1/2 Fat
Sushi	Kona Grill	Shrimp Tempura	1 full roll	290	8	n/a	49	7	2	25	610	3 Starch, 1 Medium-Fat Protein

(table continues on next page)

Healthier Bets

Category	Restaurant Name	Dish Name	Serving Size	Cal.	Total Fat (g)	Sat. Fat (g)	Carb. (g)	Pro. (g)	Fiber (g)	Chol. (mg)	Sodium (mg)	Exchanges/ Choices
Sushi	Hissho Sushi	Tempura Shrimp	1 full roll	256	1	0	54	5	2	19	507	3 Starch, 1/2 Lean Protein
Sushi	Tokyo Joe's	Spicy Tuna	1 full roll	192	7	1	24	7	1.4	n/a	138	1 1/2 Starch, 1/2 Medium-Fat Protein, 1 Fat
Sushi	Sansai Japanese Grill	Spicy Tuna	1 full roll	166	3	0.5	24	12	1	19	341	1 1/2 Starch, 1 Lean Protein
Sushi	Kona Grill	Tuna	1 full roll	160	0	n/a	26	12	0	15	370	1 1/2 Starch, 1 Lean Protein
Sashimi	Kona Grill	Tuna	1 portion	150	0.5	n/a	18	20	0	30	110	1 Starch, 2 Lean Protein
Sashimi	Kona Grill	Octopus	1 portion	120	1	n/a	18	11	0	30	80	1 Starch, 1 Lean Protein

(table continues on next page)

Healthier Bets

Category	Restaurant Name	Dish Name	Serving Size	Cal.	Total Fat (g)	Sat. Fat (g)	Carb. (g)	Pro. (g)	Fiber (g)	Chol. (mg)	Sodium (mg)	Exchanges/ Choices
Sashimi	Sansai Japanese Grill	Seared Ahi Tuna	1 portion	148	1	0	6	30	2	51	78	4 Lean Protein
Sashimi	Kona Grill	Mackerel	1 portion	150	10	n/a	1	13	0	50	70	2 Medium-Fat Protein
Salads	Sansai Japanese Grill	Sumi	1 salad	164	11	1	11	7	7	0	92	2 Vegetable, 1 Medium-Fat Protein, 1 Fat
Salads	Hissho Sushi	Octopus	1 salad	148	2	0	13	16	1	0	882	3 Vegetable, 1 1/2 Lean Protein
Salads	Zen Japanese Fast Food	Tataki & Water-cress	1 salad	250	12	1.5	13	23	3	35	620	3 Vegetable, 2 1/2 Medium-Fat Protein

(table continues on next page)

Healthier Bets

Category	Restaurant Name	Dish Name	Serving Size	Cal.	Total Fat (g)	Sat. Fat (g)	Carb. (g)	Pro. (g)	Fiber (g)	Chol. (mg)	Sodium (mg)	Exchanges/ Choices
Entrées, Teriyaki	Rice King	Char-broiled Chicken	1 portion	234	10	2	8	28		45	710	1/2 Starch, 4 Lean Protein
Entrées, Teriyaki	Teriyaki Experience	Vegetable	1 portion	318	1	0	68	8	3	0	21	4 Starch
Entrées, Teriyaki	Teriyaki Experience	Shrimp	1 portion	432	3	0.6	71	28	3	151	308	4 1/2 Starch, 2 Lean Protein
Entrées, Teriyaki	Teriyaki Experience	Chicken	1 portion	537	4	1	75	47	4	99	456	4 1/2 Starch, 4 Lean Protein
Entrées, Teriyaki	Tokyo Joe's	Kid's Noodles & Teriyaki	1 portion	520	4	0	100	20	7	n/a	966	6 1/2 Starch

✅ Green-Flag Words

Ingredients:

- ► Avocado
- ► Chicken
- ► Clear broth
- ► Cucumber
- ► Dipping sauce (high in sodium)
- ► Miso dressing (high in sodium)
- ► Pickled ginger
- ► Seafood—raw and cooked, fish and shellfish
- ► Soy sauce (high in sodium)
- ► Soybeans (edamame)
- ► Spinach
- ► Teriyaki sauce (high in sodium)
- ► Tofu
- ► Udon, rice or bean thread noodles
- ► Vinegar sauce (salt and sugar added)
- ► Vinegared, seasoned, or su rice (vinegar, salt, and sugar added)
- ► Wasabi

Cooking Methods/Menu Descriptions:

- ► Barbecued
- ► Boiled
- ► Braised
- ► Marinated
- ► Mushimono (steamed)
- ► Nabemono (one-pot meal; high in sodium)
- ► Nimono (simmered)
- ► On skewers
- ► Pickled
- ► Raw
- ► Salads
- ► Sautéed
- ► Served in broth (high in sodium)
- ► Served with vegetables

- ▶ Yaki (broiled)
- ▶ Yakimono (grilled)

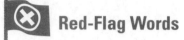 **Red-Flag Words**

Ingredients:

- ▶ Cream cheese (used in sushi such as Philadelphia rolls)
- ▶ Fried bean curd
- ▶ Mayonnaise-based sauces

Cooking Methods/Menu Descriptions:

- ▶ Agemono (deep-fried)
- ▶ Battered and fried, breaded and fried
- ▶ Katsu (fried)
- ▶ Pan-fried
- ▶ Tempura

At the Table:

- ▶ Soy sauce (high in sodium)

Healthy Eating Tips and Tactics

- ▶ Start your meal with filling, low-calorie appetizers, such as edamame or miso soup.
- ▶ Avoid the tempura dishes. There are many flavorful, low-fat options on the menu. Take advantage!
- ▶ The fancier the roll, the more calories it generally has. For example, a tempura roll or dragon roll is likely in the 500-calorie range. A simpler tuna roll or California roll will have 150–250 calories.
- ▶ Remember that rice acts like a sponge for high-sodium soy sauce. Dip and drizzle sparingly.
- ▶ Choose your own dishes, rather than ordering omakase—a method of dining in which the chef chooses your foods for you. While Japanese chefs will generally keep things light and healthy, you will better meet your health goals if you remain in the driver's seat.

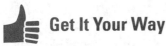

Get It Your Way

▶ Let the server know if you are carefully watching your sodium intake. Ask that less soy sauce be used in preparing a high-sodium dish, such as a teriyaki, and that no salt or soy sauce be added to your edamame or steamed spinach.

▶ Ask that the mayonnaise-based sauce be left off the sushi to lighten up on fat grams.

▶ Substitute leaner proteins, such as shrimp, scallops, or chicken, for the beef in a dish.

▶ If you're watching your cholesterol, request that egg be left out of the *donburi* (or other egg-containing dishes).

▶ Request dressing on the side of your salad.

Tips and Tactics for Gluten-Free Eating

▶ Soy, tamari, teriyaki, hoisin, plum, and Japanese barbeque sauces are used in the majority of Japanese dishes and typically contain gluten.

▶ Most tempura-based dishes, mock duck/seitan, imitation meats, fish-cakes, and miso contain gluten.

▶ Most sushi and sashimi are naturally gluten-free, except for unagi, which is cooked eel marinated in soy sauce

▶ Try rice, rice noodles, or soba noodles that are 100% buckwheat (ask to check the label to make sure soba noodles are 100% gluten-free), or spring roll wrappers made from only rice with gluten-free fillings.

▶ Edamame prepared without soy sauce; steamed, stir fried, or grilled meat, poultry, seafood; and vegetables can all be safe choices if they are prepared in a clean wok or on a clean cooking surface.

Tips and Tactics to Help Kids Eat Healthy

▶ Sushi can be very foreign to kids. If it's new to your child, start with sushi that contains more familiar ingredients, such as a cucumber roll or avocado roll. Remember, kids like to dip and that's what sushi is all about.

- Demystify sushi and offer your child cheap entertainment by grabbing a seat at the sushi bar to watch sushi being prepared. Young kids may also like to watch fish in the fish tank of some Japanese restaurants.
- Nabemonos, the one-pot meals, are kid-friendly dishes that are generally low fat. Just be prepared for your child to do some serious slurping!
- Opt for cooked seafood, not raw, for kids under the age of 5 years. Young children are particularly susceptible to food-borne illnesses.

(?) What's Your Solution?

Your boss is taking you out to a nice sushi restaurant to thank you for a job well done. Your boss has a large appetite, is a bit of a sushi aficionado, and wants to handle the ordering, so you know there will be more than enough food on the table. Two of the healthy eating strategies you have been working on to get your diabetes under better control are managing portion sizes and limiting sodium. Could be a challenging meal!

How can you enjoy your meal without sabotaging your goals or offending your boss?

a) Fill up on the bowl of miso soup your boss ordered to start your sushi feast.

b) Ask for low-sodium soy sauce and limit the amount you use as a dip.

c) Employ chopsticks to help you eat slowly.

d) Let your boss know about one or two of the healthier side items you enjoy with sushi, such as wakame salad or edamame, both of which are vegetable-based, filling, low-calorie options.

See page 499 for answers.

Menu Samplers

Light 'N' Healthy

Menu Samplers Section	Menu Item	Amount	Calories	Fat (g)	% Calories from Fat	Saturated Fat (g)	Chol. (mg)	Sodium (mg)	Carb. (g)	Fiber (g)	Protein (g)	Exchanges/ Choices
Light 'N' Healthy (Women)	Miso soup	1 cup	40	1		0	0	650	5	1	2	1/2 Other Carbohydrate
	California sushi roll	2 pieces	130	5		1	3	270	19	3	3	1 Starch, 1 Vegetable, 1 Fat
	Sushi nigiri (salmon)	2 pieces	134	4		1	16	193	17	1	7	1 Starch, 1 Lean Protein
	Cucumber roll	2 pieces	45	0		0	0	99	10	1	1	1 Starch

(table continues on next page)

Light 'N' Healthy

Menu Samplers Section	Menu Item	Amount	Calories	Fat (g)	% Calories from Fat	Saturated Fat (g)	Chol. (mg)	Sodium (mg)	Carb. (g)	Fiber (g)	Protein (g)	Exchanges/Choices
	Tuna roll	2 pieces	59	1		0	6	104	10	1	4	1/2 Starch, 1/2 Medium-Fat Protein
Totals			408	11	24	2	25	1316	61	7	17	3 1/2 Starch, 1/2 Other Carbohydrate, 1 Vegetable, 1 1/2 Medium-Fat Protein, 1 Fat
Light 'N' Healthy (Men)	Miso soup	1 cup	40	1		0	0	650	5	1	2	1/2 Other Carbohydrate
	Wakame (seaweed salad)	1/2 cup	45	0.5		0	0	650	9	0.5	3	2 Vegetable

(table continues on next page)

Light 'N' Healthy

Menu Samplers Section

Menu Item	Amount	Calories	Fat (g)	% Calories from Fat	Saturated Fat (g)	Chol. (mg)	Sodium (mg)	Carb. (g)	Fiber (g)	Protein (g)	Exchanges/Choices
Soba noodles with hibachi sauce	2 cups	226	1		0	0	500	49	3	12	2 Starch, 1/2 Other Carbohydrate, 2 Lean Protein
Tempura vegetables	2 pieces of eggplant	94	5		1	19	9	11	4	2	1/2 Starch, 1 Vegetable, 1 Fat
Hibachi steak	4 oz cooked	219	9		4	62	65	0	0	31	4 1/2 Lean Protein
Totals		**624**	**17**	**25**	**5**	**81**	**1874**	**74**	**8.5**	**50**	**2 1/2 Starch, 1 Other Carbohydrate, 3 Vegetable, 6 1/2 Lean Protein, 1 Fat**

(table continues on next page)

Hearty 'N' Healthy

Menu Samplers Section	Menu Item	Amount	Calories	Fat (g)	% Calories from Fat	Saturated Fat (g)	Chol. (mg)	Sodium (mg)	Carb. (g)	Fiber (g)	Protein (g)	Exchanges/ Choices
Hearty 'N' Healthy (Women)	Dashi stock soup	1 cup	3	0		0	0	134	1	0	0	Free Food
	Edamame	1/2 cup, shelled	188	9		1	0	19	14	5	17	3 Vegetable, 2 1/2 Lean Protein
	Hibachi chicken with mushrooms, Chinese cabbage, and eggplant	1 cup of entrée	212	7		1.5	73	664	8	0	27	1 Vegetable, 4 Lean Protein
	Brown rice	1 cup	218	2		0	0	2	46	4	5	3 Starch
Totals			**621**	**18**	**26**	**2.5**	**73**	**819**	**69**	**9**	**49**	**3 Starch, 4 Vegetable, 6 1/2 Lean Protein**

(table continues on next page)

Hearty 'N' Healthy

Menu Samplers Section	Menu Item	Amount	Calories	Fat (g)	% Calories from Fat	Saturated Fat (g)	Chol. (mg)	Sodium (mg)	Carb. (g)	Fiber (g)	Protein (g)	Exchanges/ Choices
Hearty 'N' Healthy (Men)	Edamame	1/2 cup, shelled	188	9		1	0	19	14	5	17	3 Vegetable, 2 1/2 Lean Protein
	Sukiyaki beef with peppers and cabbage	2 cups	460	14		4	50	1000	64	3	20	3 Starch, 1/2 Other Carbohydrate, 2 Vegetable, 3 Medium-Fat Protein, 1 Fat
	Brown rice	1/2 cup	109	0		0	0	1	23	2	2	1 1/2 Starch
Totals			**757**	**23**	**27**	**5**	**50**	**1020**	**101**	**10**	**39**	**4 1/2 Starch, 1/2 Other Carbohydrate, 5 Vegetable, 5 1/2 Medium-Fat Protein, 1 Fat**

(table continues on next page)

Lower Carb 'N' Healthy

Menu Samplers Section	Menu Item	Amount	Calories	Fat (g)	% Calories from Fat	Saturated Fat (g)	Chol. (mg)	Sodium (mg)	Carb. (g)	Fiber (g)	Protein (g)	Exchanges/ Choices
Lower Carb 'N' Healthy (Women)	Wakame (sea-weed salad)	1/2 cup	45	0.5		0	0	650	9	0.5	3	2 Vegetable
	Caterpillar roll sushi (crab, cucumber, avocado, rice, and nori)	8 pieces	329	5		1	23	530	60	3	9	3 1/2 Starch, 1 Vegetable, 1 Lean Protein
	Tuna sashimi	4 pieces	122	1		0	51	42	0	0	26	4 Lean Protein
Totals			**496**	**7**	**13**	**1**	**74**	**1222**	**69**	**4**	**38**	**3 1/2 Starch, 3 Vegetable, 5 Lean Protein**

(table continues on next page)

Lower Carb 'N' Healthy

Menu Samplers Section	Menu Item	Amount	Calories	Fat (g)	% Calories from Fat	Saturated Fat (g)	Chol. (mg)	Sodium (mg)	Carb. (g)	Fiber (g)	Protein (g)	Exchanges/ Choices
Lower Carb 'N' Healthy (Men)	Gyoza (pan-fried dumplings filled with beef)	3 dumplings	171	8		2	8	350	21	2	6	1 1/2 Starch, 2 Fat
	Japanese grilled vegetables with rice	1 3/4 cups	252	1		0	0	450	54	3	7	3 Starch, 2 Vegetable
	Teriyaki salmon	5 oz fillet	233	6		1	83	1000	11	0	34	1 Other Carbohydrate, 5 Lean Protein
Totals			656	15	21	3	91	1800	86	5	47	4 1/2 Starch, 1 Other Carbohydrate, 2 Vegetable, 5 Lean Protein, 2 Fat

Menu Lingo

▶ **Bonito:** a fish important in Japanese cuisine, it is a member of the mackerel family. Bonito flakes are an important ingredient in the basic Japanese stock (broth) called dashi.

▶ **Daikon:** a giant white radish. Grated daikon is mixed into tempura sauces and sliced daikon can be used in sushi.

▶ **Dashi:** an important element in Japanese cooking, dashi is a basic stock made with water, kombu (seaweed), and bonito flakes.

▶ **Edamame:** steamed or boiled soybeans served warmed and salted.

▶ **Gyuniku:** the Japanese word for beef.

▶ **Kombu:** a Japanese seaweed that is a central ingredient in the basic stock (broth) dashi. Kombu is also used in sauces and as a wrapper for certain dishes.

▶ **Mirin:** Japanese rice wine, which is used more in sauces than consumed as a beverage. It is a central ingredient in the sauces and flavors of Japanese cuisine.

▶ **Miso:** a fermented soybean paste that comes in various types, thicknesses, and degrees of saltiness. It is used in soups, sauces, and dressings; it's a basic ingredient in Japanese cooking.

▶ **Nori:** a seaweed often toasted prior to being used in dishes. It has a strong flavor and is used to wrap sushi (both rolls and hand rolls).

▶ **Sake:** fermented rice wine. Sake is the national alcoholic beverage of Japan and is most often served warm. It is also used as an ingredient in sauces.

▶ **Shiitake:** an abundant mushroom variety in Japanese cookery. It has a woody and fruity flavor and is used fresh or dried.

▶ **Shoyu:** Japanese soy sauce with both light and dark varieties. It is made from soybeans, wheat, and salt and is an essential ingredient in Japanese cooking.

▶ **Teriyaki:** a sauce used when broiling foods. It is made from shoyu and mirin. Teriyaki means "shining broil."

▶ **Tofu (soybean curd):** a major source of protein in the Japanese diet; it is used in soups, appetizers, salads, and entrées.

▶ **Ton:** the Japanese word for pork.

▶ **Tori:** the Japanese word for chicken.

▶ **Vinegar:** in Japan, it is made from rice and it's lighter and sweeter than the vinegar Americans are used to.

▶ **Wakame:** a seaweed used for its flavor and texture. It's available dried.

▶ **Wasabi:** also called Japanese horseradish, it is fragrant and sharp in taste; regularly served with sushi and sashimi.

ⓘ **What's Your Solution? Answers**

a) Soup is often a great way to start a meal, as it can be filling. Miso soup works well because it's mainly broth with bits of tofu. If there's an option on sizes, go with the small.

b) Smart move. Rice can quickly soak up soy sauce, which is high in sodium. Ask for low-sodium soy sauce to immediately cut back on the sodium, but know that it's still not really that low in sodium. Measure a small amount of low-sodium soy sauce into your dipping bowl and dip lightly to restrict your use to the amount poured—no refills.

c) Eating slowly is one of the best ways to implement portion control, especially if the dining partner(s) you are sharing your meal with are eating faster than you. Chopsticks can help slow down your eating, especially if you aren't adept with them.

d) This is a great way to share your excitement about Japanese food with your boss, while subtly requesting a few healthier options.

CHAPTER 24

Indian

The influx of people from India to the United States has increased greatly over the last several decades. According to 2010 census data, Asian Indians, also referred to as Indian Americans, are now the second-largest Asian population in the U.S., after Chinese Americans. As is common with the immigration of a population, their foods, preparation methods, and ways of serving meals, come along too. People from India have opened restaurants and today, it is quite common to find Indian restaurants among your choices when you decide to dine ethnic.

Restaurants serving Indian food are generally found in metropolitan areas. They're commonly located where there is a population or community of Asian Indian people, such as in areas of New York, New Jersey, California, and other areas between the coasts. Most Indian restaurants are sit-down establishments; a single owner might own just one or a few restaurants in the same general area or city. A few fast casual Indian restaurants are also beginning to crop up in major cities. Menus in these restaurants typically feature sandwiches, wraps, or create-your-own bowls in which you pick a base (rice, salad, bread), a protein, and various toppings and chutneys.

On the Menu

One simply has to glance at India's location on a world map for clues about the tastes and flavors the cuisine will yield. Though Indian cuisine boasts many unique qualities and dishes, it closely resembles the cuisines of its neighbors—Pakistan, Sri Lanka, Thailand, and Burma. There are also a few similarities with the foods and tastes of China, which is geographically a bit further off. However, Indian food is most similar to that of Thailand in terms of the spices and ingredients used. The dishes of both countries can be hot and spicy and are often accompanied by rice (though flavorful steamed white basmati rice is most common in Indian restaurants). Plus, curry dishes are popular in both Thai and Indian cooking.

India is one of the world's largest countries. Regional cuisines have developed because of the vast size of the country and because different areas grow and produce different foods and ingredients. Northern Indian dishes tend to be cooler to the taste buds than southern cuisine, which makes use of chilies and peppers. The North uses more wheat products, teas, and eggs, whereas the South features more rice, vegetables, and coffee. More seafood is eaten in the South, which abuts the sea, as well as hot pickles and chutneys. Yogurt (plain) is a common ingredient used in both northern and southern Indian cooking. The food served in Indian restaurants in America bends toward northern Indian cuisine.

As with most ethnic cuisines, there are pros and cons to Indian cooking when it comes to health. The pros include smaller portion sizes, the focus on starches and vegetables, the de-emphasis of proteins, and the heavy use of spices and seasonings that can add flavor without adding fat.

Basmati rice, the premier flavorful rice, is a main element of Indian cuisine. Breads are also considered an important and regular element of the meal. (Do watch out for the fried varieties of bread, like paratha and poori.) Legumes, including lentils and chickpeas, are often found in Indian dishes and their accompaniments. Legumes are healthy for a variety of reasons, including the fact that they're a good source of several types of fiber and non-animal protein. Vegetables are easily incorporated into most Indian dishes: curry dishes, biryani (a rice dish), and pulao (basmati rice with bits of saffron, which give the rice a yellow hue, that is served with entrées). Commonly served Indian vegetables include eggplant, cabbage, potatoes, and peas. Onions, green peppers, and tomatoes are often found in the stewed entrées. Plain yogurt is frequently used in sauces.

Another positive aspect of Indian cuisine is the wide availability of chicken and seafood. Beef and lamb are commonly found on the menu too, but can easily be limited. Pork and pork products are rarely found on Indian menus. Generally, only small quantities of protein are used in Indian dishes. If two people share a chicken or shrimp masala, one won't eat much more than 2–3 ounces of protein—just the right amount. It's also easy to eat vegetarian if you desire. It is a great idea to order one chicken or seafood dish and one vegetable dish to split and share, maybe a biryani or aloo chole, a mixture of potatoes and chickpeas, to keep the portions and thus calories, protein, and fat low.

Spices are used heavily in Indian cooking. A garam masala, a fragrant mix of ground spices, produces many of the wonderful tastes of Indian cuisine. Some spices frequently found in the garam masala are cardamom, coriander, cumin, cloves, and cinnamon—the "C" spices. Several of these spices are referred to as "fragrant" spices. In the southern regions, you might find peppers and chilies added to raise the "heat" of the mixture. Mint, garlic, ginger, yogurt (plain), and coconut milk are other common ingredients in Indian cooking. Find more of these spices and ingredients defined in the *Menu Lingo* section at the end of this chapter (page 515).

The negative health and nutrition aspect of Indian cuisine can be the high fat content of many dishes. Fat finds its way into Indian foods by way of preparation. Ghee, defined as clarified butter, is a common ingredient used in food preparation. It's a hidden item that makes small amounts of Indian food seem quite filling. Frying and sautéing are common preparation methods in Indian kitchens. For example, most appetizers, such as samosa and pakora, are fried. Some breads, such as paratha and poori, are deep fried, and others are brushed with oil or butter.

The oils most frequently used in Indian cooking are sesame and coconut oil. Sesame oil is mainly a polyunsaturated fat. However, coconut oil contains some saturated fat. You might want to ask about the type of oil in use at the Indian restaurant your visit, and if it is coconut oil, it's particularly wise to limit fried food there. This will help you reduce calories as well as saturated fat. In fact, avoiding fried foods is good idea, regardless of the type of oil used. Coconut milk is also widely used in Indian cooking, especially in soups and curry dishes. This ingredient, too, contributes calories, fat, and saturated fat. Look for the words coconut milk, coconut cream, or simply shredded coconut in the descriptions of menu items and try to limit these.

The sodium content of an Indian meal can be kept within bounds by navigating around the menu carefully. It is best to avoid the soups, which tend to be high in sodium. Many dishes have small amounts of added salt, but if the dish you choose is divided into a number of servings and you keep the portions small, you will consume a minimal quantity.

The Menu Profile

Appetizers

A healthy appetizer is a rarity in Indian restaurants. Most appetizer options are deep-fried: samosas, a turnover stuffed with peas and potatoes, then fried; cheese, chicken, or vegetable pakoras, all fried; and fried shrimp with poori (a deep-fried bread). You may find a nonfried option, such as a chicken tikka kebab, which is healthier. If you have calories to spare, sample one appetizer. Share it with your dining partner. If you're with a group and you order several appetizers or a combination plate (pu pu platter, Indian style), decide what's healthiest and take one piece or half pieces of two different appetizers.

Ordering bread can present difficulties, but there are a few healthy choices available. Or you can just skip it. There are plenty of other interesting foods to try. Papadum, also seen abbreviated as "papad," is a crisp, baked lentil wafer, which is fairly low in fat. It is, however, spicy. Chapati is a flat disk of unleavened bread resembling pita bread. It may even be made with whole-wheat flour. Naan is leavened bread made with white flour, and it is available plain, seasoned with garlic, or stuffed with cheese or meat. Stick with the plain or garlic varieties. Three more options are kulcha, a baked bread stuffed with vegetables, such as onions, or fruit and nuts; roti, a bread made with whole-wheat flour and baked; and paratha, a multilayered unleavened bread (which also may be whole wheat). Request that they not top the bread with clarified butter (aka ghee). Poori, a light, puffed fried bread should be left alone for obvious reasons.

Soups

Two healthier soups that make nice starters or entrées (when paired with a healthier bread or side item) are mulligatawny and lentil soup. They both combine very healthy legumes and are seasoned with Indian spices, which make them low in fat and calories. Creamy soups such as poppy seed and coconut should be avoided.

Entrées

You'll find similar cooking styles used for chicken, fish, shrimp, beef, and lamb dishes. To keep total fat, saturated fat, and calories on the decline, stick with fish, chicken, or shrimp. Try these healthy cooking preparations: masala, cooked with a combination of Indian spices, sautéed tomatoes, and onions; bhuna, another dish similar to masala; jalpharezi, cooked with vegetables and hot peppers; saag, cooked with spinach and spices; matar, cooked with green peas; and vindaloo, cooked with a mixture of Indian spices with potatoes. Preparations done in a clay oven, called a tandoor, are known as tandoori and tikka; they are healthy preparations, too. Steer away from the murg makhani (butter chicken), malai, and korma dishes, which are creamy and, therefore, higher in calories and fat.

In most restaurants you'll get plain pulao (basmati rice touched with saffron) with your entrée without asking. If you want more rice or want to order a different type of rice dish, there's an entrée called biryani that is an option (but your waitperson will probably still bring the plain rice for protein-focused main dishes). Biryani works well as an entrée if you're trying to eat more carbohydrate and less protein. It is made with chicken, lamb, beef, shrimp, or just vegetables (though there aren't that many vegetables to speak of in this dish). A chicken masala, for instance, nicely complements a shrimp biryani. Pairing these two dishes can help you keep the protein and fat content of your meal down. But this still won't give you enough vegetables. Don't forget to ask them not to bring the pulao (rice for entrées), unless you're with a crowd. Or, have them bring it ready to take home if you can. Having both the pulao and the biryani will be too much rice (carbohydrate).

Vegetable dishes can easily be a main course. From a nutrition standpoint, this is a great option as long as you steer clear of fried items. Vegetable dishes in Indian cuisine use a variety of legumes and vegetables, including chickpeas, lentils, potatoes, spinach, cauliflower, onions, peppers, and/or tomatoes. Often these vegetables are in curry or cheese (paneer) sauces. Paneer, which is called "cheese" in Indian cookery, is not like cheese in America. Paneer is made from milk and lemon juice. The milk is curdled by the lemon juice to create a thick cheese-like mixture, which is then formed into small cubes. Go ahead and enjoy paneer in small amounts, but watch your portion size as it does contain a small amount of saturated fat.

Accompaniments

A fun and unique aspect of Indian cuisine is the array of accompaniments. Several usually come with the meal in small amounts and others can be ordered as small side dishes. Raita, a combination of plain yogurt, cucumbers, and onions (though it can have tomatoes or fruit added in), is quite healthy. Its role is actually to cool the mouth after eating hot curry. Use it as a side dish or a dip for bread or appetizers rather than using sweet mango chutney, which you should avoid—it's pure, concentrated carbohydrate. Dahl is a low-fat, spicy, lentil-based side sauce that is served warm. Onion chutney, sometimes called relish, might arrive without request. It is quite low in calories and adds zip to Indian foods. Three other sauces you'll regularly see on the table in Indian restaurants are tamarind, cilantro chile (green sauce), and lemon rind with peppers. The cilantro-chile sauce traditionally doesn't have sugar added, but some restaurants add a bit. The tamarind and lemon chutneys are often quite high in sugar, as is the popular mango chutney, which usually can be ordered as a side item. Limit your use of these higher-sugar accompaniments by eating them in very small quantities and opting instead for the chile or onion chutneys. If in doubt about whether or not your favorite accompaniment contains hidden sugar, ask your server.

Desserts

There are more dessert options at Indian restaurants than you'll typically find at other Asian restaurants. Many are deep-fried. It's best to say no to these options. Rice puddings are also popular at Indian restaurants. These are typically made with whole milk, sugar, nuts, often some fruit, and, of course, rice. A bite or two should be plenty to satisfy your sweet tooth and curiosity if you must indulge. Other small dessert bites are sadesh, made with cottage cheese, cardamom, and saffron, and modak, a sweet flour dumpling that is stuffed with coconut, nutmeg, and saffron, and then steamed. The benefit of these desserts is that they are usually each just a bite or two, but they are certainly carbohydrate dense.

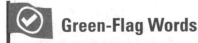 **Green-Flag Words**

Ingredients:

- ► Baked, leavened bread made with whole-wheat flour
- ► Basmati rice (pulao)

- ▶ Dried fruit
- ▶ Ginger and garlic
- ▶ Indian spices and spice combinations (curry, garam masala, saffron)
- ▶ Lentils, chickpeas, and peas (matta)
- ▶ Nuts
- ▶ Papadum
- ▶ Potatoes
- ▶ Saag
- ▶ Shrimp and other seafood—not fried
- ▶ Skinless chicken
- ▶ Vegetables (tomatoes, onions, spinach, and potatoes)

Cooking Methods/Menu Descriptions:

- ▶ Chutneys (mint, onion, chile)
- ▶ Cooked with onions, tomatoes, spinach, peppers, potatoes, or peas
- ▶ Cooked with or marinated in yogurt
- ▶ Dahl (lentils)
- ▶ Garnished with dried fruits
- ▶ Indian hot spices
- ▶ Kebab
- ▶ Marinated or cooked in Indian spices
- ▶ Masala
- ▶ Paneer (homemade cheese)
- ▶ Pickle
- ▶ Raita
- ▶ Tandoori
- ▶ Tikka

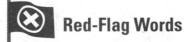 **Red-Flag Words**

Ingredients:

- ▶ Coconut milk
- ▶ Ghee (clarified butter)
- ▶ Molee (stew)

Cooking Methods/Menu Descriptions:

- ▶ Chutneys (mango, tamarind, lemon pepper; all are high in sugar)
- ▶ Creamy curry sauce
- ▶ Dipped in batter or chickpea batter
- ▶ Fried, deep-fried
- ▶ Fritters (particularly appetizers)
- ▶ Korma (cream sauce)
- ▶ Sautéed in butter, served in butter sauce
- ▶ Stuffed and fried

🍎 Healthy Eating Tips and Tactics

- ▶ Start off with a healthy and filling soup, such as lentil soup or mulligatawny.
- ▶ Enjoy small portions of rice. If you order a biryani, request that the plain pulao not be brought to the table.
- ▶ Fill up on the plethora of vegetables and vegetarian options available. Just be sure to choose vegetable dishes that aren't fried or cooked in a cream-based sauce.
- ▶ Opt for lean sources of protein, such as lentils, chickpeas, chicken, or seafood. Accompany them with flavorful sides like raita, dahl, and onion chutney.
- ▶ Skip traditional desserts. Opt for a cup of Darjeeling tea or perhaps even some mango slices if you see them being served.

👍 Get It Your Way

- ▶ Many dishes can be made with your choice of protein. If you see a dish you'd like to order, but it features a higher-fat meat, ask if it can be prepared with chicken instead or skip the protein altogether and go vegetarian.
- ▶ Request that no salt be added to your dish in the kitchen.
- ▶ Specify that you don't want any butter (ghee) added on top of your bread (kulcha, naan, or paratha).

▶ Ask that less paneer be used in vegetable dishes, such as saag paneer (spinach with fresh Indian cheese). This will give you more healthy greens with less fat.

Tips and Tactics for Gluten-Free Eating

▶ Authentic Indian restaurants offer a wide variety of naturally gluten-free dishes such as tandoori chicken, fish, and shrimp. Watch for skewered meats that may have been dusted in flour or marinades. Sauces made with maida flour or suji, and chutneys and curries may contain wheat. Other sauces may also contain wheat, so be sure to ask about the ingredients.

▶ The Indian breads chapatti, naan, roti, and poori all contain gluten.

▶ The appetizer samosas contain gluten.

▶ Most vegetable and lentil or bean side dishes are gluten-free. Coconut milk is gluten-free.

▶ Gluten-free starches include rice, potatoes, sweet potatoes, papadum (an Indian flatbread made from lentils), bhajis, and pakoras (made with 100% chickpea flour or garbanzo flour). Make sure they have a dedicated fryer for gluten-free grains and other fried gluten-free foods.

Tips and Tactics to Help Kids Eat Healthy

▶ Order à la carte to construct a meal that is kid-friendly both in flavor and portion size. Order several dishes, such as chicken tikka, saag paneer, and a masala dish, and eat them family style so that everyone can get a small taste of several items.

▶ Ask for mild preparation of dishes to share with your children.

▶ Take advantage of the plethora of vegetarian choices. Try matta paneer (peas with paneer) or dahl, both of which are popular choices among children.

▶ Help your child expand his or her repertoire of accepted foods and flavors by ordering a new-to-your-child dish. If it ends up being a flop, the pulao and bread will always be there to help satiate or you can order up a chicken tikka appetizer (aka Indian chicken fingers).

⑦ What's Your Solution?

You and your significant other are eating at your favorite Indian restaurant. You typically order among a few dishes that you are most familiar with: samosas, butter chicken, saag paneer, buttered naan, and of course, pulao (rice). As you strive to improve your eating out habits, you want to shake up your ordering routine at this Indian restaurant. But your significant other isn't so sure about or supportive of this concept.

What are a few changes you can make to improve the overall healthfulness of your meal that won't make your significant other feel like he or she is missing familiar great tastes or sufficient food to eat?

a) Cut down on fat by skipping the samosas in favor of a cup of lentil soup and ordering plain naan (instead of the buttered kind). If your spouse wants a samosa, ask if you can order just one. If not, take the second one home for him or her to eat later.

b) Opt for chicken masala instead of butter chicken to further cut down on fat.

c) Get your greens another way. Instead of saag paneer, try chaan saag, which is spinach with chickpeas. To up your servings of vegetables even more, take advantage of the offer to order a half or side serving of vegetables.

d) Share all the dishes with your significant other. Compensate for the decrease in food by adding a few healthy accompaniments, such as raita and onion chutney.

See page 516 for answers.

Menu Samplers

Light 'N' Healthy

Menu Samplers Section	Menu Item	Amount	Calories	Fat (g)	% Calories from Fat	Saturated Fat (g)	Chol. (mg)	Sodium (mg)	Carb. (g)	Fiber (g)	Protein (g)	Exchanges/ Choices
Light 'N' Healthy (Women)	Tandoori salmon	2 oz	180	11		1.5	40	160	8	1	13	1/2 Other Carbohydrate, 2 Medium-Fat Protein
	Palak paneer	1/2 cup	87	4		0	0	294	8	2	5	2 Vegetable, 1 Fat
	Madras curry asparagus	1 cup	120	8		0	0	525	9	4	4	2 Vegetable, 2 Fat
	Basmati rice	1/2 cup	170	1		0	0	200	38	0	4	2 1/2 Starch
Totals			557	24	39	1.5	40	1179	63	7	26	2 1/2 Starch, 1/2 Other Carbohydrate, 4 Vegetable, 2 Medium-Fat Protein, 3 Fat

(table continues on next page)

Light 'N' Healthy

Menu Samplers Section	Menu Item	Amount	Calories	Fat (g)	% Calories from Fat	Saturated Fat (g)	Chol. (mg)	Sodium (mg)	Carb. (g)	Fiber (g)	Protein (g)	Exchanges/ Choices
Light 'N' Healthy (Men)	Samosas	1 piece	308	18		4	9	600	32	2	5	2 Starch, 1/2 Medium-Fat Protein, 3 Fat
	Mixed curried vegetables	1/2 cup	124	5		0.5	0	198	17	2	2	1/2 Other Carbohydrate, 2 Vegetable, 1 Fat
	Chicken tikka masala	1 cup	291	10		1	100	400	4	1	42	1/2 Other Carbohydrate, 6 Lean Protein
	Basmati rice	1/2 cup	170	1		0	0	200	38	0	4	2 1/2 Starch
Totals			**893**	**34**	**34**	**5.5**	**109**	**1398**	**91**	**5**	**53**	**4 1/2 Starch, 1 Other Carbohydrate, 2 Vegetable, 6 1/2 Medium-Fat Protein, 3 Fat**

(table continues on next page)

Hearty 'N' Healthy

Menu Samplers Section	Menu Item	Amount	Calories	Fat (g)	% Calories from Fat	Saturated Fat (g)	Chol. (mg)	Sodium (mg)	Carb. (g)	Fiber (g)	Protein (g)	Exchanges/ Choices
Hearty 'N' Healthy (Women)	Naan (bread)	1/2 piece	86	2		0.5	2	194	14	1	2	1 Starch
	Vegetable korma	1 cup	188	4		0	0	420	33	2	5	1 1/2 Starch, 2 Vegetable, 1 Fat
	Tandoori chicken with spinach (saag)	1 entrée	170	5		1	30	840	19	3	14	1 Other Carbohydrate, 2 Lean Protein
	Basmati rice	1/2 cup	170	1		0	0	200	38	0	4	2 1/2 Starch
Totals			**614**	**12**	**18**	**1.5**	**32**	**1654**	**104**	**6**	**25**	**5 Starch, 1 Other Carbohydrate, 2 Vegetable, 2 Lean Protein, 1 Fat**

(table continues on next page)

Hearty 'N' Healthy

Menu Samplers Section	Menu Item	Amount	Calories	Fat (g)	% Calories from Fat	Saturated Fat (g)	Chol. (mg)	Sodium (mg)	Carb. (g)	Fiber (g)	Protein (g)	Exchanges/ Choices
Hearty 'N' Healthy (Men)	Papadum	2 whole pieces	80	1		0	0	600	4	0	4	1/2 Starch
	Guferati (Indian spiced green beans)	1 cup	160	14		2	0	350	9	4	2	2 Vegetable, 3 Fat
	Lamb vindaloo	1 cup	360	15		0	80	600	32	0	26	2 Other Carbohydrate, 3 Medium-Fat Protein
	Basmati rice	1/2 cup	170	1		0	0	200	38	0	4	2 1/2 Starch
Totals			**770**	**31**	**36**	**2**	**80**	**1750**	**83**	**4**	**36**	**3 Starch, 2 Other Carbohydrate, 2 Vegetable, 3 Medium-Fat Protein, 3 Fat**

(table continues on next page)

Lower Carb 'N' Healthy

Menu Samplers Section	Menu Item	Amount	Calories	Fat (g)	% Calories from Fat	Saturated Fat (g)	Chol. (mg)	Sodium (mg)	Carb. (g)	Fiber (g)	Protein (g)	Exchanges/ Choices
Lower Carb 'N' Healthy (Women)	Mixed curried vegetables	1 1/2 cups	375	15		2	0	600	52	7	7	2 1/2 Starch, 2 Vegetable, 3 Fat
	Chicken biryani	1/2 entrée	165	6		0.5	10	400	17	2	13	1 Starch, 2 Lean Protein
Totals			**540**	**21**	**35**	**2.5**	**10**	**1000**	**69**	**9**	**20**	**3 1/2 Starch, 2 Vegetable, 2 Lean Protein, 3 Fat**
Lower Carb 'N' Healthy (Men)	Roti	1 piece (7 inch)	115	3		1	0	190	11	3	4	1 Starch, 1/2 Fat
	Chicken kebab	1 skewer	180	5		1	66	200	4	0	26	4 Lean Protein
	Chana masala (stewed, spiced chickpeas)	1 entrée	261	7		0	0	500	22	9	9	1 1/2 Starch, 1 Lean Protein, 1 Fat
	Basmati rice	1/4 cup	85	1		0	0	100	19	0	2	1 1/2 Starch
	Mango lassi	1 cup	138	1		1	4	47	31	2	4	1 Fat-Free Milk, 1 Fruit
Totals			**779**	**17**	**20**	**3**	**70**	**1037**	**87**	**14**	**45**	**4 Starch, 1 Fruit, 1 Fat-Free Milk, 5 Lean Protein, 1 1/2 Fat**

Menu Lingo

- **Bombay duck:** this term does not describe a bird, but rather fish served sautéed, fried, or dried, along with curries and rice. It is not often seen on U.S. Indian menus.
- **Cardamom:** an expensive spice native to India that is part of the ginger family. Either the whole cardamom pod or only the seeds are used. This is one of the most common spices found in garam masalas (curry mixtures).
- **Cinnamon:** a delicate spice commonly found in curries and spice combinations. It is often dry roasted before use to release more flavor. Both cinnamon sticks and ground cinnamon are used in Indian cuisine.
- **Clove:** another commonly used spice in curry dishes, it is the dried flower bud of an evergreen tropical tree found in Southeast Asia.
- **Coconut milk:** this does not refer to the liquid found inside the coconut, rather the creamy fluid is extracted from the flesh of the coconut.
- **Coriander:** a fragrant spice that is often the main ingredient in curries. Both ground coriander or the whole coriander leaf (also known as cilantro) are used in Indian cooking. It is also called Chinese parsley.
- **Cumin:** another fragrant spice important to curry dishes. It is used either in seed form or ground.
- **Curry:** is not an individual spice used in Indian cooking. The word "curry" means sauce, and many spices, individually roasted, make up a curry mixture (also known as garam masala).
- **Fennel:** another spice used in curries. It is a member of the cumin family and, on occasion, it is referred to as sweet cumin.
- **Ghee:** clarified butter. It contains no milk solids. This is the ingredient that adds some of the richness and calories to Indian foods.
- **Malai:** a thick cream made by separating and collecting the top part of boiled milk. It is used in entrées for a thick, creamy sauce.
- **Mint:** used to add flavor to curry dishes and also as a main ingredient in mint chutney and mint sambal. It can also be used in biryani and as a dipping sauce for appetizers.
- **Paneer:** often referred to as homemade cream cheese or cottage cheese and made from milk curdled with lemon juice and then strained through cheesecloth. Paneer is used in vegetable and rice dishes. For vegetarians, it is a complete protein source.

► **Poppy seeds:** seeds that are ground to a powder and used in curry dishes to thicken the sauces.

► **Rose water:** a flavoring agent used in Indian desserts. It is extracted from rose petals by steaming them and then diluting the essence.

► **Saffron:** known as the most expensive spice in the world, small quantities are used commonly in Indian cooking. It is obtained by drying the stamens of saffron crocus. Saffron strands are thread-like and deep orange in color.

► **Tamarind:** used for its acidic quality, it is a fruit from a large tropical tree. Tamarind is a commonly used Indian spice and food.

► **Turmeric:** a spice that lends the yellow-orange color to commercial curry powder. It is a member of the ginger family and is commonly used in Indian cooking.

► **Yogurt:** a common ingredient in Indian cooking; it is always plain and unflavored.

(i) What's Your Solution? Answers

a) Small changes like these can add up to a big difference in the overall fat and calorie content of your meal. After a serving of tasty soup you'll be fuller as your entrée is delivered and you won't even miss the samosa.

b) Smart move choosing a tomato-based chicken dish over a cream-based one! If the butter chicken remains a favorite, go ahead and order it next time, but be sure to share it and/or take some home.

c) Chaan saag is a great way to get two healthy vegetables—spinach and chickpeas—in your meal. And ordering a side dish or half portion of another vegetable dish is a terrific way to help fill up on healthful vegetables.

d) Portion control is always an important healthy eating strategy. Adding extra healthful accompaniments, such as raita or onion chutneys, can help ease you into eating less food without feeling deprived.

CHAPTER 25

Middle Eastern

Middle Eastern restaurants vary significantly in type. They range from mall eateries that confine their menus to gyros, souvlaki sandwiches, or platters to upscale white-tablecloth restaurants that serve the breadth of traditional Middle Eastern fare. You'll also see Middle Eastern family-style restaurants. Many of the upscale restaurants specialize in the cuisine of a specific Middle Eastern country, like Morocco or Lebanon, rather than offering a fusion of cuisines from the Middle East. The Middle Eastern cuisine best known and enjoyed in the U.S. at this point is Greek. Greece is not a Middle Eastern country but, because of culinary similarities, Greek food is often categorized as Middle Eastern cuisine.

The majority of Middle Eastern restaurants in America fall into one of two categories: the sandwich shop or the family-style restaurant. The casual sandwich shop is where you can go to order a gyro, falafel, or shawarma sandwich. Soups, salads, potatoes (fried or roasted), and various dips may be offered as sides. At family-style Middle Eastern restaurants you'll be able to choose from a full menu of options—appetizers, soups, salads, entrées, and desserts.

As with most ethnic restaurants, the majority of Middle Eastern restaurants are independently owned and operated. However, a few national chains are taking root. Garbanzo Mediterranean Grill has several locations across the country, mainly in California, Colorado, Arizona, and the Southeast and Mid-Atlantic areas. This chain is on a growth curve and features salads and build-your-own entrées, for which you can choose a base, protein, salads, and sauces. Aladdin's Eatery in the Midwest and Southeast features fast casual Lebanese fare with an Americanized spin. Zoës Kitchen, a walk-up-and-order restaurant where the food is delivered to your table, has locations mainly in the South and the East and offers a healthy Mediterranean-inspired menu. And as small plates continue to grow in popularity, you find a few more upscale restaurants that specialize in high-quality mezze, the Middle Eastern version of appetizers.

As Middle Eastern food has inched its way into our culinary repertoire, you'll also find some Middle Eastern foods integrated into "American" restaurant menus. It's common to see gyros and Greek salads on the menus of sandwich shops or family-style restaurants. And several Middle Eastern items, such as hummus, baba ghanoush, feta cheese, and Greek-style yogurt, are stocked in just about every supermarket.

On the Menu

Middle Eastern restaurants represent the cuisines from many Middle Eastern countries, including Lebanon, Israel, Turkey, Iran, Morocco, Syria, and more. While there are similarities among the cuisines of each of these countries, preparation methods and seasonings differ slightly. It's common to see items such as pita bread, hummus, baba ghanoush, and chickpeas on the menu in all kinds of Middle Eastern restaurants. Commonly used spices in Middle Eastern cuisine are parsley, mint, cilantro, and oregano, plus a host of others that are also mainstays in Indian cooking—cumin, coriander, cinnamon, and ginger. Long ago, the Middle East was a major link on the spice route between the East and Europe (the Silk Road), so it makes sense that a wide variety of spices are used in Middle Eastern cuisine.

As with other cuisines, the foods that play a predominant role in Middle Eastern cooking are those that are naturally plentiful in the region—wheat, other grains, legumes, olives, dates, figs, lamb, and eggplant, to name a few. Grains are a big part of Middle Eastern cuisine. Rice, combined with a variety of ingredients to make rice pilaf, is commonly served in Greece and the Middle East, whereas couscous, made with granules of wheat, is indigenous to North African countries. Tabouli, a cold cracked wheat or bulgur salad tossed with raw vegetables and lots of parsley, is most familiar in Lebanese cuisine; however, it is commonly served throughout the Middle East.

Pita bread, or pockets as they're sometimes called in America, is flat, round, slightly leavened bread. Due to the very hot oven in which it is cooked, steam is created, and the process results in a hollow center. This "pocket" in the bread is perfect for stuffing. Though whole-wheat pita breads are available in most supermarkets, the pita bread served in restaurants is typically made with white flour.

It is common to find stuffed dishes in Middle Eastern restaurants. Probably the best known of these dishes is dolmades, or stuffed grape leaves. You may also see stuffed cabbage or stuffed eggplant on Middle Eastern menus. The stuffings in these foods are usually meat, rice, and/or vegetarian mixtures.

Chickpeas, fava beans, and other legumes are indigenous to the Middle East and, thus, are central to Middle Eastern cuisine. Chickpeas and/or fava beans can be puréed to make falafel or ta'amia. Chickpeas are mashed and mixed with tahini (sesame seed paste or purée) to make the familiar hummus.

Due to the plentitude of olives in the Middle East, olive oil is frequently the fat/oil of choice in this type of cuisine. It is often used in cold dishes. Olives, both green and black, are frequently served. The fact that olive oil is the predominant fat used in Middle Eastern cuisine (rather than butter, which is higher in saturated fat) is good news. However, remember that there are just as many calories in olive oil as there are in equal amounts of butter. (Learn more about olives and olive oil in Chapter 19: Italian on page 368.)

There are minimal seafood dishes in Middle Eastern cookery. Lamb is the most familiar protein option, and beef is also served but to a lesser degree. Eggs are used quite a bit in dishes such as avgolemono (soup made from chicken broth, rice, egg yolks, and lemon juice), shakshuka (eggs poached in tomato sauce), and in many variations of omelets.

Milk is not frequently consumed in the Middle East due in part to the high incidence of lactose intolerance. Yogurt is frequently used, however; the same Greek yogurt that has taken this country by storm. Yogurt is served plain or mixed with cucumber, garlic, mint, and/or salt to make a sauce or side dish called tzatziki. Or it may be strained to create labneh, which has a consistency akin to the Greek yogurt you can find in your supermarket. The purpose of yogurt in Middle Eastern cuisine, as in Indian cuisine, is to act as a palate refresher, or soother, after the spiciness of the cuisine. (However, Middle Eastern cuisine isn't as spicy as Indian cuisine.) Two cheeses, feta and kasseri, are commonly used in Middle Eastern cookery. They may be served alone in chunks or incorporated into appetizers, salads, and entrées, such as spinach cheese pie (spanakopita) or a Greek salad.

Phyllo (also filo or fila), which literally means leaf, is a paper-thin Middle Eastern dough. It is used to make sweet desserts, such as baklava, and dinner pies, such as spanakopita, the well-known spinach and feta cheese dish.

When eating Middle Eastern fare, one of the best strategies for eating healthy is to choose from the plethora of vegetarian options, when possible, as protein portions can be large. Also be on the lookout for fried food and excessive olive oil; you should avoid or limit these. Again, even though olive oil is a healthy fat, the calories add up. Oftentimes, even rice dishes are made with a generous pour of olive oil mixed in, so be cautious.

The Menu Profile

Mezze (Appetizers)

Middle Eastern appetizers, or mezze as they may be called, are traditionally eaten leisurely. This leisurely pace is a good strategy to follow when trying to eat healthy in Middle Eastern restaurants. Several appetizers are high in fat and should be limited: spanakopita, taramosalata, and cheese casserole.

Healthier options are baba ghanoush and hummus, but they definitely aren't fat free. They contain olive oil and tahini (sesame seed paste), which boost the fat content of these dishes (though these ingredients are mostly healthy fat). You'll find baba ghanoush and hummus served with pita bread and in small quantities. If you can hold back, eating these in small amounts is fine. Dolmades (stuffed grape leaves) are also healthy options, especially when you opt for the vegetarian stuffing.

Soups and Salads

A few soups are common on Middle Eastern menus. Lemon-egg soup, avgolemono, is a regular. It is light and relatively low in calories. If cholesterol is a concern for you, it is best to skip this soup. You might also find lentil, vegetable, and/or yogurt-based soup on the menu, all of which are quite healthy.

There are many salad options. Greek or house salads are lettuce-based with cucumbers, tomatoes, onion, and cheese and olives (both of which are high-sodium ingredients). Don't forget to order the dressing on the side. You might find fattoush with cucumbers, tomatoes, onions, and toasted pieces of pita bread. This option might be dressed with olive oil, lemon, and seasonings prior to serving, because it usually marinates for a while. Tabouli, cracked-wheat salad, and tomato and cucumber salad are also regulars on Middle Eastern menus. All of these range from very to relatively healthy, so enjoy.

Sandwiches and Wraps

You'll find several popular sandwich options on many Middle Eastern menus. The style and toppings of these sandwiches vary, based on the country's specific cuisine, but the concept is the same: grill the meat (often on a spit), slice it, then stuff or roll it into pita bread and top it with vegetables and sauces.

Gyros meat, hailing from Greece, is a spicy combination of lamb and beef, and is perhaps the most well-known of Middle Eastern sandwiches. It is usually wrapped in pita bread, along with lettuce, tomato, onion, and a sauce called tzatziki. Tzatziki is made either with sour cream or yogurt. When it comes to tzatziki, the best advice is to ask at each restaurant to find out whether it's low-calorie yogurt or high-fat sour cream. Try to limit or avoid tzatziki made with sour cream. Souvlaki, the Greek version of shish kebabs, is often offered in the same sandwich-style fashion.

Falafel, another well-known sandwich stuffer, is made from mashed chickpeas that are formed into balls and deep-fried. While chickpeas are inherently healthy, the deep-fried method takes away somewhat from its health value. However, all foods considered, falafel is still a reasonably healthy choice. If you are craving falafel, it's best, based on the fat and carbohydrate content, to enjoy only a small portion. Perhaps a falafel pita sandwich loaded with fresh vegetables, such as lettuce and tomato.

Shawarma, which is popular in Lebanese, Syrian, and Turkish cuisines, among others, is a protein preparation in which chicken, lamb, or beef (or a mixture) are minced and spit-roasted. Shavings are then cut off and served on a platter or sandwich style—wrapped in a pita with toppings such as tahini, hummus, and pickled turnips.

Oftentimes, places that specialize in gyros or shawarma sandwiches also offer some type of potato dish. It may be french fries, as we know them in America, or a thicker cut of potato. Sometimes, the potatoes are placed directly in the pita to help soak up the sauces and keep them from draining off. As always, it's better to load up your sandwich with vegetables such as tomatoes and cucumbers, rather than fried potatoes.

Entrées

When it comes to Middle Eastern entrées, there are plenty of options. It's possible to order seafood or to go vegetarian, but beef and lamb are the predominant sources of protein in this cuisine. Some popular dishes are kibbeh, consisting of meat (sometimes raw) and cracked wheat with vegetables and spices tossed in, as well as kafta, which is made with ground beef, onions, parsley, and spices. If desired, it's easy to eat vegetarian when consuming Middle Eastern food; order stuffed eggplant or a vegetarian appetizer and several à la carte salads. Grilling, stovetop cooking, and baking are the preparation methods of choice.

A very familiar entrée is shish kebab. Its origins relate to the time when the Ottoman armies camped outdoors and had to cook quickly. They devised the method of putting chunks of meat and vegetables on skewers and cooking them quickly over an open outdoor oven. Today, they are cooked on a grill. In most restaurants you can order shish kebab with lamb, beef, chicken, shrimp, or just vegetables. Sometimes a combination is available. The meats are marinated in olive oil, lemon, wine, and spices, then they're grilled on a skewer with vegetables, such as bell peppers, onions, and tomatoes.

Eggplant is an ingredient in several Middle Eastern dishes, moussaka being a familiar one, which consists of an eggplant and tomato casserole with a white sauce topping known as a béchamel sauce (butter, flour, and milk). Yes, a thick béchamel layer can layer on the fat and calories. Or you might find sheikh el mahshi—eggplant stuffed with meat. It's important to realize that eggplant absorbs lots of oil and that prior to cooking eggplant, it is sometimes salted to remove the bitter taste. So, eggplant dishes are probably not as low in fat and sodium as you think.

Lahmajun is the Armenian answer to pizza. It's dough that is topped with ground meat, parsley, tomatoes, onions, and Middle Eastern spices. This is a reasonably healthy choice as long as you practice portion control. It's light on fat, contains some vegetables and a balance of protein and carbohydrate. Omelets made with feta cheese or loukaniko (sausage) and three eggs are offered on Middle Eastern menus. Avoid or split. Adding cheese or sauce to three eggs gives you enough cholesterol for several days, not to mention the fat load it contains.

Dinners in Middle Eastern restaurants are usually served with a small salad, pita bread, rice pilaf, and/or a steamed vegetable. All of these are relatively low-fat additions to your meal, except for the rice pilaf, which may have a fair share of olive oil mixed in (as is often the case with the Lebanese version of this dish). If you closely watch your calories, pick and choose which of these sides you want to eat. The salad and pita bread are good options.

When eating at a Middle Eastern restaurant, don't feel compelled to include an entrée. Unless you can split or complement two dishes by sharing with a dining partner, ordering multiple dishes (to create a well-balanced meal) might be too much food and an invitation to overeat. Mix and match à la carte appetizers, salads, and side dishes to create a healthy, balanced meal that will allow you to taste more foods. Middle Eastern restaurants make ordering à la carte from the list of great-tasting and healthy appetizers quite easy. Complement a couple of these appetizers with a healthy Greek salad. Another approach is to split everything with a dining partner, from appetizer to—if you must and it tastes absolutely great—dessert. Or, once again, eat family style by ordering and dividing a number of dishes. But don't forget—when eating family style, always order fewer dishes than there are people at the table or be ready to store some food away for tomorrow's eats.

Dessert

Dessert in the Middle East is traditionally just a bowl of fruit, but this is not so in Middle Eastern restaurants in America. You'll often have the sweet choices of baklava, kataif, and rice pudding. Kataif is a small pancake filled with either sweet items (served for dessert) or savory items (served with the meal). The sweet pancakes may be filled with a white cheese, topped with ground pistachios, and dipped in or served with simple sugar syrup. They may be baked or deep-fried. Baklava is traditionally made with phyllo dough, plenty of butter, walnuts, honey, and spices. A number of other varieties of baklava may be available using different nuts and seasonings. Regardless of the variety, baklava is always high in fat and sugar and that translates to calories. It's best to avoid high-fat, high-calorie desserts. Or, at most, nibble a few bites to quench your sweet tooth. It might take care of sweet cravings for a week or so.

The other half of enjoying pastries in the Middle East is sipping a cup of Turkish or Greek coffee, which resembles and is served like espresso in Italian restaurants and upscale dining establishments. It is strong and sometimes thick or muddy. Small portions are served in demitasse cups. The coffee alone might be a new taste treat for you and, best yet, it has almost zero calories. Do make sure they don't add sugar to it before serving.

Nutrition Snapshot

Health Busters

Category	Restaurant Name	Dish Name	Serving Size	Cal.	Total Fat (g)	Carb. (g)	Sod. (mg)
Appetizers	Shiraz	Falafel	1 portion	649	19	94	1211
Appetizers	T.G.I. Friday's	Classic Mediterranean Hummus	1 portion	1010	42	133	1830
Appetizers	Yard House	Hummus w/Oven Grilled Pita Bread	1 portion	818	32	101	2160
Appetizers	Zoës Kitchen	Hummus & Pita	1 portion	830	34	102	1600
Appetizers	Olga's Kitchen	Mediterranean Olives & Peppers	1 portion	250	20	11	1810
Salads	Chickpea	Greek w/Grilled Chicken	1 portion	680	33	20	1560
Salads	Olga's Kitchen	Mediterranean Spinach	1 portion	710	52	18	1410
Salads	Zoës Kitchen	Tossed Greek (no dressing)	1 portion	710	30	47	2520
Salads	Daphne's Greek Cafe	Classic Greek w/Fresh-Carved Gyros	1 portion	620	47	28	1270
Entrées	Zoës Kitchen	Chicken Kabob	1 portion	870	31	89	2460
Entrées	Zoës Kitchen	Shrimp Kabob	1 portion	800	31	88	3560
Entrées	Daphne's Greek Cafe	Fresh-Carved Gyros Entrée	1 portion	740	64	16	1200
Entrées	Sticks Kebob Shop	Falafel Platter	1 portion	650	24	94	1620
Sandwiches	Pita Pit	Gyro	1 pita	560	29	49	1110
Sandwiches	Daphne's Greek Cafe	Classic Gyros Pita	1 pita	660	47	40	1025

Healthier Bets

Category	Restaurant Name	Dish Name	Serving Size	Cal.	Total Fat (g)	Sat. Fat (g)	Carb. (g)	Pro. (g)	Fiber (g)	Chol. (mg)	Sodium (mg)	Exchanges/ Choices
Appetizers	Olga's Kitchen	Spinach & Cheese Pie	1 portion	300	15	8	28	13	2	55	630	2 Starch, 1 High-Fat Protein, 1 Fat
Appetizers	Sticks Kebob Shop	Falafel	1 portion	240	13	1	24	9	7	0	600	1 1/2 Starch, 1 Lean Protein, 2 Fat
Appetizers	Daphne's Greek Cafe	Falafel	1 portion	180	11	2	16	5	5	0	320	1 Starch, 1/2 Lean Protein, 1 1/2 Fat
Appetizers	Sticks Kebob Shop	Hummus	1 portion	190	13	2	16	4	3	0	390	1 Starch, 2 1/2 Fat
Appetizers	Zoës Kitchen	Hummus (4 oz or 1/2 cup)	1 portion	550	36	4	44	17	11	0	1170	3 Starch, 1 Lean Protein, 6 Fat

(table continues on next page)

Healthier Bets

Category	Restaurant Name	Dish Name	Serving Size	Cal.	Total Fat (g)	Sat. Fat (g)	Carb. (g)	Pro. (g)	Fiber (g)	Chol. (mg)	Sodium (mg)	Exchanges/ Choices
Appetizers	Daphne's Greek Cafe	Roasted Red Pepper Hummus and Multigrain Pita Chips	1 portion	320	14	1	40	9	6	0	740	2 1/2 Starch, 1/2 Lean Protein, 2 1/2 Fat
Appetizers	Daphne's Greek Cafe	Original Hummus and Pita Bread	1 portion	300	15	2	37	6	3	0	520	2 1/2 Starch, 2 1/2 Fat
Appetizers	Daphne's Greek Cafe	Original Hummus (only)	1 portion	180	13	2	13	4	2	0	390	1 Starch, 2 1/2 Fat
Soups	Au Bon Pain	Mediter-ranean Pepper (small)	1 portion	120	4	0	19	5	5	0	430	3 Vegetable, 1 Fat

(table continues on next page)

Healthier Bets

Category	Restaurant Name	Dish Name	Serving Size	Cal.	Total Fat (g)	Sat. Fat (g)	Carb. (g)	Pro. (g)	Fiber (g)	Chol. (mg)	Sodium (mg)	Exchanges/ Choices
Soups	Olga's Kitchen	Peasant (7 oz)	1 portion	160	7	3	14	10	2	30	840	1 Starch, 1 Lean Protein, 1 Fat
Soups	Zoës Kitchen	Chicken Orzo (cup)	1 portion	140	6	1.5	12	11	2	30	1270	1 Starch, 1 Lean Protein, 1/2 Fat
Soups	Daphne's Greek Cafe	Lemon Chicken w/Pita	1 portion	230	13	4	24	5	1	56	1160	1 1/2 Starch, 1/2 Lean Protein, 2 Fat
Soups	Nanoosh	Lentil (8 oz)	1 portion	122	3	0	18	6	n/a	0	349	1 Starch, 1/2 Lean Protein, 1/2 Fat
Salads	Nanoosh	Tabouleh	1 portion	230	9	1	36	5	n/a	0	401	2 Starch, 2 Fat
Salads	Nanoosh	Quinoa Salad	1 portion	238	8	1	36	6	n/a	0	190	2 Starch, 2 Fat

(table continues on next page)

Healthier Bets

Category	Restaurant Name	Dish Name	Serving Size	Cal.	Total Fat (g)	Sat. Fat (g)	Carb. (g)	Pro. (g)	Fiber (g)	Chol. (mg)	Sodium (mg)	Exchanges/ Choices
Salads	Nanoosh	Nanoosh Green	1 portion	129	7	1	16	3	n/a	0	37	1 Starch, 1 1/2 Fat
Salads	Shiraz	Fatoosh	1 portion	259	17	3.7	22	6.9	3	14	409	1 1/2 Starch, 3 Fat
Salads	Sticks Kebob Shop	Tabouleh	1 portion	100	8	1	8	1	2	0	320	1/2 Starch, 1 1/2 Fat
Salads	Sticks Kebob Shop	Roasted Eggplant	1 portion	60	4	0.5	7	1	3	0	380	1 Vegetable, 1 Fat
Salads	Sticks Kebob Shop	Cucumber, Tomato, and Red Onion	1 portion	40	3	0	3	1	1	0	220	1 Vegetable, 1/2 Fat
Salads	Daphne's Greek Cafe	Side Greek w/Dressing	1 portion	70	4	2	7	3	2	13	230	1 Vegetable, 1 Fat
Salads	Daphne's Greek Cafe	Side Greek w/Classic Dressing	1 portion	150	12	3	8	3	2	13	380	1 1/2 Vegetable, 2 1/2 Fat

(table continues on next page)

Healthier Bets

Category	Restaurant Name	Dish Name	Serving Size	Cal.	Total Fat (g)	Sat. Fat (g)	Carb. (g)	Pro. (g)	Fiber (g)	Chol. (mg)	Sodium (mg)	Exchanges/ Choices
Salads	Sticks Kebob Shop	Lamb	1 portion	280	10	2.5	25	23	6	55	260	1/2 Starch, 3 Vegetable, 2 1/2 Lean Protein, 1/2 Fat
Salads	Sticks Kebob Shop	Kibbeh	1 portion	330	14	5	31	22	7	35	810	1 Starch, 3 Vegetable, 2 1/2 Medium-Fat Protein
Salads	Sticks Kebob Shop	Falafel	1 portion	360	14	1	49	14	13	0	750	2 Starch, 3 Vegetable, 3 Fat
Salads	Zoës Kitchen	Greek (no dressing)	1 portion	420	21	8.5	33	15	10	40	1850	1 Starch, 3 1/2 Vegetable, 2 High-Fat Protein, 1 Fat

(table continues on next page)

Healthier Bets

Category	Restaurant Name	Dish Name	Serving Size	Cal.	Total Fat (g)	Sat. Fat (g)	Carb. (g)	Pro. (g)	Fiber (g)	Chol. (mg)	Sodium (mg)	Exchanges/ Choices
Salads	Daphne's Greek Cafe	Classic Greek w/ Grilled Chicken	1 portion	330	15	6	21	32	5	90	1130	1/2 Starch, 3 Vegetable, 3 1/2 Lean Protein, 1 Fat
Salads	Daphne's Greek Cafe	Classic Greek w/ Crispy Shrimp	1 portion	350	19	6	28	19	5	105	1130	1 Starch, 3 Vegetable, 1 1/2 Lean Protein, 3 Fat
Salads	Daphne's Greek Cafe	Classic Greek (no protein)	1 portion	190	11	5	19	8	5	25	590	1/2 Starch, 2 1/2 Vegetable, 2 Fat
Pita Chips	Sticks Kebob Shop	Pita Chips	1 portion	210	2	0	39	8	3	0	410	2 1/2 Starch
Pita Chips	Daphne's Greek Cafe	Multigrain Pita Chips	1 portion	170	5	0	27	6	5	0	270	2 Starch, 1 Fat

(table continues on next page)

Healthier Bets

Category	Restaurant Name	Dish Name	Serving Size	Cal.	Total Fat (g)	Sat. Fat (g)	Carb. (g)	Pro. (g)	Fiber (g)	Chol. (mg)	Sodium (mg)	Exchanges/ Choices
Sides	Daphne's Greek Cafe	Seasoned Rice Pilaf	1 portion	250	6	1	47	5	1	0	400	3 Starch, 1 Fat
Entrées	Shiraz	Salmon Kabob	1 portion	271	12	1.76	0	37.9	0	105	617	5 1/2 Lean Protein
Entrées	Shiraz	Lamb Kabob	1 portion	257	16	7	0	25	0	93	599	3 1/2 Medium-Fat Protein
Entrées	Shiraz	Jumbo Shrimp Kabob	1 portion	348	18	4	22	26	3	189	1142	1 1/2 Starch, 3 Medium-Fat Protein
Entrées	Sticks Kebob Shop	Rosemary-Rubbed Leg of Lamb Kebob	1 portion	160	9	2.5	0	18	0	55	110	2 1/2 Medium-Fat Protein
Entrées	Sticks Kebob Shop	Lemon-Garlic Shrimp Kebob	1 portion	130	6	1	0	18	0	170	250	2 1/2 Lean Protein

(table continues on next page)

Healthier Bets

Category	Restaurant Name	Dish Name	Serving Size	Cal.	Total Fat (g)	Sat. Fat (g)	Carb. (g)	Pro. (g)	Fiber (g)	Chol. (mg)	Sodium (mg)	Exchanges/ Choices
Entrées	Zoës Kitchen	Veggie Kabob Dinner	1 portion	560	24	2	69	17	17	0	1750	3 Starch, 4 1/2 Vegetable, 4 1/2 Fat
Entrées	Zoës Kitchen	Shrimp Kabobs (without dressing or pita bread)	1 portion	580	24	11	52	33	6	220	3240	2 Starch, 4 Vegetable, 4 Lean Protein, 3 Fat
Entrées	Daphne's Greek Cafe	Kid's Falafel Street Pita	1 portion	340	19	4	33	9	5	11	590	2 Starch, 1 Lean Protein, 3 Fat

✓ Green-Flag Words

Ingredients:

- ► Chickpeas
- ► Cracked wheat (tabouli)
- ► Cucumber
- ► Eggplant—not fried or drenched in oil
- ► Fava beans
- ► Grape leaves
- ► Green beans, spinach
- ► Gyro meat
- ► Herbs and spices
- ► Lemon juice
- ► Mint
- ► Onions
- ► Parsley
- ► Pine nuts
- ► Shrimp, squid (calamari)
- ► Souvlaki
- ► Spiced ground beef or lamb
- ► Tomatoes, onions, and green peppers
- ► Yogurt

Cooking Methods/Menu Descriptions:

- ► Baked
- ► Charcoal broiled
- ► Dolmas, dolmades
- ► Grilled on a skewer (kebab)
- ► Lemon dressing
- ► Marinated and barbecued
- ► Simmered
- ► Stewed
- ► Stuffed with ground lamb or meat
- ► Stuffed with rice and meat
- ► Tomato sauce

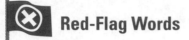

Red-Flag Words

Ingredients:

- ▶ Caviar (high in sodium and cholesterol)
- ▶ Egg
- ▶ Feta cheese, kasseri cheese (high in sodium and fat)
- ▶ Kalamata olives, Greek olives (high in sodium and fat)
- ▶ Loukaniko (pork sausage; high in sodium and fat)
- ▶ Olive oil
- ▶ Sesame seed paste or purée
- ▶ Tahini (ground sesame seeds)

Cooking Methods/Menu Descriptions:

- ▶ Béchamel sauce (white sauce)
- ▶ Cheese pie
- ▶ Golden fried
- ▶ In pastry crust
- ▶ Lemon and butter sauce
- ▶ Pan-fried, deep-fried
- ▶ Phyllo dough (problem is the butter used between the layers)
- ▶ Spanakopita
- ▶ Tarator sauce (made with yogurt, shredded cucumber, garlic, walnut, dill, vegetable oil, and water)
- ▶ Topped with creamy sauce

Healthy Eating Tips and Tactics

- ▶ Order à la carte. Rather than ordering a large entrée, which can be heavy on the rice and protein (meat), opt for a cup of soup, a salad, and perhaps an appetizer.
- ▶ Go vegetarian. Lamb and chicken often get center stage at Middle Eastern restaurants in America, but vegetarian options are bountiful and make it easy to enjoy a flavorful meatless meal.
- ▶ Opt for soup or salad, instead of a heavier appetizer.
- ▶ Watch portion sizes, which can be large. Share with your dining companion(s) or ask for a box to take half of your meal home.

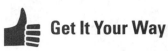 **Get It Your Way**

▶ Request salad dressing on the side. Or ask for some lemon slices to add extra flavor to your salad along with a small drizzle of olive oil.

▶ Many dips and spreads, like hummus, labneh, and baba ghanoush, are drizzled with olive oil before they hit your table. Ask that this extra olive oil be left off to shave a few calories and grams of fat from your meal.

▶ Watch out for high-fat additions—such as feta cheese, olives, or fried pita chips—to otherwise healthy salads.

▶ Tahini, hummus, and/or tzatziki are often spooned onto sandwiches with a heavy hand. Ask for these to be served on the side so you can control how much goes on your sandwich.

Tips and Tactics for Gluten-Free Eating

▶ All bread, bulgur, tabouli, pita, couscous, and falafel made with wheat flour contain gluten.

▶ Meat kebabs that have been marinated or dusted in flour contain gluten. Moussaka (the white béchamel sauce is made with wheat flour) and spanakopita (cheese and spinach pie) contain gluten. Ground meat patties (kafta) and meat pastries (sambousik) contain wheat. And gyro lamb contains gluten.

▶ Rice, hummus, baba ghanoush, and traditional Middle Eastern vegetables are typically gluten-free.

▶ Greek salads with feta, olives, tomatoes, and cucumbers with vinegar and olive oil dressing are gluten-free.

▶ Grilled meat, poultry, and seafood kebabs without marinades are a good choice.

▶ Marinades that contain fresh herbs, olives, capers, tomatoes, lemon, and olive oil are safe.

▶ Dolmades (stuffed grape leaves) and tzatziki (Greek yogurt and cucumber dip) typically are gluten-free.

▶ Stuffed peppers and cabbage rolls in a gluten-free sauce are good choices.

▶ Fresh yogurt and fruit is an excellent choice for dessert if they're on the menu.

Tips and Tactics to Help Kids Eat Healthy

▶ Skip the kids' menu if there is one, such as in more Americanized versions of Middle Eastern restaurants.

▶ It's no surprise that kids' menus items, when they appear in Middle Eastern restaurants, are often higher in saturated fat—featuring more cheese and deep-fried options—than the foods you traditionally find in Middle Eastern cuisine.

▶ Split a sandwich with your child. Gyro and shawarma sandwiches are often quite large, offering enough to share. Supplement the sandwich with a healthy side, like a cup of soup, a Greek salad, or rice.

▶ Experiment with dips, since kids love to dunk, dip, and drizzle whenever they can. Hummus, baba ghanoush, and tzatziki may be new to your child, but they are generally healthy and are often well liked by children.

What's Your Solution?

You and your family are spending the day in the city and decide to have dinner at a new-to-you Greek restaurant. You typically don't eat Greek food, so you aren't immediately familiar with all the menu options. You take a look around and notice that everyone is ordering a flaming cheese, which the servers make a big deal about. You also cast your eyes upon large entrée portions.

Which of the following options can help you stick to your health goals of managing your weight and glucose?

a) Control calories by asking for a takeout container at the start of your meal.

b) Order the sagnaki (flaming cheese), but enjoy just a few bites.

c) Start with a soup and salad, then share an entrée with your dining partner(s).

d) Split and share several vegetarian options on the menu.

See page 546 for answers.

Menu Samplers

Light 'N' Healthy

Menu Samplers Section	Menu Item	Amount	Calories	Fat (g)	% Calories from Fat	Saturated Fat (g)	Chol. (mg)	Sodium (mg)	Carb. (g)	Fiber (g)	Protein (g)	Exchanges/ Choices
Light 'N' Healthy (Women)	Hummus	1/2 cup	208	12		2	0	470	18	8	10	1 Starch, 1 Lean Protein, 2 Fat
	Whole-wheat pita	1/2 large pita	74	1		0	0	140	15	2	3	1 Starch
	Lentil soup	1 cup	140	3		0	0	900	24	9	8	1 1/2 Other Carbohydrate, 1 Lean Protein
	Greek salad (lettuce, feta, cucumber, red onion)	1 cup	93	4		1	2	66	13	1	2	2 Vegetable, 1 Fat

(table continues on next page)

Light 'N' Healthy

Menu Samplers Section	Menu Item	Amount	Calories	Fat (g)	% Calories from Fat	Saturated Fat (g)	Chol. (mg)	Sodium (mg)	Carb. (g)	Fiber (g)	Protein (g)	Exchanges/ Choices
	Oil and vinegar dressing	1 teaspoon oil	39	5		0.5	0	0	0	0	0	1 Fat
Totals			554	25	41	3.5	2	1576	70	20	23	1 Starch, 1 1/2 Other Carbohydrate, 2 Vegetable, 2 Lean Protein, 4 Fat
Light 'N' Healthy (Men)	Baba ghanoush	1/4 cup	208	23		5	19	340	2	0	2	1 Vegetable, 4 Fat
	Whole-wheat pita	3/4 large pita	111	2		0	0	210	22	3	5	1 1/2 Starch

(table continues on next page)

Light 'N' Healthy

Menu Samplers Section	Menu Item	Amount	Calories	Fat (g)	% Calories from Fat	Saturated Fat (g)	Chol. (mg)	Sodium (mg)	Carb. (g)	Fiber (g)	Protein (g)	Exchanges/ Choices
	Ful (fava beans)	1/2 cup	94	1		0	0	55	17	5	7	1 Starch, 1/2 Lean Protein
	Lamb kabob with onions, peppers, and tomatoes	2 (4-inch) sticks	210	8		3	92	60	5	0	29	1 Vegetable, 4 Lean Protein
	Rice	1/2 cup	110	2		0	0	8	22	1	3	1 1/2 Starch
Totals			**733**	**36**	**44**	**8**	**111**	**673**	**68**	**9**	**46**	**4 Starch, 2 Vegetable, 4 1/2 Lean Protein, 4 Fat**

(table continues on next page)

Hearty 'N' Healthy

Menu Samplers Section	Menu Item	Amount	Calories	Fat (g)	% Calories from Fat	Saturated Fat (g)	Chol. (mg)	Sodium (mg)	Carb. (g)	Fiber (g)	Protein (g)	Exchanges/ Choices
Hearty 'N' Healthy (Women)	Labneh (strained yogurt)	1/4 cup	70	4		3	15	100	4	0	4	1/2 Reduced-Fat Milk
	Spanakopita	4-inch square	200	7		1	20	450	23	5	10	1 Starch, 2 Vegetable, 1 Fat
	Tabbouleh	1 cup	204	15		0	0	800	23	8	8	1 Starch, 1 Vegetable, 3 Fat
	Greek salad (lettuce, feta, cucumber, red onion)	1 cup	93	4		1	2	66	13	1	2	2 Vegetable, 1 Fat
	Oil and vinegar dressing	1 teaspoon oil	39	5		0.5	0	0	0	0	0	1 Fat
Totals			**606**	**35**	**52**	**5.5**	**37**	**1416**	**63**	**14**	**24**	**2 Starch, 1/2 Reduced-Fat Milk, 5 Vegetable, 6 Fat**

(table continues on next page)

Hearty 'N' Healthy

Menu Samplers Section	Menu Item	Amount	Calories	Fat (g)	% Calories from Fat	Saturated Fat (g)	Chol. (mg)	Sodium (mg)	Carb. (g)	Fiber (g)	Protein (g)	Exchanges/ Choices
Hearty 'N' Healthy (Men)	Dolmades	5 pieces	205	11		1	0	570	23	3	5	1 Starch, 1 Vegetable, 2 Fat
	Gyro pita platter with falafel, chicken, onion, lettuce, cucumber, and tomato	3 small falafel, 1/2 cup chopped chicken, 1 (6 1/2" diameter) pita	646	31		5	70	852	59	8	34	3 Starch, 2 Vegetable, 3 Medium-Fat Protein, 3 Fat
Totals			**851**	**42**	**44**	**6**	**70**	**1422**	**82**	**11**	**39**	**4 Starch, 3 Vegetable, 3 Medium-Fat Protein, 5 Fat**

(Table continues on next page)

Lower Carb 'N' Healthy

Menu Samplers Section	Menu Item	Amount	Calories	Fat (g)	% Calories from Fat	Saturated Fat (g)	Chol. (mg)	Sodium (mg)	Carb. (g)	Fiber (g)	Protein (g)	Exchanges/ Choices
Lower Carb 'N' Healthy (Women)	Hummus	1/2 cup	208	12		2	0	470	18	8	10	1 Starch, 1 Lean Protein, 2 Fat
	Whole-wheat pita	1 large pita	74	1		0	0	140	15	2	3	1 Starch
	Moussaka	4-inch square	184	8		3	16	471	18	5	10	1/2 Starch, 2 Vegetable, 1 1/2 Medium-Fat Protein
	Greek salad	1 cup	93	4		1	2	66	13	1	2	2 Vegetable, 1 Fat
	Oil and vinegar dressing	1 teaspoon oil	39	5		0.5	0	0	0	0	0	1 Fat
Totals			**598**	**30**	**45**	**6.5**	**18**	**1147**	**64**	**16**	**25**	**2 1/2 Starch, 4 Vegetable, 2 1/2 Medium-Fat Protein, 4 Fat**

(table continues on next page)

Lower Carb 'N' Healthy

Menu Samplers Section	Menu Item	Amount	Calories	Fat (g)	% Calories from Fat	Saturated Fat (g)	Chol. (mg)	Sodium (mg)	Carb. (g)	Fiber (g)	Protein (g)	Exchanges/ Choices
Lower Carb 'N' Healthy (Men)	Lamb gyro sandwich (with yogurt dressing, shredded lettuce, onions, and cucumber)	1 medium sandwich (12 oz)	562	27		10	60	1200	52	5	29	3 Starch, 1 Vegetable, 3 Medium-Fat Protein, 1 Fat
	Seasoned ful (fava beans)	1/2 cup	94	0		0	0	55	17	5	7	1 Starch
Totals			**656**	**27**	**37**	**10**	**60**	**1255**	**69**	**10**	**36**	**4 Starch, 1 Vegetable, 3 Medium-Fat Protein, 1 Fat**

Menu Lingo

- **Avgolemono:** Greek soup made from chicken broth, rice, egg yolks, and lemon juice.
- **Baba ghanoush:** a purée of eggplant, tahini, olive oil, lemon juice, and garlic. It is used as a spread or dip for pita.
- **Baklava:** a sweet dessert consisting of layers of butter-drenched phyllo pastry, spices, rose water, and chopped nuts. After it's baked, a honey syrup is poured over to soak into the layers.
- **Dolma (plural: dolmades):** this term technically means "something stuffed," but often refers to stuffed grape leaves, filled with rice, onions, pine nuts, seasonings, and (sometimes) a ground meat.
- **Falafel:** small, deep-fried balls made of spiced, ground chickpeas. Generally served inside pita bread as a sandwich, but it can also be served as an appetizer.
- **Fattoush:** a salad made from mixed greens, cucumber, tomatoes, onions, toasted or fried pieces of pita bread, olive oil, and lemon juice. It is seasoned with sumac, which lends it a tart flavor.
- **Ful medames:** cooked and mashed fava beans (a very large bean) served with vegetable oil and flavorings such as cumin, garlic, onion, chopped parsley, and lemon juice.
- **Gyro:** a Greek specialty consisting of lamb (and sometimes beef) that is minced, molded around a spit, and vertically roasted. The meat is then sliced, folded into a pita, and topped with grilled onions, sweet peppers, and a cucumber-yogurt sauce.
- **Hummus:** a mixture of mashed or puréed chickpeas, tahini, lemon juice, garlic, and olive oil. It is usually served as a dip with pieces of pita bread.
- **Kafta:** the Middle Eastern version of meatballs, which are made from ground meat (usually lamb or beef), onions, and spices.
- **Kasseri cheese:** a Greek cheese made from sheep or goat milk that has a sharp, salty flavor. Kasseri is the cheese used in the famous Greek dish, Saganaki, in which it is sautéed in butter and flamed with brandy.
- **Kibbeh:** popular in Lebanon and Syria, this dish combines ground meat (usually lamb), bulgur wheat, and various flavorings. Multiple variations exist and the meat may be raw or cooked.

- **Lahmajun:** a thin, pizza-like crust topped with minced meat, and minced vegetables and herbs, including onions, tomatoes, and parsley.
- **Moussaka:** sliced eggplant and ground lamb or beef that are layered, then baked. The eggplant may be deep-fried prior to being put into the casserole. This dish is often covered with a béchamel sauce. Other variations include the addition of onions, tomatoes, or potatoes.
- **Shawarma:** a protein preparation in which chicken, lamb, or beef (or mixed meats) are minced and placed on a spit where they are grilled. Shavings are cut off and often served sandwich style—wrapped in a pita with toppings such as tahini, hummus, and pickled turnips.
- **Shish kebab:** chunks of meat, fish, and/or vegetables that are threaded on a skewer and grilled or broiled.
- **Souvlaki:** a traditional Greek dish of lamb that has been marinated in oil, lemon juice, and seasonings, then threaded on a skewer and grilled. This dish sometimes includes vegetables such as green pepper or onion.
- **Spanakopita:** a savory phyllo pie filled with a mixture of sautéed spinach, onions, feta cheese, eggs, and seasonings.
- **Tabouli:** a salad made of finely chopped parsley, tomatoes, onions, mint, bulgur wheat, olive oil, and lemon juice.
- **Taramosalata:** a thick, creamy Greek specialty made with fish roe, lemon juice, milk-soaked bread crumbs, olive oil, and seasonings. It is often served with bread or crackers as an appetizer, but may be used as a vegetable dip also.
- **Tzatziki:** strained yogurt mixed with cucumber, lemon, and garlic. It may be made with sour cream. Tzatziki is used as a condiment or dip.

(i) What's Your Solution? Answers

a) Portion sizes at Greek restaurants are often quite large. Ask for a couple of takeout containers at the start of your meal to immediately create more reasonable portion sizes for yourself when the food arrives. The bonus: you'll have another meal to enjoy the next day.

b) It is a special outing for your family, so you can indulge in this festive dish if you can't resist. You are smart to have just a few bites. Here's another tip: request that your salad arrives at the same time as the fried cheese so you have something else to fill up on. You can also make an effort to limit the saturated fat in the rest of your meal by limiting cheese and red meat.

c) The popular Greek soup, avgolemono, is a great start to your meal, as is a Greek salad. Other healthy strategies you may want to consider are asking for the salad dressing on the side and omitting either the feta or olives from the salad.

d) Middle Eastern vegetarian options are often very healthy, but be sure to read the menu descriptions. At Greek restaurants, the vegetarian options are often deep-fried or stuffed with cheese, as with the popular spanakopita. Healthy options are vegetables stuffed with rice, braised eggplant, and green bean and tomato casserole.

Hungry for more information?

Get the App!

Download the
Eat Out Well—Restaurant Nutrition Finder
from the American Diabetes Association
mobile app today!

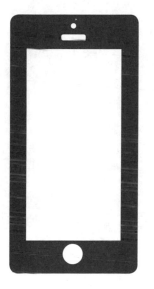

You've read the book, now practice healthy reastaurant eating on the go! This easy-to-use app companion to *Eat Out, Eat Well* puts the nutrition information for hundreds of independent and chain restaurants at your fingertips. You can search for restaurants near you and save your favorite healthy dishes. Keeping up with restaurant nutrition has never been easier!

Eat Out Well—Restaurant Nutrition Finder from the American Diabetes Association. Available from the iTunes App Store and, coming soon, Google Play.

Index

N